Comprehensive Review on Upper Tract Urothelial Carcinoma: An Update in 2023

Comprehensive Review on Upper Tract Urothelial Carcinoma: An Update in 2023

Guest Editors

Hooman Djaladat
Alireza Ghoreifi

MDPI

Basel • Beijing • Wuhan • Barcelona • Belgrade • Novi Sad • Cluj • Manchester

Guest Editors

Hooman Djaladat
Institute of Urology
University of Southern California
Los Angeles
USA

Alireza Ghoreifi
Institute of Urology
University of Southern California
Los Angeles
USA

Editorial Office
MDPI AG
Grosspeteranlage 5
4052 Basel, Switzerland

This is a reprint of the Special Issue, published open access by the journal *Cancers* (ISSN 2072-6694), freely accessible at: https://www.mdpi.com/journal/cancers/special_issues/4OVRM62K2P.

For citation purposes, cite each article independently as indicated on the article page online and as indicated below:

Lastname, A.A.; Lastname, B.B. Article Title. *Journal Name* **Year**, *Volume Number*, Page Range.

ISBN 978-3-7258-4727-3 (Hbk)
ISBN 978-3-7258-4728-0 (PDF)
https://doi.org/10.3390/books978-3-7258-4728-0

Contents

About the Editors

Hooman Djaladat

Hooman Djaladat, MD, MS, is Dean's Professor of Clinical Urology at the Institute of Urology, University of Southern California (USC), Los Angeles, USA. Dr. Djaladat went to medical school at Tehran University of Medical Sciences in Tehran, Iran. He was in the top 1% of his class and completed a urology residency in Sina Hospital, a well-known urology center at Tehran University of Medical Sciences. Before finishing his residency, Dr. Djaladat underwent training in endo-uro-oncology in Medway Hospital, affiliated with the University College of London in the United Kingdom. In 2004, Dr. Djaladat started his academic career in urology as an Assistant Professor of Urology. From 2007 to 2009, he completed his endourology and uro-laparoscopy clinical fellowship at the Labbafinejad Medical Center, which is one of the most prestigious centers pioneering modern urology in the Middle East. Subsequently, he moved to the United States and completed his SUO-accredited urologic oncology fellowship at the Keck School of Medicine of USC in 2012 and immediately joined the USC Institute of Urology. Dr. Djaladat has published more than 200 peer-reviewed articles and book chapters, some of which resulted from impressive surgical clinical trials. He has also been selected as a reviewer for many urology journals. Dr. Djaladat also invented a new Foley catheter for prostatectomy patients, and the patent for this has been filed with the US Patent and Trade Organization.

Alireza Ghoreifi

Alireza Ghoreifi, MD, is a Society of Urologic Oncology (SUO) fellow at the Department of Urology at Duke University. He earned his medical degree from Hormozgan University of Medical Sciences and completed his urology residency in 2014 at Mashhad University of Medical Sciences in Mashhad, Iran. He subsequently served as an Assistant Professor of Urology at Mashhad University for four years. In 2018, Dr. Ghoreifi joined the University of Southern California (USC) Institute of Urology as a research fellow in Urologic Oncology. In July 2024, he began a SUO fellowship at the Duke University Department of Urology. Dr. Ghoreifi's primary research interests include bladder and upper tract urothelial carcinoma, as well as advanced kidney cancer. He has received research grants from the AUA Urology Care Foundation and the USC Urology Research Council to study urine-based methylation markers and blood-based liquid biopsies in patients with upper tract urothelial carcinoma. He has presented over 200 abstracts at national and international scientific meetings, earning the Grand Prize at the Western Section AUA in 2022 and the Best Poster Presentation at the AUA in 2023. Dr. Ghoreifi has authored more than 120 peer-reviewed original articles, reviews, and book chapters. He also serves as a reviewer for multiple urology journals and was recognized with the Best Reviewer awards from the *SIU Journal* and *Current Urology Journal* in 2023, as well as from *The Journal of Urology* in 2024.

Preface

It is our honor to serve as Guest Editors for this Special Issue of *Cancers*, titled *"Comprehensive Review on Upper Tract Urothelial Carcinoma: An Update in 2023"*. This Special Issue brings together a curated collection of high-quality manuscripts authored by leading experts in the field, offering a multifaceted exploration of the latest developments in upper tract urothelial carcinoma (UTUC).

UTUC continues to evolve rapidly, driven by innovations in diagnostics, therapeutics, and interdisciplinary collaboration. The articles in this issue reflect the breadth and depth of current research, spanning from foundational biological insights to clinical applications and emerging technologies. Several contributions delve into novel diagnostic modalities, while others examine risk stratification tools, surgical advancements, and systemic therapies. Together, these works provide a holistic view of the state of the art in UTUC, as well as a roadmap for future research and clinical practice.

We are confident that this Special Issue will serve as a valuable resource for clinicians, researchers, and healthcare professionals seeking to deepen their understanding of UTUC. We extend our sincere gratitude to all the authors for their outstanding contributions and to the reviewers for their thoughtful evaluations. We hope this collection will inspire continued innovation and collaboration in the pursuit of improved outcomes for patients worldwide.

Hooman Djaladat and Alireza Ghoreifi
Guest Editors

cancers

MDPI

Editorial

A Comprehensive Review on Upper Tract Urothelial Carcinoma: An Update in 2023

Alireza Ghoreifi * and Hooman Djaladat *

Institute of Urology, University of Southern California, Los Angeles, CA 90089, USA
* Correspondence: alireza.ghoreifi@med.usc.edu (A.G.); djaladat@med.usc.edu (H.D.)

It is our pleasure to serve as the guest editors for the *Cancers* journal for this Special Issue, titled "Comprehensive Review on Upper Tract Urothelial Carcinoma: An Update in 2023". This Special Issue comprises nine manuscripts authored by experts in the field, covering various aspects of the diagnosis and management of upper tract urothelial carcinoma (UTUC).

UTUC is a relatively uncommon type of cancer, which shares similarities with urothelial bladder cancer. Nevertheless, significant differences exist between these two cancer types in terms of epidemiological, clinical, pathological, and biological features. In a review article, Lefort et al. extensively explored these differences and their clinical implications [1]. The key steps in the management of patients with UTUC include precise diagnosis and risk stratification. Tsikitas et al. presented the latest advancements in imaging for UTUC [2]. The authors reviewed the strengths and weaknesses of conventional imaging techniques, including CT urography and magnetic resonance imaging (MRI), as well as other promising modalities, such as contrast-enhanced ultrasound (CEUS) and positron emission tomography (PET). They also highlighted the role of artificial intelligence and multiomics in the classification and prognostication of UTUC. In another paper, Bitaraf et al. reviewed other diagnostic tools (i.e., urine cytology and ureteroscopy), as well as patient- and disease-related prognostic factors that affect the outcomes of patients with UTUC [3]. They emphasized the substantial role of preoperative risk stratification tools and nomograms, which have been developed to guide surgical management and perioperative systemic therapy in UTUC. A real-world study in this context was presented by Huang et al., who reviewed the outcomes of 476 patients with pT2N0M0 UTUC undergoing radical nephroureterectomy (RNU) or ureterectomy [4]. They found that age >60 years, previous bladder cancer history, ureteral involvement, and positive surgical margins were independently associated with negative oncological outcomes.

The gold standard for the management of UTUC is RNU with bladder cuff excision. During the recent two decades, there has been a major shift from open RNU towards minimally invasive techniques. Franco et al. presented the latest evidence regarding surgical techniques and outcomes of minimally invasive RNU, focusing on robotic RNU [5]. The authors reviewed novel robotic techniques, including single-stage transperitoneal, retroperitoneal, and single-port RNUs. Another evolution in the management of UTUC has been kidney-sparing surgery, which emerged as the preferred option for select patients, particularly those with a low-risk disease. Ghoreifi et al. reviewed the outcomes of these techniques, including endoscopic ablation and segmental ureterectomy [6]. Several retrospective comparative studies have confirmed the feasibility and efficacy of kidney-sparing management approaches for UTUC, yet the only level I evidence so far in this setting is mitomycin gel therapy in low-risk patients.

Despite the technical advancements in the management of UTUC, oncologic outcomes are still not optimal. A multidisciplinary approach, incorporating perioperative intravesical and systemic therapy, has shown to improve these outcomes. Wang et al. comprehensively reviewed the medications, dosage, and timing of intravesical therapy for UTUC, and reported a reduced risk of intravesical recurrence and improved patient survival among those receiving this type of therapy [7]. In another study, Kolawa et al. reviewed the importance of perioperative systemic therapy in these patients and emphasized that neoadjuvant cisplatin-based therapy is preferred by clinicians over adjuvant therapy in high-risk patients, due to the potential decline in renal function following RNU [8]. The results of the ongoing trials have the potential to establish adjuvant immunotherapy as a potential new standard of care of UTUC.

All patients with UTUC require a close follow-up after a surgical intervention with curative intent. Klemm et al. presented surveillance protocols following definitive therapy for UTUC [9]. The surveillance modalities included urine cytology, cystoscopy, and CT/MR urography, and ureteroscopy (in kidney-sparing surgeries), with intervals varying according to risk stratification and the surgical approach used.

The management of UTUC has seen notable advancements in the recent decade. Nonetheless, this area is undergoing rapid evolution, and future studies will provide insights into the optimal approach for managing these patients.

Conflicts of Interest: The authors declare no conflict of interest.

References

1. Lefort, F.; Rhanine, Y.; Larroquette, M.; Domblides, C.; Heraudet, L.; Sionneau, B.; Lambert, S.; Lasserre, M.; Robert, G.; Ravaud, A.; et al. Clinical and Biological Differences between Upper Tract Carcinoma and Bladder Urothelial Cancer, Including Implications for Clinical Practice. *Cancers* **2023**, *15*, 5558. [CrossRef] [PubMed]
2. Tsikitas, L.A.; Hopstone, M.D.; Raman, A.; Duddalwar, V. Imaging in Upper Tract Urothelial Carcinoma: A Review. *Cancers* **2023**, *15*, 5040. [CrossRef] [PubMed]
3. Bitaraf, M.; Ghafoori Yazdi, M.; Amini, E. Upper Tract Urothelial Carcinoma (UTUC) Diagnosis and Risk Stratification: A Comprehensive Review. *Cancers* **2023**, *15*, 4987. [CrossRef] [PubMed]
4. Huang, Y.-C.; Liu, J.-M.; Liu, H.-Y.; Chang, Y.-L.; Chen, C.-S.; Ho, D.-R.; Wu, C.-T.; Chen, M.-F.; Wang, H.-J.; Luo, H.-L. Clinical Determinants of Extraurinary Tract Recurrence and Survival after Radical Surgery for pT2 Upper Tract Urothelial Carcinoma. *Cancers* **2023**, *15*, 1858. [CrossRef] [PubMed]
5. Franco, A.; Ditonno, F.; Feng, C.; Manfredi, C.; Sturgis, M.R.; Farooqi, M.; Del Giudice, F.; Coogan, C.; Ferro, M.; Zhang, C.; et al. Minimally Invasive Radical Nephroureterectomy: 5-Year Update of Techniques and Outcomes. *Cancers* **2023**, *15*, 4585. [CrossRef] [PubMed]
6. Ghoreifi, A.; Sari Motlagh, R.; Fuchs, G. Modern Kidney-Sparing Management of Upper Tract Urothelial Carcinoma. *Cancers* **2023**, *15*, 4495. [CrossRef] [PubMed]
7. Wang, Z.; Shi, H.; Xu, Y.; Fang, Y.; Song, J.; Jiang, W.; Xia, D.; Wu, Z.; Wang, L. Intravesical Therapy for Upper Urinary Tract Urothelial Carcinoma: A Comprehensive Review. *Cancers* **2023**, *15*, 5020. [CrossRef] [PubMed]
8. Kolawa, A.; D'Souza, A.; Tulpule, V. Overview, Diagnosis, and Perioperative Systemic Therapy of Upper Tract Urothelial Carcinoma. *Cancers* **2023**, *5*, 4813. [CrossRef] [PubMed]
9. Klemm, J.; Bekku, K.; Abufaraj, M.; Laukhtina, E.; Matsukawa, A.; Parizi, M.K.; Karakiewicz, P.I.; Shariat, S.F. Upper Tract Urothelial Carcinoma: A Narrative Review of Current Surveillance Strategies for Non-Metastatic Disease. *Cancers* **2023**, *16*, 44. [CrossRef] [PubMed]

cancers

MDPI

Review

Imaging in Upper Tract Urothelial Carcinoma: A Review

Lucas A. Tsikitas, Michelle Diamond Hopstone, Alex Raman and Vinay Duddalwar *

Department of Radiology, Keck School of Medicine, University of Southern California,
Los Angeles, CA 90033, USA; lucas.tsikitas@med.usc.edu (L.A.T.); michelle.hopstone@med.usc.edu (M.D.H.); alex.raman@med.usc.edu (A.R.)
* Correspondence: vinay.duddalwar@med.usc.edu

Simple Summary: Urothelial carcinoma, a cancer of the urinary tract, is relatively common in the urinary bladder, termed the lower urinary tract. However, it is much less common in the upper urinary tract, which consists of the pelvicalyceal system and ureters. Medical imaging plays an important role in detection, diagnosis, and treatment planning of this uncommon disease. We aim to review the imaging methods currently available and future directions in the field of radiology to aid clinicians in treatment planning.

Abstract: Medical imaging is a critical tool in the detection, staging, and treatment planning of upper urinary tract urothelial carcinoma (UTUC). This article reviews the strengths and weaknesses of the different imaging techniques and modalities available clinically. This includes multidetector computed tomography (CT), multiparametric magnetic resonance imaging (MRI), ultrasound (US), and positron emission tomography (PET) for the detection, staging, and management of UTUC. In addition, we review the imaging techniques that are being developed and are on the horizon but have not yet made it to clinical practice. Firstly, we review the imaging findings of primary UTUC and the techniques across multiple modalities. We then discuss imaging findings of metastatic disease. Lastly, we describe the role of imaging in the surveillance after resection of primary UTUC based upon current guidelines.

Keywords: upper tract urothelial carcinoma; imaging

1. Introduction

UTUC is a type of cancer that arises from the urothelial cells lining the renal pelvicalyceal system and ureters. It is far less common than lower tract urothelial carcinoma, making up for only 5–7% of all urothelial carcinomas [1]. Detection is usually incidental or in the clinical setting of hematuria or flank pain [2]. UTUC is most often detected in the renal pelvis [3]. It is then most commonly detected in the distal third of the ureter, then mid ureter, and lastly proximal ureter occurring at rates of 73%, 24%, and 3%, respectively [3]. As UTUC is much rarer than lower urinary tract urothelial carcinoma, there are limited epidemiologic data; the overall incidence of UTUC is reported as 1–2 cases per 100,000 people [1,4,5]. Approximately 11–13% of patients with UTUC develop metachronous UTUC tumors, underscoring the importance of optimized imaging techniques in primary detection and surveillance [1,6]. Treatment of UTUC widely varies depending on the location and number of masses, presence of metastatic disease, and whether the patient is high- or low-risk. Surgical management ranges from kidney-sparing resection or chemoablation in localized low-risk disease to open radical ureteronephrectomy with lymph node dissection in localized high-risk disease [1]. Additionally, patients over the age of 70 who undergo radial nephrectomy may have worse outcomes than those who have noninvasive treatment [7]. As such, detection of the full disease extent is crucial prior to developing the clinical treatment plan.

2. Detection and Diagnosis

UTUC typically presents on imaging in one of three ways: a filling defect within the renal pelvicalyceal system or ureter; focal thickening of a segment of urothelial lining, often with prominent focal enhancement; or as an infiltrative mass [2,3]. Of note, one general feature of an infiltrative renal urothelial carcinoma is that the contour of the involved kidney is preserved, helping to differentiate itself from RCC [8].

2.1. UTUC Staging

The staging of UC is based on the tumor, node, and metastasis (TNM) system, which considers the size and extent of the tumor, lymph node involvement, and presence of distant metastases [9]. The staging system for UTUC ranges from Tis (carcinoma in situ) to T4 (tumor invades adjacent organs or structures) [9].

If there is a fat plane or layer of excreted contrast that separates a pelvicalyceal mass from the normal renal parenchyma, the tumor can be classified as T1 or T2 [8]. Although desirable for treatment planning, differentiation between T1 and T2 on imaging is difficult. A T3 lesion will lose this fat plane or layer of contrast and may show enhancement in the adjacent renal parenchyma [8]. Invasion into the renal parenchymal is designated as T4 disease [8].

In a study of 188 patients with UTUC treated using radical nephroureterectomy, distant metastatic disease was found to occur most commonly in multiple organs sites, in 30% of cases [6]. Single-organ metastatic disease was then highest in the lungs at 28% of cases, followed by both liver and bone at 13%, and distant lymph nodes at 10% [6]. Lung metastases typically present as multiple pulmonary nodules [10]. Cystic lung nodules have also been reported, although less commonly [11]. Metastatic disease in the liver is typically seen as multiple hypoattenuating masses, although solitary masses are reported in approximately 10% of cases [10]. Osseous metastatic disease can present as sclerotic, lytic, or mixed picture masses, only rarely resulting in vertebral body compression fractures or spinal cord compression [10]. Metastatic lymph nodes are often enlarged and bulky conglomerates in various locations based on where the primary tumor originated. Regional lymph nodes for primary intrarenal and proximal ureteral UTUC occur in the perihilar and retroperitoneal stations. For the distal ureters, regional lymph nodes include the hypogastric, obturator, iliac (internal, external), perivesical, pelvic (not otherwise specified), sacral, and presacral lymph node stations [6,10]. Common iliac nodes are not included as regional nodes and are considered distant metastases (M1). Single lymph node metastases are associated with better clinical outcomes when compared to an increased number of nodes or increased nodal density [6]. Less commonly, pleural, adrenal gland, brain, peritoneal, and bowel metastases have also been reported [10].

2.2. Computed Tomography

CT urography (CTU) is a technique that combines multiple CT acquisitions typically with and without contrast [2,3]. While UTUC is an uncommon local for urothelial carcinoma, the upper urinary tract is considered the second most common site of involvement after the bladder, and multifocality is a hallmark of the disease. Therefore, proper distention of the renal pelvis and ureters is essential for detection, and the optimization of CTU protocols is essential. Suboptimal technique can lead to poor urinary tract distention, making the detection of subtle tumors impossible. CTU has a sensitivity of over 90% in patients with painless hematuria and is accepted as routine evaluation for this clinical indication [2]. Meta-analysis has demonstrated the best diagnostic accuracy for UTUC of all non-invasive medical imaging with CTU [5]. Specifically, CT urography has been found to have a pooled sensitivity of 92% for the detection of UTUC (95% CI; 0.85–0.96), and pooled specificity of 95% (95% CI; 0.88–0.98) in a meta-analysis of 13 studies comprising 1233 patients [5]. Additionally, CTU has sufficient sensitivity for the detection of additional common causes of hematuria [2,3]. Below, we discuss the various CT acquisitions encountered in CTU.

Noncontrast CT has very limited to no utility for the identification of primary UTUC, as there is no natural contrast attenuation difference between the primary tumor and the normal renal collecting system and ureters. It is primarily useful in patients presenting with hematuria by elucidating hyperattenuating renal calculi. Occasionally, primary UTUC may show fine encrusted calcifications, which are difficult to differentiate from renal calculi with just noncontrast imaging [8]. Additionally, space-occupying lesions, if detected, are difficult to differentiate from other renal masses in a noncontrast-enhanced study.

Following the administration of intravenous contrast, few additional etiologies of hematuria can be evaluated (Figure 1). In the corticomedullary phase of contrast (approximately 25–30 s post injection), UTUC can be seen as an infiltrative mass with arterial hyperenhancement [1,2]. Small urothelial carcinomas in the ureters tend to demonstrate early arterial enhancement, which helps differentiate them from benign entities such as blood clots or sloughed papillae in papillary necrosis as well as having a more central intraluminal position rather than asymmetrically on the ureteral wall [1–3]. Renal cell carcinoma can also be identified using early arterial enhancement but tends to exhibit a mass effect and deform the normal renal contour [1–3].

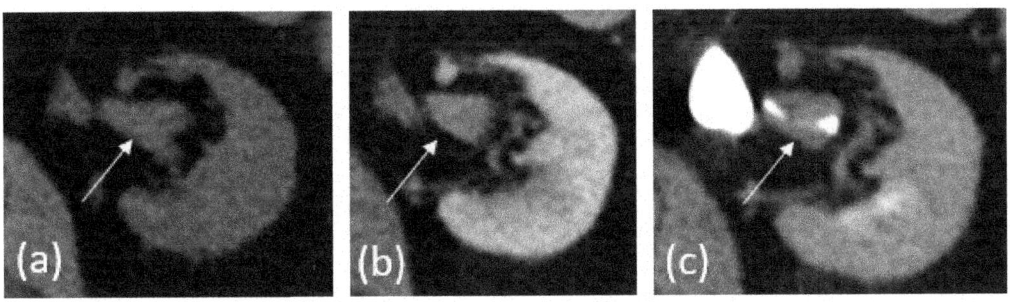

Figure 1. An 81-year-old male with history of bladder UC presenting for surveillance. (**a**) Pre-contrast images demonstrate no significant abnormality. (**b**) Corticomedullary phase demonstrates unequivocal enhancement in tumor (measuring 75 HU compared to 30 HU on pre-contrast images). (**c**) Excretory phase reveals the tumor as a filling defect, outlined by excreted iodinated contrast.

The nephrographic phase of contrast allows for the detection of some urothelial carcinomas, as well as renal cell carcinomas [2,3]. The detection of primary pelvicalyceal UTUC remains limited, however, as the ureters are not well opacified and the renal collecting systems are isoattenuating to adjacent renal parenchyma. This makes soft tissue masses, flat epithelial lesions, or focal urothelial thickening extremely difficult to detect [1].

Imaging obtained during the excretory phase of contrast administration (approximately 4–8 min post injection) allows for optimal opacification and distention of the ureters, resulting in maximum opacification of the collecting system and ureters [2,3]. On excretory imaging, UTUC appears as ureteral filling defects or irregularities of the calyx or infundibular narrowing [2,3]. The addition of image reconstruction techniques such as excretory maximum-intensity projections (MIPs) and 3D reconstructions helps reveal UTUC in the intrarenal collecting systems as calyceal amputation or destruction can be easier to visualize [2]. A careful review of the imaging dataset using a combination of multiple viewing windows and reconstructions is critical for an accurate imaging review. The use of three-dimensional (3D) imaging techniques has also been found helpful, as it can make a conspicuous lesion stand out more than relying on the evaluation of axial images alone [2,3].

CTU is performed in one of two techniques, depending on the clinical scenario, institutional volume, and staffing: the single bolus technique and split bolus technique. The single bolus technique involves a noncontrast image acquisition followed by injection of a single contrast agent bolus, followed by multiple CT acquisitions during the corticomedullary, nephrogenic, and delayed excretory phases, leading to the highest sensitivity for all etiologies of hematuria. The delayed excretory phase of the single bolus technique provides excellent visualization of the urinary tract as the entire contrast bolus contributes to opacification/distension of the collection system [2,3]. Additionally, the single bolus technique is simpler and quicker to perform compared to the split bolus technique [2,3]. The largest downside of the single bolus technique is its undesirably high radiation dose [2,3].

The split bolus technique can include a noncontrast image acquisition, although this is sometimes omitted. During a split bolus exam, the same contrast volume is administered, but in two separately timed boluses, achieving a combined nephrographic and excretory phase, decreasing the number of image acquisitions and thus radiation dose [2,3]. While decreasing radiation dose, especially over a patient's lifetime, this technique provides questionable visualization of the bladder and distal ureters, particularly for small UCs, as only half the volume of contrast contributes to collecting system opacification/distension [2,3]. Additionally, the lack of a corticomedullary phase decreases the sensitivity for detection of renal cell carcinomas and small flat epithelial lesions.

Several other imaging techniques aimed to enhance distention of the distal ureters include the administration of IV furosemide prior to the study, and the administration of IV or oral hydration. Both have been shown to increase distention of the distal ureters, and thus sensitivity for detection; however, the administration of IV furosemide has workflow implications including the need for nursing staff to place IVs and administer medications [2]. Additional techniques have been historically used such as using compression belts and scanning the patient in the prone position, but there is a lack of data to support their effectiveness.

Another emerging CT technique for the detection of UTUC is dual-energy CT (DECT). DECT takes advantage of the attenuation phenomenon, or the amount of X-ray energy that is attenuated by individual tissues at different X-ray energies, determined by the physical properties of the tissues such as atomic number and density. By collecting data at two different X-ray energies, it allows for the creation of iodine attenuation curves specific to each tissue. By using this technique, it is possible to subtract the attenuation solely caused by the iodinated contrast material, thus creating virtual noncontrast images. This technique is thus able to maintain a noncontrast image from a contrast-enhanced dataset, removing the need to acquire a noncontrast image, resulting in radiation dose reduction to the patient. Another useful DECT strategy is the creation of virtual monochrome images (VMI), which allow for higher contrast images using a reduced contrast bolus dose at the cost of increased image noise, which is reduced through mathematical algorithms. DECT additionally allows for an improved reduction in beam hardening artifacts, which is often present due to post-surgical hardware. Lastly, DECT allows for the evaluation of images using post-processing color-coded displays based upon the iodine uptake of tissues, greatly improving the detection of renal and urothelial lesions and differentiating solid and cystic renal masses. While DECT can greatly aid in the detection of UTUC, as a newer technology, it comes at a higher equipment cost and greater post-construction complexity, and little literature is currently available in the field of UTUC [12,13].

2.3. MRI

MRI urography (MRU) has been found to have a sensitivity of 75% after the administration of contrast for the detection of UTUC, but it has been shown to have equal specificity for UTUC detection compared to CTU [5,14,15]. MRU is limited in the detection of small nephrolithiasis and has decreased diagnostic accuracy in patients with ureteral stents or nephrostomy tubes [14]. Compared with CTU, MRU provides decreased spatial resolution and the susceptibility to motion artifacts from both patient movement and ureteral peristalsis. Additionally, the T2* effect seen with dense gadolinium can lower the sensitivity for detection in contrast-enhanced excretory phase sequences [8,16]. As CTU has a higher sensitivity, faster imaging times, and increased patient throughput, MRU is typically reserved for patients with contraindications to iodinated contrast administration or radiation [5].

MRU is composed of multiple sequences (Figure 2). T2-weighted sequences are performed at standard and very long echo times to allow for quick hydrographic images. This sequence allows for the detection of filling defects or truncation of the pelvicalyceal system, ureters, and bladder, without the need for IV contrast administration [5,16]. Similar to the CTU technique, oral or IV hydration, and IV furosemide administration help distend the ureters [16]. These sequences are somewhat limited, however, as the ureters may not be fully distended and are prone to motion artifacts from peristalsis [16].

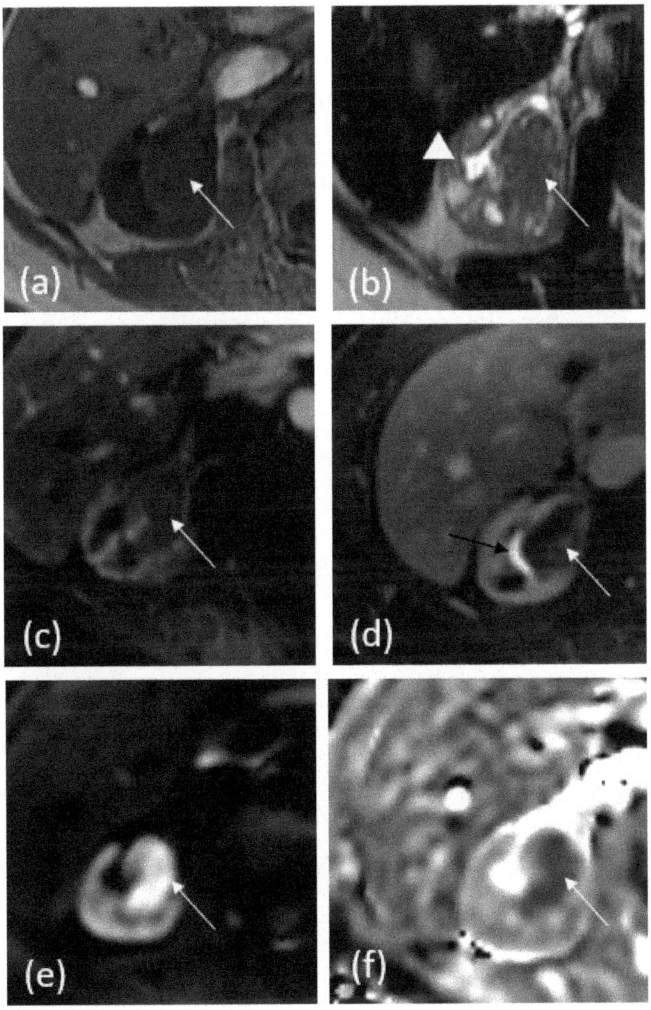

Figure 2. A 64-year-old female with history of right renal mass. (**a**) T1 pre-contrast demonstrates isoechoic mass (white arrow) in the renal pelvis with obliteration of multiple calyces. (**b**) T2-weighted image demonstrates iso- to hypoechoic mass signal again with obliteration of normal calyces and mild associated hydronephrosis (white arrowhead). (**c**) Fat-saturated T1 post-contrast corticomedullary phase demonstrates subtle heterogeneous enhancement within the mass. (**d**) Fat-saturated T1 post-contrast 5 min delayed phase delineates the tumor better, which is enhanced less than adjacent renal parenchyma is. Excreted contrast is noted in the collecting system (black arrow). (**e**) Diffusion-weighted images show increased signal within the mass. (**f**) ADC map shows dark signal in the mass, confirming restricted diffusion.

Pre-contrast T1 sequences demonstrated T1 hypointense signals in tumor cells, and chemical shift imaging enables the evaluation of intravoxel fat. After the administration of IV gadolinium, T1-weighted dynamic post-contrast sequences are obtained in the corticomedullary, nephrographic, and excretory pyelographic phases, allowing for the detection of enhancing masses, urothelial linings, and filling defects [16]. Similar to CTU, papillary lesions and infiltrative disease demonstrate diffuse contrast enhancement, differentiating themselves from benign differential diagnoses such as sloughed papillae and blood clots [15].

Diffusion-weighted imaging demonstrates increased signals in tumors with decreased apparent diffusion coefficient (ADC) values, due to the greater restriction of water movement in tumor cells [17].

The modern MRU technique is generally composed of T2-weighted sequences at standard and very long echo times, T1-weighted dual-echo chemical shift sequences, fat-saturated pre- and post-contrast T1-weighted sequences, and diffusion-weighted imaging sequences. Alternatively, MRU can be obtained without the administration of intravenous contrast in certain patient populations, like those who are pregnant or have chronic renal failure, at a significantly decreased sensitivity [18].

2.4. US/CEUS

Although less sensitive than CTU and MRU in identifying upper tract urothelial carcinoma, ultrasound remains a useful tool in the detection of UTUC (Figure 3), especially in cases of renal failure, contrast allergies, or in the setting of limited medical resources.

On grayscale ultrasound, pelvicalyceal tumors are solid masses that can appear hypo, iso, or hyperechoic to the adjacent echogenic renal sinus fat and may occur with or without the associated hydronephrosis. Ureteral lesions are seen as intraluminal soft-tissue masses with or without hydroureteronephrosis. Small, nonobstructive tumors may be difficult to differentiate from the renal sinus fat in the absence of the associated hydronephrosis. Large, diffuse infiltrative tumors may also be difficult to distinguish from adjacent renal parenchyma on grayscale ultrasound. Color Doppler ultrasound may show vascular flow; however, upper tract tumors frequently show low or no-flow and may be difficult to distinguish from clot or debris [19–21].

Contrast-enhanced ultrasound is emerging as a promising technique to aid in the diagnosis of upper tract tumors. As of this writing, no clear sonographic enhancement pattern has been established for UTUC, with variable enhancement characteristics likely dependent on tumor grade [19,21]. Nevertheless, multiple studies have found that many urothelial tumors demonstrate early washout relative to the renal cortex [19,20]. Contrast-enhanced ultrasound can accurately differentiate solid, enhancing tumors from non-solid, non-enhancing material such as blood clot, debris, or pus. As a result, CEUS appears to be more accurate in estimating tumor size when compared to CTU/MRU and grayscale ultrasound, which can overestimate tumor size by 15–20% and 25%, respectively [21]. Conducted in real-time, CEUS is more sensitive than CTU in the detection of tumor microvascularization [19].

Limitations remain, however, as contrast-enhanced ultrasound cannot distinguish UTUC from other, less common types of upper tract tumors including epidermoid tumors, adenocarcinoma, or lymphoma [19]. Ultrasound evaluation of the ureter remains limited, as the ureter cannot be seen in its entirety.

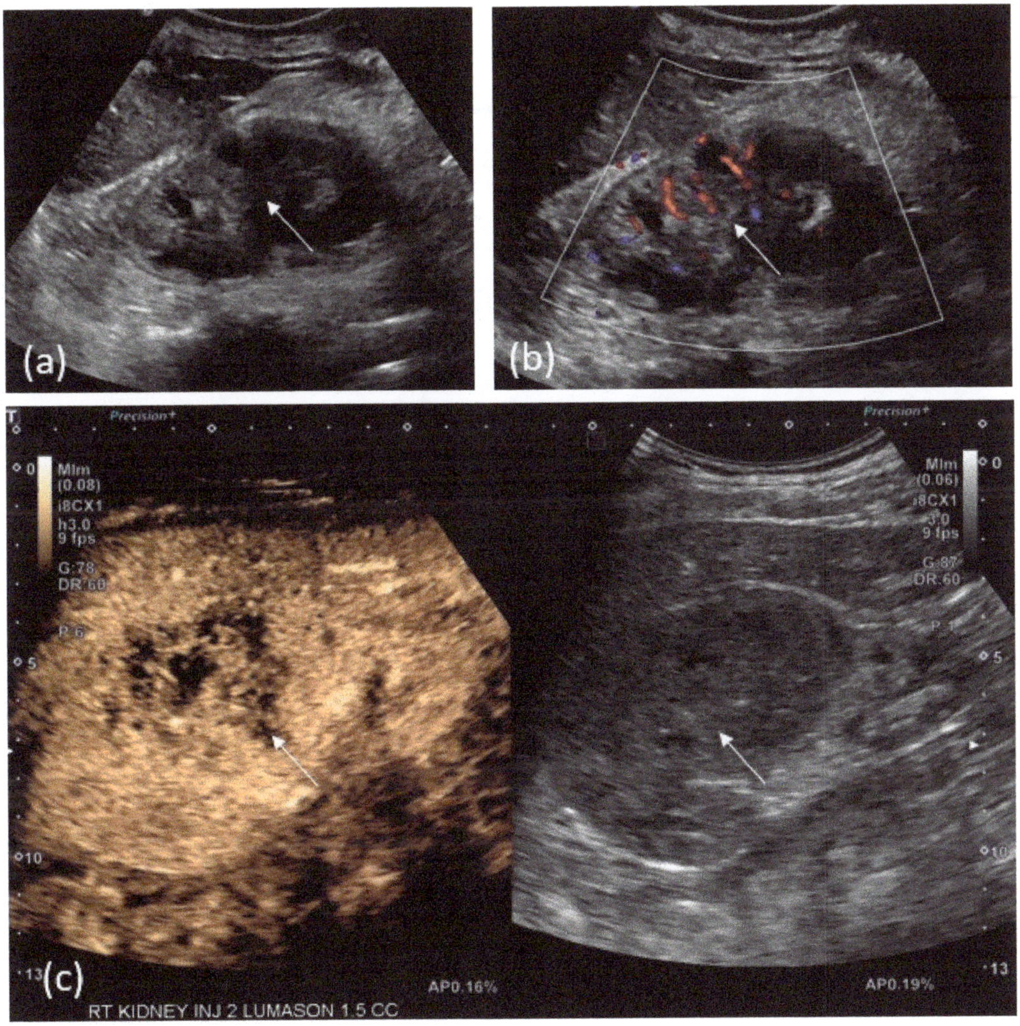

Figure 3. A 71-year-old-woman with right renal mass. (**a**) Grey-scale ultrasound image shows a mass-like hyperechoic area involving the renal pelvis. (**b**) Color Doppler reveals only mild vascularity. (**c**) After injection of 1.5 cc of Lumason, post-contrast images confirm a hypoenhancing mass in that location.

2.5. PET/CT

18F-fluorodeoxyglucose positron emission tomography with computed tomography (FDG-PET/CT) is commonly used in cancer staging; however, its use in the evaluation of primary tumors of the urinary tract in general is limited due to physiologic excretion of the radiotracer through the urinary system. Nevertheless, multiple studies have shown that FDG-PET/CT has high diagnostic accuracy in the detection of lymph nodes and distant metastases during initial staging and restaging of urothelial carcinoma (Figure 4) [22–24].

11C-choline is a PET radiotracer with very late urinary excretion, allowing the urinary tract to be free from urinary radioactivity at the time of image acquisition [25]. Multiple small series studies have shown that urothelial carcinoma demonstrates 11C-choline uptake [25,26]. The results of these studies show that 11C-choline PET/CT is highly sensitive in detecting primary tumors and metastases, as well as CT occult metastases, and can potentially provide valuable prognostic information in preoperative staging.

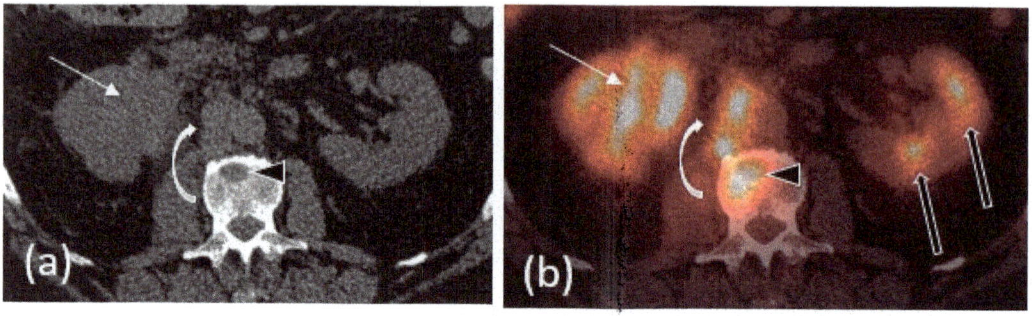

Figure 4. A 63-year-old male with metastatic UTUC. (**a**) Non-contrast CT images demonstrate an infiltrative right renal mass (white arrow) with obliteration of the renal pelvis. (**b**) Fusion PET/CT images demonstrate intense FDG uptake in the mass. FDG avid retroperitoneal lymph node metastases (curved white arrow) and osseous metastases (black arrowhead) are also included in this image. Note the physiologic radiotracer activity in the left renal collecting system (black arrows).

Additional novel PET tracers are being studied to improve the diagnostic accuracy of staging urothelial cancer. Examples include a pilot clinical trial at Thomas Jefferson University studying copper CU-64 TP3805 in patients with urothelial bladder cancer [27] and a study at Hadassah-Hebrew University Medical Center comparing the radiotracer uptake of 11C-acetate to the radiotracer uptake of 11C-choline in patients with urothelial carcinoma of the bladder [28]. Further research must be performed to determine whether these radiotracers can be useful in the staging of UTUC.

3. AI and Multiomics in the Classification and Prognostication of Upper Urothelial Tract Urothelial Carcinoma

Machine learning and multiomics can be useful tools in the classification and prognostication of upper urothelial tract carcinomas. Although no algorithms are routinely used in the clinical setting at this time, work has been carried out to predict the staging and grading of UTUC using deep learning, predict protein-based UTUC subtypes based on hematoxylin and eosin (H&E) slides, and predict overall survival based on inflammatory markers [29–31].

He et al. used a dataset of 884 patients with UTUC who underwent radical nephroureterectomy and collected clinical data including past medical history and laboratory tests, along with data derived from radiologic imaging, including the presence of hydronephrosis and the longest diameter of the tumor. Their primary prediction endpoints were T-staging and grading based on both 1973 and 2004 WHO Classifications. They trained five different neural network architectures and achieved maximum AUCs of 0.76, 0.804, and 0.824 for T-staging, 1973 grading, and 2004 grading, respectively.

Another group directly used H&E slides to predict the immunohistochemical expression of UTUC. Using 163 samples, a RESNET50 model was trained to predict the underlying expression of relevant biomarkers. Their model achieved an AUC of 0.62–0.99 (95% confidence interval) and presents a potentially useful tool in guiding therapeutic options for UTUC.

Lastly, Liu et al. developed a prognostic model for survival, using five inflammatory markers from 483 patients with UTUC. These five markers included neutrophil-to-lymphocyte ratio, monocyte-to-lymphocyte ratio, platelet-to-lymphocyte ratio, systemic immune inflammation index, and systemic inflammation response index. After computing a "systemic immune inflammation score" based on these markers, the authors used random forest and Cox regression models to achieve AUCs of 0.872 and 0.801, respectively, for predicting overall survival at 5 years.

There has been promising recent work applying deep learning and multiomics methods to UTUC. Future work may incorporate the direct use of radiologic imaging in these machine learning models for UTUC detection, subtyping, and prognostication, as has been performed in abundance for urothelial cancer of the bladder [32,33].

3. Image-Guided Percutaneous Biopsy

Percutaneous biopsy of UTUS is rarely performed due to the perceived risk of biopsy tract tumor seeding carried over from case reports of tumor tract seeding for percutaneous biopsy of renal cell carcinoma. While there are a few case reports of UTUC biopsy tract tumor seeding, Huang et al. have shown that percutaneous-image-guided biopsy can be performed safely with no additional risk [34,35]. Thus, in patients for which ureteroscopic biopsy cannot be performed, percutaneous-image-guided biopsy remains a safe option for tissue diagnosis [35]. Multidisciplinary discussion of the risks and benefits of the procedure is recommended prior to percutaneous biopsy.

4. Surveillance

After treatment of UTUC, follow-up is recommended to evaluate for recurrent tumor or local/distant metastatic disease. Current European Association of Urology (EAU) guidelines suggest different follow-up imaging pathways depending on whether the primary tumor is high- versus low-risk and if the tumor was treated using radical nephroureterectomy (RNU) or kidney sparing management or partial ureteral resection [1]. Of note, the risk for the development of metachronous bladder tumors is higher than that of metachronous UTUC tumors [6]. Roughly 40% of patients with UTUC go on to develop lower tract UC [8]. This risk decreases 4 years after RNU [6].

In low-risk primary UTUC following RNU, CTU is management or partial ureteral resection, postoperative CTU is recommended at 3 months, 6 months, and then yearly for 5 years [6].

In high-risk primary UTUC, postoperative CTU is recommended every 6 months for 2 years and then yearly following RNU. Following kidney sparing management or partial ureteral resection, postoperative CTU is recommended at 3 months, 6 months, and then yearly.

These guidelines generally have weak strength ratings, however, and more data are needed to increase the effectiveness of surveillance guidelines [6].

5. Discussion

Multiple imaging modalities are available to the referring clinician for detection of UTUC. CTU demonstrates the highest sensitivity and specificity for evaluation of hematuria including those caused by UTUC. Many factors influence an institution's choice of single bolus or split bolus technique. Both techniques have similar sensitivity and specificity, each with their own drawbacks: the single bolus technique increases the radiation dose, and the split bolus technique has a higher chance of suboptimal opacification of the distal collecting system. PO or IV hydration prior to imaging is generally favorable, whereas prone imaging or an abdominal belt has not shown to be useful. In younger patients with hematuria with low risk of UTUC, the single bolus technique is likely best as the chances of having to repeat imaging is low. In high-risk patients or those undergoing surveillance, a split bolus technique will likely reduce the patients' lifetime radiation dose. Additionally, a single bolus technique using DECT will likely provide the best results with reasonable radiation dose. As machine learning algorithms are developed using pathological specimens, improved detection and prognostication are likely possible with first imaging.

In patients unable to undergo CTU, MRU remains a promising alternative, with decreased but still high sensitivity and specificity. Given that the potential treatment plan of UTUC is based on staging, while there are studies evaluating the role of imaging in differentiating between T1 and T2 disease, this has not yet translated to clinical practice. With further trials or through the development of new sequencing and the development of scoring systems similar to VIRADS, MRU sensitivity and specificity may approach that of CTU [36].

While demonstrating lower sensitivity and specificity, CEUS remains a promising modality in detection due to its lack of ionizing radiation. CEUS could be used for contrast evaluation of the kidneys in the setting of hematuria in patients who may not be able to receive contrast.

PET/CT, while currently limited, shows a promising future in its detection role through the development of new radiotracers with very delayed urinary excretion such as 11C-Choline, although radiation dose will still likely remain a limiting factor.

With the future development of algorithms and deep machine learning, it may be possible to obtain diagnostic imaging of equal sensitivity and specificity with single-phase contrast CT or noncontrast MRI.

6. Conclusions

While UTUC is a rare disease, the proper detection and staging of tumor burden are crucial in treatment planning. In clinical practice, CTU has been shown to be the most effective and widely available imaging modality available for the detection of UTUC and all-cause microscopic hematuria. MRU remains an effective detection modality at slightly decreased sensitivity and specificity. Advancements in imaging techniques and artificial intelligence continue to offer a promising future in the detection of UTUC with decreased radiation dose.

Author Contributions: Conceptualization, V.D., M.D.H. and L.A.T.; writing—original draft preparation, L.A.T.; writing of CEUS and PET/CT imaging section, M.D.H.; writing of AI and multiomics section, A.R.; image selection and annotation, M.D.H.; writing—review and editing, L.A.T.; supervision and project administration, V.D. All authors have read and agreed to the published version of the manuscript.

Funding: This research received no external funding.

Conflicts of Interest: The authors declare no conflict of interest.

References

1. Rouprêt, M.; Seisen, T.; Birtle, A.J.; Capoun, O.; Compérat, E.M.; Dominguez-Escrig, J.L.; Andersson, I.G.; Liedberg, F.; Mariappan, P.; Mostafid, A.H.; et al. European association of urology guidelines on upper urinary tract urothelial carcinoma: 2023 Update. *Eur. Urol.* **2023**, *84*, 49–64. [CrossRef] [PubMed]
2. Raman, S.P.; Fishman, E.K. Upper and lower tract urothelial imaging using computed tomography urography. *Urol. Clin. N. Am.* **2018**, *45*, 389–405. [CrossRef] [PubMed]
3. Ali, O.; Fishman, E.K.; Sheth, S. Upper urinary tract urothelial carcinoma on multidetector CT: Spectrum of disease. *Abdom. Imaging* **2019**, *44*, 3874–3885. [CrossRef] [PubMed]
4. Burger, M.; Grossman, H.B.; Droller, M.; Schmidbauer, J.; Hermann, G.; Drăgoescu, O.; Ray, E.; Fradet, Y.; Karl, A.; Burgués, J.P.; et al. Photodynamic diagnosis of non–muscle-invasive bladder cancer with hexaminolevulinate cystoscopy: A meta-analysis of detection and recurrence based on raw data. *Eur. Urol.* **2013**, *64*, 846–854. [CrossRef] [PubMed]
5. Takahashi, N.; Kawashima, A.; Glockner, J.F.; Hartman, R.P.; Kim, B.; King, B.F. MR urography for suspected upper tract urothelial carcinoma. *Eur. Radiol.* **2008**, *19*, 912–923. [CrossRef] [PubMed]
6. Cheaib, J.G.; Claus, L.E.; Patel, H.D.; Kates, M.R.; Matoso, A.; Hahn, N.M.; Bivalacqua, T.J.; Hoffman-Censits, J.H.; Pierorazio, P.M. Site of metastatic recurrence impacts prognosis in patients with high-grade upper tract urothelial carcinoma. *Urol. Oncol. Semin. Orig. Investig.* **2021**, *39*, 74.e9–74.e16. [CrossRef] [PubMed]
7. Ferro, M.; Chiujdea, S.; Vartolomei, M.D.; Bove, P.; Porreca, A.; Busetto, G.M.; del Giudice, F.; Antonelli, A.; Foschi, N.; Racioppi, M.; et al. Advanced Age Impacts Survival After Radical Nephroureterectomy for Upper Tract Urothelial Carcinoma. *Clin. Genitourin. Cancer* **2023**, *9*, 1–11. [CrossRef] [PubMed]
8. Vikram, R.; Sandler, C.M.; Ng, C.S. Imaging and Staging of Transitional Cell Carcinoma: Part 2, Upper Urinary Tract. *Am. J. Roentgenol.* **2009**, *192*, 1488–1493. [CrossRef]
9. Bray, F.; Ferlay, J.; Soerjomataram, I.; Siegel, R.L.; Torre, L.A.; Jemal, A. Global cancer statistics 2018: GLOBOCAN estimates of incidence and mortality worldwide for 36 cancers in 185 countries. *CA Cancer J. Clin.* **2018**, *68*, 394–424. [CrossRef]

10. Alessandrino, F.; Ghaith, O.; Williams, K.; Sonpavde, G.P.; Silverman, S.G.; Shinagare, A.B. Advanced urothelial cancer: A radiology update. *Abdom. Radiol.* **2019**, *44*, 3858–3873. [CrossRef]
11. Imokawa, S.; Uehara, M.; Uto, T.; Sagisaka, S.; Sato, J.; Yasuda, K.; Matsushita, K.; Oi, S.; Tanioka, F.; Suda, T.; et al. Pulmonary metastasis from urothelial carcinoma showing progressive multiple cystic lesions. *Am. J. Respir. Crit. Care Med.* **2013**, *188*, 1267–1268. [CrossRef] [PubMed]
12. Galluzzo, A.; Danti, G.; Bicci, E.; Mastrorosato, M.; Bertelli, E.; Miele, V. The role of Dual-Energy CT in the study of urinary tract tumours: Review of recent literature. *Semin. Ultrasound CT MRI* **2023**, *44*, 136–144. [CrossRef] [PubMed]
13. Bicci, E.; Mastrorosato, M.; Danti, G.; Lattavo, L.; Bertelli, E.; Cozzi, D.; Pradella, S.; Agostini, S.; Miele, V. Dual-Energy CT applications in urinary tract cancers: An update. *Tumori J.* **2022**, *109*, 148–156. [CrossRef] [PubMed]
14. Razavi, S.A.; Sadigh, G.; Kelly, A.M.; Cronin, P. Comparative effectiveness of imaging modalities for the diagnosis of upper and lower urinary tract malignancy: A critically appraised topic. *Acad. Radiol.* **2012**, *19*, 1134–1140. [CrossRef] [PubMed]
15. Abreu-Gomez, J.; Udare, A.; Shanbhogue, K.P.; Schieda, N. Update on MR urography (MRU): Technique and clinical applications. *Abdom. Radiol.* **2019**, *44*, 3800–3810. [CrossRef] [PubMed]
16. O'Connor, O.J.; McLaughlin, P.; Maher, M.M. MR Urography. *Am. J. Roentgenol.* **2010**, *195*, 201–206. [CrossRef] [PubMed]
17. Iancu, A.S.; Colin, P.; Puech, P.; Villers, A.; Ouzzane, A.; Fantoni, J.C.; Leroy, X.; Lemaitre, L. Significance of ADC value for detection and characterization of urothelial carcinoma of upper urinary tract using diffusion-weighted MRI. *World J. Urol.* **2012**, *31*, 13–19. [CrossRef] [PubMed]
18. Lonati, C.; Simeone, C.; Suardi, N.; Spiess, P.E.; Necchi, A.; Moschini, M. Genitourinary manifestations of Lynch syndrome in the urological practice. *Asian J. Urol.* **2022**, *9*, 443–450. [CrossRef]
19. Seguel, A.P.; Pérez, M.M.; González, T.R.; Gómez, D.; del Río, J.V.; Benítez, G.M. Evaluation of upper tract urothelial carcinomas by contrast-enhanced ultrasound. *Radiol. (Eng. Ed.)* **2018**, *60*, 496–503. [CrossRef]
20. Xue, L.-Y.; Lu, Q.; Huang, B.-J.; Li, C.-L.; Yan, C.-J.; Wen, J.-X.; Wang, W.-P. Evaluation of renal urothelial carcinoma by contrast-enhanced ultrasonography. *Eur. J. Radiol.* **2013**, *82*, e151–e157. [CrossRef]
21. Drudi, F.M.; Di Candio, G.; Di Leo, N.; Malpassini, F.; Gnecchi, M.; Cantisani, V.; Iori, F.; Liberatore, M. Contrast-enhanced ultrasonography in the diagnosis of upper urinary tract urothelial cell carcinoma: A preliminary study. *Ultraschall Med.—Eur. J. Ultrasound* **2012**, *34*, 30–37. [CrossRef]
22. Tanaka, H.; Yoshida, S.; Komai, Y.; Sakai, Y.; Urakami, S.; Yuasa, T.; Yamamoto, S.; Masuda, H.; Koizumi, M.; Kohno, A.; et al. Clinical value of 18F-fluorodeoxyglucose positron emission tomography/computed tomography in upper tract urothelial carcinoma: Impact on detection of metastases and patient management. *Urol. Int.* **2015**, *96*, 65–72. [CrossRef] [PubMed]
23. Voskuilen, C.S.; Schweitzer, D.; Jensen, J.B.; Nielsen, A.M.; Joniau, S.; Muilwijk, T.; Necchi, A.; Azizi, M.; Spiess, P.E.; Briganti, A.; et al. Diagnostic value of 18F-fluorodeoxyglucose positron emission tomography with computed tomography for lymph node staging in patients with upper tract urothelial carcinoma. *Eur. Urol. Oncol.* **2020**, *3*, 73–79. [CrossRef] [PubMed]
24. Zattoni, F.; Incerti, E.; Moro, F.D.; Moschini, M.; Castellucci, P.; Panareo, S.; Picchio, M.; Fallanca, F.; Briganti, A.; Gallina, A.; et al. 18F-FDG PET/CT and urothelial carcinoma: Impact on management and prognosis—A multicenter retrospective study. *Cancers* **2019**, *11*, 700. [CrossRef] [PubMed]
25. Sassa, N.; Kato, K.; Abe, S.; Iwano, S.; Ito, S.; Ikeda, M.; Shimamoto, K.; Yamamoto, S.; Yamamoto, T.; Gotoh, M.; et al. Evaluation of 11C-choline PET/CT for primary diagnosis and staging of urothelial carcinoma of the upper urinary tract: A pilot study. *Eur. J. Nucl. Med.* **2014**, *41*, 2232–2241. [CrossRef] [PubMed]
26. Gofrit, O.N.; Mishani, E.; Orevi, M.; Klein, M.; Freedman, N.; Pode, D.; Shapiro, A.; Katz, R.; Libson, E.; Chisin, R. Contribution of 11C-Choline Positron Emission Tomography/Computerized Tomography to Preoperative Staging of Advanced Transitional Cell Carcinoma. *J. Urol.* **2006**, *176*, 940–944. [CrossRef] [PubMed]
27. Thakur, M.L.; Tripathi, S.K.; Gomella, L.G.; Salmanoglu, E.; Kim, S.; Kelly, W.K.; Keith, S.W.; Intenzo, C.; McCue, P.; Hoffman-Censits, J.; et al. Imaging urothelial bladder cancer: A VPAC PET targeted approach. *Can. J. Urol.* **2021**, *28*, 10596–10602. [PubMed]
28. Orevi, M.; Klein, M.; Mishani, E.; Chisin, R.; Freedman, N.; Gofrit, O.N. 11C-Acetate PET/CT in Bladder Urothelial Carcinoma: Intraindividual Comparison with: 11: C-Choline. *Clin. Nucl. Med.* **2012**, *37*, e67–e72. [CrossRef]
29. He, Y.; Gao, W.; Ying, W.; Feng, N.; Wang, Y.; Jiang, P.; Gong, Y.; Li, X. A Novel Preoperative Prediction Model Based on Deep Learning to Predict Neoplasm T Staging and Grading in Patients with Upper Tract Urothelial Carcinoma. *J. Clin. Med.* **2022**, *11*, 5815. [CrossRef]
30. Angeloni, M.; van Doeveren, T.; Lindner, S.; Volland, P.; Schmelmer, J.; Foersch, S.; Matek, C.; Stoehr, R.; Geppert, C.I.; Heers, H.; et al. A deep-learning workflow to predict upper tract urothelial cancer subtypes supporting the prioritization of patients for molecular testing. *medRxiv* **2023**. [CrossRef]
31. Liu, J.; Wu, P.; Lai, S.; Wang, J.; Hou, H.; Zhang, Y. Prognostic models for upper urinary tract urothelial carcinoma patients after radical nephroureterectomy based on a novel systemic immune-inflammation score with machine learning. *BMC Cancer* **2023**, *23*, 574. [CrossRef] [PubMed]
32. Deng, Z.; Dong, W.; Xiong, S.; Jin, D.; Zhou, H.; Zhang, L.; Xie, L.; Deng, Y.; Xu, R.; Fan, B. Machine learning models combining computed tomography semantic features and selected clinical variables for accurate prediction of the pathological grade of bladder cancer. *Front. Oncol.* **2023**, *13*, 1166245. [CrossRef] [PubMed]

33. Sarkar, S.; Min, K.; Ikram, W.; Tatton, R.W.; Riaz, I.B.; Silva, A.C.; Bryce, A.H.; Moore, C.; Ho, T.H.; Sonpavde, G.; et al. Performing Automatic Identification and Staging of Urothelial Carcinoma in Bladder Cancer Patients Using a Hybrid Deep-Machine Learning Approach. *Cancers* **2023**, *15*, 1673. [CrossRef] [PubMed]
34. Slywotzky, C.; Maya, M. Needle tract seeding of transitional cell carcinoma following fine-needle aspiration of a renal mass *Abdom. Imaging* **1994**, *19*, 174–176. [CrossRef]
35. Huang, S.Y.; Ahrar, K.; Gupta, S.; Wallace, M.J.; Ensor, J.E.; Krishnamurthy, S.; Matin, S.F. Safety and diagnostic accurary of percutaneous biopsy in upper tract urothelial carcinoma. *BJUI Int.* **2015**, *115*, 625–632. [CrossRef] [PubMed]
36. Messina, E.; Pisciotti, M.L.; Pecoraro, M.; Borrelli, A.; Del Giudice, F.; Panebianco, V. The use of MRI in urothelial carcinoma. *Curr. Opin. Urol.* **2022**, *32*, 536–544. [CrossRef]

cancers

Review

Upper Tract Urothelial Carcinoma (UTUC) Diagnosis and Risk Stratification: A Comprehensive Review

Masoud Bitaraf, Mahmood Ghafoori Yazdi and Erfan Amini *

Uro-Oncology Research Center, Tehran University of Medical Sciences, Tehran 1419733141, Iran; sm-bitaraf@alumnus.tums.ac.ir (M.B.); ghafoori5@gmail.com (M.G.Y.)
* Correspondence: e-amini@sina.tums.ac.ir; Tel./Fax: +98-21-66903063

Simple Summary: To choose the appropriate treatment for patients with upper tract urothelial carcinoma (UTUC), proper diagnosis and risk assessment of the disease is mandatory. This study reviews some of the diagnostic tools, and the patient- and disease-related prognostic factors that affect the outcome. Predictive tools designed by these factors help determine which patients should undergo radical nephroureterectomy. Other tools help post-operative decisions regarding the use of chemotherapy and planning follow-up sessions. The available pre-operative predictive tools and post-operative nomograms are discussed. A revision of the current classification of patients to low- and high-risk groups is recommended, to expand the number of patients benefiting from kidney-sparing surgeries.

Abstract: Diagnosis and risk stratification are cornerstones of therapeutic decisions in the management of patients with upper tract urothelial carcinoma (UTUC). Diagnostic modalities provide data that can be integrated, to provide nomograms and stratification tools to predict survival and adverse outcomes. This study reviews cytology, ureterorenoscopy and the novel tools and techniques used with it (including photodynamic diagnosis, narrow-band imaging, optical coherence tomography, and confocal laser endomicroscopy), and biopsy. Imaging modalities and novel biomarkers are discussed in another article. Patient- and tumor-related prognostic factors, their association with survival indices, and their roles in different scores and predictive tools are discussed. Patient-related factors include age, sex, ethnicity, tobacco consumption, surgical delay, sarcopenia, nutritional status, and several blood-based markers. Tumor-related prognosticators comprise stage, grade, presentation, location, multifocality, size, lymphovascular invasion, surgical margins, lymph node status, mutational landscape, architecture, histologic variants, and tumor-stroma ratio. The accuracy and validation of pre-operative predictive tools, which incorporate various prognosticators to predict the risk of muscle-invasive or non-organ confined disease, and help to decide on the surgery type (radical nephroureterectomy, or kidney-sparing procedures) are also investigated. Post-operative nomograms, which help decide on adjuvant chemotherapy and plan follow-up are explored. Finally, a revision of the current stratification of UTUC patients is endorsed.

Keywords: upper tract urothelial carcinoma; UTUC; diagnosis; risk stratification; nomogram; prognosis

1. Introduction

Upper tract urothelial carcinoma (UTUC) is a rare and heterogeneous disease that accounts for up to 5% of all urothelial neoplasms [1]. Accurate diagnosis and risk stratification are indispensable for determining the optimal therapeutic management for each individual patient. While the standard therapy for UTUC used to be radical nephroureterectomy (RNU), kidney-sparing surgeries (KSS) have emerged as an alternative and are increasingly being utilized. KSS includes endoscopic management, such as ureteroscopy or a percutaneous approach, as well as segmental ureterectomy that preserves the ipsilateral renal unit [2].

Diagnostic tools guide stratification, which in turn, leads to decisions regarding type of surgery, chemotherapy, and follow-up strategy. However, UTUC diagnosis and risk stratification can be challenging, and various prognostic models, nomograms, and new diagnostic tools have been developed to guide risk stratification and improve UTUC diagnosis accuracy. This review aims to provide a comprehensive overview of the current state of UTUC diagnosis and risk stratification, including the use of cytology, endoscopic evaluation, prognostic factors, and nomograms. Imaging modalities and novel biomarkers are discussed in another article from the same issue. Pre- and post-operative predictive tools are discussed and the need for novel classifications is highlighted.

2. Methods

This is a narrative review. Medline was searched through Pubmed from commencement to 22 April 2023. Studies on diagnosis and risk stratification of UTUC were included only after assessment of methodological rigor, and conceptual consistency. No language or article type limit was applied. Data on imaging and novel biomarkers were excluded.

3. Diagnostic Tests

3.1. Urine Cytology

Once carcinomas of the bladder and prostatic urethra are ruled out, abnormal cytology may point to high-grade UTUC. Voided urinary cytology has a sensitivity of 11% to 71.1%. Performing selective cytology, or combining cytology with biopsy improves its detection rates [3]. Selective urinary cytology is the process of obtaining urine samples from ureters separately. It is highly sensitive to high-grade tumors, including carcinoma in situ (CIS) [4]. Zhao et al. suggested that biopsy or cytology alone yields a sensitivity of about 60% for high-grade UTUC. While combining the two, increases the sensitivity to 85% [3]. Barbotage cytology is the process of infusing saline into the urinary tract, using a flexible ureteroscope and gently flushing the fluid in and out, to obtain mucosal cells. Barbotage cytology is accurate in diagnosing UTUC with a detection rate of up to 91% [5]. Overall, urine cytology is an available, cost-effective and simple test that has retained its application in UTUC diagnosis despite its limitations.

3.2. Ureterorenoscopy and Biopsy

Formerly, UTUC diagnosis was mainly based on imaging. Emerging new kidney-sparing and neo-adjuvant treatments, highlighted the importance of ureterorenoscopy (URS). It is now an integral part of UTUC workup, which helps determine the size, location, and architecture of the suspicious lesions, and obtain biopsy samples [6]. However, concerns remain regarding diagnostic URS's impact on oncological outcomes. A meta-analysis on 5489 patients indicated that URS plus biopsy is associated with worse intravesical recurrence-free survival (IVRFS) following RNU (Hazard ratio (HR): 1.44, 95% Confidence interval (CI): 1.29–1.61, $p < 0.001$), but it does not affect long-term survival outcomes. Diagnostic URS without biopsy was not associated with worse IVRFS [7]. Table 1 summarizes the studies assessing the association between URS, IVR (intravesical recurrence), and RFS (recurrence-free survival) [8–22]. A study on 143 patients demonstrated a pathological phenotype-specific association between pre-operation URS and oncological outcomes, as the subgroup of patients with non-papillary and ≥pT3 UTUC had poorer overall and progression-free survival [23].

Table 1. Summary of studies reporting the association between URS and IVR, and RFS.

Study	Patient Population/Study Duration	No. of Patients	Median Follow Up	Urinary Bladder Recurrence	Recurrence Free Survival	Median Time to Recurrence	Cancer-Specific Death	Comments
Liedberg F, et al. (2023) [8]	Sweden 2015–2019	1038 IDM+: 536 IDM−: 502	1.3 yrs	220 (21.2%) IDM+: 120 (22.38%) IDM−: 100 (19.20%)			IDM+: HR: 1.56 95% CI: (1.12–2.18)	IDM increases risk of IVR in ureteric tumor and not in the renal pelvis
Luo Z, et al. (2023) [9]	China 2009–2020	220 1-session URS: 22 (10%) 2-session URS: 112 (51%) No URS: 86 (39%)	41 mos	58 (26.4%) 1-session URS: 5 (22.7%) 2-session URS: 36 (32.1%) No URS:17 (19.8%)				Delayed RNU following URS (2-session) could increase the IVR risk, but not immediate RNU after URS (1-session)
Anbarasan T, et al. (2023) [10]	UK 1998–2015	267		73 (27.3%)	5-yr RFS 64.7% URS + Bx: 49.9% URS−: 76.4%			Identical mutational changes in genes (TP53 and FGFR3) between primary UTUC and subsequent IVR.
Douglawi A, et al. (2022) [11]	USC-USA 2005–2019	143 URS+: 104 (73%) Access sheath+: 36 (25%) No URS: 39 (27%)	27 mos	36 (25%) URS+: 30.8% (Access sheath+: 11.5% Access sheath−: 39.7%) No URS: 7.7%		URS+: 9.0 mos No URS: 12.1 mos		URS increases IVR but using an access sheath may mitigate this effect
Ha JS, et al. (2022) [12]	R Korea 2016–2019	396 Rigid URS: 178 (45%) Flexible URS: 111 (28%) No URS: 107 (27%)	1 yr	99 (25%) Rigid URS: 41 Flexible URS: 37 No URS: 21				Rigid URS may not increase the risk of IVR, whereas flexible URS appears to be associated with a higher risk of IVR.
Sharma V. et al. (2021) [13]	USA 1995–2019	834 no URS: 210 (25.2%) Percutaneous Bx: 57 (6.6%) URS-Bx: 125 (15%) URS + BX: 442 (53%)	2 yrs	No URS: 15% Percutaneous Bx: 12.7% URS-Bx: 18.7% URS + BX: 21.9%				URS + Bx but not percutaneous Bx or URS-Bx increases IVR risk
İzol V et al. (2021) [14]	Turkey 2005–2019	194 URS+: 95 (49% URS−: 99 (51%)	39.17 mos	54 (27.8%) URS+: 38.9% URS−: 17.2%	URS+: 60 mos URS−: 111 mos	10 mos		URS was associated with poor recurrence free survival
Shsm H, et al. (2021) [15]	UK 2012–2019	69 URS+: 49 (71%) URS−: 20 (29%)	48.5 mos	URS+: 28.3% URS−: 5.9%				Diagnostic URS delays definitive treatment and is associated with higher IVR
Chung Y, et al. (2020) [16]	Korea 2003–2018	453 URS+: 226 (49.9%) URS−: 227 (50.1%)	15 mos	URS+: 99 (43.8%) URS−: 61 (26.9%)	5-yr URS+: 56.2% URS−: 73.1%			Preoperative URS increases IVR. It is better not to perform URS before surgery
Baboudjian M, et al. (2020) [17]	France 2005–2017	93 URS+: 70 No URS: 23	35 mos	47 (50%) URS+: 41 (87%)		URS+: 226 days No URS: 427 days		High IVR rate after URS

Table 1. *Cont.*

Study	Patient Population/Study Duration	No. of Patients	Median Follow Up	Urinary Bladder Recurrence	Recurrence Free Survival	Median Time to Recurrence	Cancer-Specific Death	Comments
Lee HY, et al. (2018) [18]	Taiwan 1990–2013	502 URS + Bx: 206, 41% No URS: 296, 59%	6.4 yrs	138 (27.5%) URS+ Bx did not increase IVR (p = 0.609)	URS+ = no URS (p = 0.829)			URS + Bx is not associated with higher risk of IVR
Lee HY, et al. (2018) [18]	Taiwan 1996–2013	5713 URS+: 3079 No URS: 2634		No URS: 392 (14.88%) URS + Bx: 515 (16.73%)	URS + Bx = no URS p = 0.442 in low grade p = 0.292 in high grade			URS + Bx do not increase IVR irrespective of the tumor location
Sankin A, et al. (2016) [19]	New York, USA 1994–2012	201 URS+: 144 (72%) URS−: 57 (28%)	5.4 yrs	89 URS+: HR 2.58; 95% CI 1.47, 4.54	3-yr RFS URS+: 42% URS−:71%			URS increases the risk for IVR but does not have an effect on disease progression or survival
Liu P, et al. (2016) [20]	Beijing, China 2000–2011	664 URS+: 81 No URS: 583	48 mos	223 (33.6%)	2-yr RFS URS+: 71.4% No URS: 79.3%	17 months		URS is independently associated with IVR
Sung HH, et al. (2015) [21]	Korea 1994–2013	630 URS+: 282 (44.7%) No URS: 348 (55.3%)	34.3 mos	268 (42.5%)	5-yr RFS URS+: 42.6 ± 8.0% No URS: 63.6 ± 6.9%			URS increases IVR but URS with manipulation does not have an effect IVR
Ishikawa S, et al. (2010) [22]	Japan 1990–2005	208 URS+: 55 (26.5) No URS: 153 (73.5%)	44 mos	86 (41.3%)	2-yr RFS URS+: 60% No URS: 58.7%			Diagnostic URS does not have an effect on IVR or cancer specific survival

IDM: Invasive Diagnostic Modalities, including all invasive workup tools such as antegrade/retrograde uretero-pyelography and/or selective urine cytology/barbotage, and URS with or without concomitant biopsy.

Due to limitations of white light URS, novel tools are being experimented with the aim of improving the detection rate and increasing sensitivity and specificity. Photodynamic diagnosis (PDD), using 5-aminolevulinic acid (ALA), is one of these tools. In this method, ALA is administered orally, and a high concentration of ALA in cancer cells, results in their red appearance in blue light URS [24]. The most common side effect of this method is hypotension, which is mild in nature [25]. PDD has shown improvements in detecting CIS but its application in UTUC diagnosis is limited since it requires dedicated ureteroscopes, and its highest quality is achieved when the tissue being observed is positioned at a perpendicular angle to the ureteroscope, while in URS, the mucosa is mainly parallel to the probe [25,26].

Narrow band imaging (NBI) is a technique that uses two narrow bands of white light, which are taken up by hemoglobin in the blood vessels, and theoretically, makes identification of tumors easier. Only two papers have been published on its application at UTUC [27,28]. In 2011, Traxer et al. published a series of 27 patients that were simultaneously inspected by both NBI and white light. NBI improved visualization and tumor detection by 22.7% [27]. In 2018, Lordache et al. used NBI on 87 patients and concluded that NBI improves the detection rate of pTa and CIS [28].

Optical coherence tomography (OCT) is a tool that is used in ophthalmology to visualize retinal layers. It is based on light emission, reflection and scattering. It has been used with flexible URS to assess the depth and penetration of the tumor. Its main drawback is that it is limited to approximately 2 mm of depth. Although it discriminates between invasive and non-invasive tumors, it is not helpful in cases of more advanced disease. It can also assess tumor grade by measuring the decrease in light intensity [29]. When compared to biopsy, it has shown superior results in terms of staging and grading of the tumors [30].

Confocal laser endomicroscopy (CLE) is a novel tool that is implemented in UTUC diagnosis. After introducing fluorescein to the tissue (either intravenously or topically), a probe is introduced to the urothelium through the URS. Excited fluorescein emits light that is absorbed through a pinhole, which ultimately gives a picture almost identical to histology. The main difference is that fluorescein cannot cross cell membranes, so it does not show nuclear features. It is also applicable to biopsied tissues [31]. Currently, there are three small patient series published on in-vivo use to diagnose UTUC [32–34]. Taken all together, CLE can correctly assess low-grade UTUC in a high percentage of patients but is less accurate in high-grade disease. Despite excellent results, more studies with bigger patient populations need to be executed.

Although great results have been documented with novel diagnostic tools, their place in the diagnostic spectrum of UTUC is not well established yet.

Since ureteroscopic biopsy can be inaccurate in assessing tumor stage, and is associated with an increased risk of post-RNU IVR, the EAU guideline favors performing URS without biopsy [6]. In terms of biopsy devices, the largest specimens are obtained using BIGopsy backloading biopsy forceps in flat and sessile lesions, and by using Nitinol basket biopsy in papillary tumors [35,36]. However, one study questioned the BIGopsy forceps utility, considering its huge size, backloading requirement, and blocking the field of view [37]. The standard 3F forceps (Piranha) is considered inferior to both of them [35,36].

Novel techniques are proposed to increase the quality of specimens obtained through biopsy. Cryobiopsy involves using a cryoprobe to create an ice ball around the tissue of interest through sudden decompression of carbon dioxide. This technique allows for effective biopsy as the ice ball adheres more strongly to the probe than to the surrounding tissue. Compared to standard biopsy tools, the use of cryoprobes have been found to produce larger and higher-quality biopsies, more representative of the original tissue structure. The implementation of this technique in clinical settings has the potential to yield promising results, as shown by an ex-vivo study. However, it requires to be confirmed by rigorous in-vivo studies [38].

In the "form tackle" technique, a cold cup biopsy forcep is introduced through the ureteroscope. It is opened and pressed at the base of the lesion to include the submucosal tissue. The forceps are advanced 3–10 mm, and then pulled. The preliminary data based on fourteen patients who went through this procedure indicated that this method provides larger specimens [39].

Obtaining a biopsy without URS has been investigated as well. Percutaneous core-needle biopsy (PCNB) was shown to be feasible, accurate, and safe for UTUC diagnosis [40]. Joseph et al. reported the results of PCNB, guided by computed tomography (CT) or ultrasonography (US), prior to RNU. PCNB provided tumor grade in 69% of the cases, and of these, 89.7% were concordant with the final pathology. No tract seeding was identified during the 28 month follow-up [41].

3.3. *Risk Stratification*

Risk stratification aims to guide therapeutic decisions regarding the type of surgery (radical vs. kidney sparing) and peri-operative systemic therapy (neo- and adjuvant chemotherapy). Patient- and tumor-related prognosticators along with various biomarkers are used for this purpose.

4. Patient-Related Prognosticators

4.1. *Age and Sex*

A meta-analysis revealed a weak significant association between advanced age and overall survival (OS) (HR: 1.05), progression-free survival (PFS) (HR: 1.01), and cancer-specific survival (CSS) (HR: 1.02) [42]. Another meta-analysis on post-operative nomograms revealed a significant negative predictive value of age for CSS [1]. Although several studies have shown the association between age and survival indices [43,44], no association was found after adjustment for performance status (PS) [45]. However, age is found to be a predictor of muscle-invasive disease [46–49].

Unlike bladder cancer, UTUC prognosis is not associated with gender [50].

4.2. *Ethnicity*

One study indicates differences in clinicopathological features and OS between United States and Chinese patients, with US patients having a worse OS ($p = 0.049$) [51]. Another study suggests worse cancer-specific mortality (CSM) in Asian ethnicity compared to Caucasians (HR: 1.29, $p < 0.01$), after PS-matching. This study did not find any difference in tumor grade or T-stage between studied ethnicities (Asian, Caucasian, Hispanic, and African American) [52]. A shorter survival is suggested for African Americans, without a clear explanation of whether it is related to access to care or biological differences [53].

4.3. *Tobacco Consumption*

While smoking ≥20 cigarettes per day for ≥20 years, increases the chance of advanced disease stage, disease recurrence, IVR after RNU, and mortality; its detrimental effects are mitigated after 10 years of cessation [54,55]. A meta-analysis with 2259 patients showed a strong association between smoking and disease recurrence (HR: 1.57, 95% CI = 1.19–1.95), and CSM (HR: 1.53, 95% CI: 1.13–1.92) [56].

4.4. *Surgical Delay*

Waiting more than 120 days between diagnosis and definitive surgery was associated with lower OS in 3581 UTUC patients who underwent RNU [57]. Sundi et al. found no significant difference in survival outcomes in their group of 186 patients who were divided into early (<3 months) and late (≥3 months) surgery groups [58]. Considering studies on surgical waiting time, the EAU recommendation remains to perform definitive surgery within the first 12 weeks of diagnosis [6].

4.5. *Other Factors*

A meta-analysis of 81,814 patients with solid tumors indicates a prevalence of 35.3% for sarcopenia [59]. A recent cohort of 142 patients found that sarcopenia is a common finding in UTUC (prevalence: 37.3%). This suggests that its prevalence in UTUC does not differ from other solid tumors. Moreover, the study found sarcopenia as a comorbidity-independent predictive factor for OS (HR: 1.77; 95% CI: 1.02–3.07; $p = 0.042$) and CSS (HR, 2.17; 95% CI 1.18–3.99; $p = 0.012$) in UTUC patients following RNU. The authors also suggested that a high visceral adipose tissue index measured on a CT-scan at the height of third lumbar vertebra is associated with better outcomes after RNU. However, this finding was not statistically significant [60].

Pre-operative nutritional status is a significant determinant of survival outcomes. The preoperative prognostic nutritional index (PNI) is calculated by the following formula: PNI = 10 × serum albumin concentration (g/dL) + 0.005 × lymphocyte counts (number/mm^3). Low PNI is associated with poorer OS and PFS. Nutritional support and possible postponement of surgery until better general status is achieved is suggested in patients with low PNI [61,62]. Albumin level is used to calculate the HALP (hemoglobin, albumin, lymphocyte, and platelets) score as well. Gao et al. divided 533 UTUC patients who underwent RNU into low- and high-HALP groups. Lower HALP score was associated with poorer OS (HR = 1.54, 95% CI, 1.14–2.01, $p = 0.006$) and PFS (HR = 1.44, 95% CI, 1.07–1.93, $p = 0.020$) [63]. A negative correlation of low pre-operative Albumin (<39.8 g/L) with OS, PFS, and CSS was reported by Zhao et al. [64].

Zhao et al. also combined decreased albumin with elevated neutrophil-to-lymphocyte ratio (NLR) and divided patients into three groups of having none, either one, or both of these factors. The 5-year PFS rate dropped from 77.8% to 52.6% to 32.3%, the 5-year CSS rate dropped from 97.7% to 71.4% to 32.9%, the 5-year OS rate dropped from 92.7% to 70.4% to 29.2%, in respective groups (all $p < 0.0001$) [64]. Increased pre-operative NLR was shown to be predictive of poor OS (HR: 1.72, 95% CI: 1.45–2.05), PFS (HR: 1.68, 95% CI: 1.44–1.96), and CSS (HR: 1.64, 95% CI: 1.39–1.93), in a meta-analysis on 11,538 patients from 32 studies [65].

Elevated pre-operative fibrinogen is another marker associated with worse OS (HR: 2.09; $p < 0.001$), RFS (HR: 2.09; $p < 0.001$), and CSS (hazard ratio [HR]: 2.33; $p < 0.001$) [66]. Egger et al. combined elevated fibrinogen with high C-reactive protein and showed that concomitant elevation of both factors is associated with adverse histological characteristics. The score based on these factors was predictive of worse CSS in multivariate analysis and of OS in univariate analysis [67].

Traditional habits such as the use of herbs and plant food supplements, especially common in eastern societies, are known as an important risk factor contributing to the disproportionately high incidence of UTUC in Taiwan. Aristolochic acid (AA)-containing Chinese herbal preparations was banned in 2003. However, a recent study showed an increasing trend in the incidence of UTUC in Taiwan that may be attributed to the consumption of unknown sources of AA. This highlights the importance of vigorous surveillance of phytotherapy and herbal products, as they are gaining popularity in the modern world [68]. AA exposure results in aristolactam (AL)-DNA adduct formation. AL-DNA adducts are poorly repaired, hence remaining in target organs for years. These adducts can be used as biomarkers of AA exposure, and are found in a high proportion of Taiwanese UTUC patients [69–71]. The AL-DNA adducts result in A:T to T:A transversion, as a mutational signature [72]. AA-related UTUC was shown to be associated with higher grade, and stage of the tumor. However, it was not associated with increased IVR [73].

5. Tumor-Related Prognosticators

5.1. Tumor Stage and Grade

Tumor stage and grade are two well-established prognostic factors of UTUC. High-grade is associated with advanced stage, loco-regional and distant recurrence, and non-organ-confined (NOC) disease [74]. It is also associated with worse RFS (HR: 2.0, $p < 0.001$) and CSS (HR: 1.7, $p = 0.001$) [75]. In a Dutch series of 13,314 UTUC patients, the 5-year relative survival rates for superficial, organ-confined, and NOC disease were 85.7%, 69.6%, and 43.6%, respectively [76]. Both uni- and multi-variate analyses on 374 patients with primary localized UTUC revealed a higher risk of IVR in patients with higher-grade tumors (Relative risk (RR): 3.776, $p < 0.0001$) [77].

Katayama et al. argued that factors used in current risk stratification models (including that of EAU and National Comprehensive Cancer Network (NCCN)) other than clinical tumor stage and grade, do not add significant predictive value in clinically low-stage low-grade tumors. However, they limit the adoption of KSS. They proposed a model solely based on grade and stage (GS model), from the data of URS biopsy and imaging, that yielded comparable accuracy to that of EAU and NCCN and considered a higher portion of patients as candidates for KSS [78].

5.2. Tumor Presentation, Location, Multifocality, and Size

A recent study assessed the association between flank pain (FP), gross hematuria (GH), and survival outcomes in UTUC patients who underwent RNU. Unlike GH, the presence of FP was associated with worse 5-year OS (47.2% vs. 81.2% (FP+ vs. FP−), $p = 0.001$) and CSS (50.2% vs. 83.9%, $p < 0.001$). Multivariate analysis revealed FP, multifocality, and pathological stage as independent prognostic factors for OS and CSS. On subgroup analysis, the patients in group 'FP without GH' had the worst oncological outcomes. Patients with FP had a 2.95 times higher hazard ratio for cancer-specific death (CSD), compared to those without FP [79]. In a cohort of 2662 patients, 80% presented with hematuria (microscopic or gross), while only 15% presented with symptomatic hydronephrosis (i.e., hydronephrosis and FP). Hematuria was associated with less hydronephrosis, renal pelvic tumors, and early pathological tumor stage. Meanwhile, symptomatic hydronephrosis was associated with ureteral tumors and advanced pathological stage. On multivariate analysis, hematuria was linked with better OS (HR 0.789, 95% CI 0.661–0.942) and CSS (HR 0.772, 95% CI 0.607–0.980), while symptomatic hydronephrosis was a predictor of poorer OS (HR 1.387, 95% CI 1.142–1.683) and CSS (HR 1.587, 95% CI 1.229–2.050) [80]. One possible explanation is that the obstruction caused by ureteral tumors, results in asymptomatic hydronephrosis and the absence of hematuria, leading to tumor upstaging. Pre-operative hydronephrosis, irrespective of pain, was shown to be associated with advanced pathological and poor survival outcomes [81,82].

A meta-analysis of 14,895 patients indicated a pooled hazard ratio of 1.52 ($p < 0.001$) and 1.39 ($p = 0.004$) for CSS and OS in patients with ureteral involvement [83]. Another study on 11,922 patients revealed lower median OS for patients with ureteral involvement compared to pelvicalyceal tumors (66.8 vs. 71.1 months; $p = 0.01$) [84]. Moreover, the microenvironment of tumors arising from either of the two locations differs in immunological profile [85]. Miyake et al. proposed a site-specific risk stratification model for ureteral and renal pelvis tumors to predict extraurinary tract recurrence (EUTR), CSD, and IVR after RNU. They found that the site-specific models yielded a higher discriminative accuracy, compared to the overall UTUC risk model for all three end-points [86]. Multifocal tumors are associated with worse CSS [79]. In the study of Miyake et al., multifocality was a common risk factor in both ureteral and pelvicalyceal models [86].

A meta-analysis of 35 studies and 32,292 patients found that an increase in tumor size is significantly associated with decreased OS, CSS, RFS, and IVR rates (HR: 1.42, 95% CI: 1.28–1.58, $p < 0.00001$; HR: 1.66, 95% CI: 1.47–1. 88, $p < 0.00001$; HR: 1.25, 95% CI: 1.13–1.38, $p < 0.0001$; HR: 1.12, 95% CI: 1.04–1.20, $p = 0.003$; respectively). The authors attributed the positive associations between tumor size and poor outcomes in UTUC to several theories on the biological mechanisms. Large tumor size correlates with aggressive tumor behavior including advanced-stage, lymphovascular invasion (LVI), lymph node metastasis, tumor necrosis, and tumor multifocality. Larger tumors are more susceptible to LVI, a prerequisite for lymph node metastases, which significantly increases the risk of disease recurrence, and cancer-specific and overall mortality even after RNU. Moreover, extensive tumor necrosis (>10% of tumor area) has been reported to be associated with metastasis- and cancer-related deaths. Lastly, patients with larger tumor sizes are more likely to involve both the ureter and the renal pelvis, making open RNU necessary, and putting the patient at risk of poorer surgical outcomes [87–89].

Although, in one study, the tumor size with the cutoff of >2 cm was shown to be associated with muscle invasion (OR 2.38, 95% CI 1.70–3.32; $p < 0.001$) [90], several studies did not show tumor size as a predictive factor for muscle-invasive disease [47,91,92].

5.3. Lymphovascular Invasion

A recent meta-analysis of 58 studies comprising 29829 UTUC patients who underwent RNU, showed that LVI was present in 26.2% of patients, which makes it a common histopathologic finding in RNU specimens. LVI was found to be a significant predictor of disease recurrence (pooled HR: 1.43, 95% CI: 1.31–1.55, $p = 0.000$; I(2) = 76.3%), CSS (pooled HR: 1.53, 95% CI: 1.41–1.66, $p = 0.000$; I(2) = 72.3%), and OSS (HR: 1.56, 95% CI 1.45–1.69, $p = 0.000$; I(2) = 62.9%) [93]. Another study indicated an association between LVI and OS (HR 4.980 CI 95%1.763–14.064, $p = 0.002$), and PFS (HR 2.687 CI 95%1.172–6.163, $p = 0.020$) [94].

The systemic immune inflammation index (SII) is calculated by multiplying NLR by platelet count. Positive LVI was found to be significantly associated with advanced tumor stage, high tumor grade, tumor necrosis, lymph node metastasis, and high SII levels. The co-existence of positive LVI and high-level SII was further found to be a significant predictor of poorer OS, CSS, and PFS (with hazards ratios and 95% confidence intervals of 3.918 [2.168–7.078], 5.623 [2.679–11.801], and 3.377 [2.138–5.334], respectively). However, on further analysis, the effect of co-occurrence of LVI and SII on survival outcomes was significant only in NOC disease [95]. LVI is also predicted by increased NLR (HR = 1.29, 95% CI = 1.17–1.43). Increased NLR also predicts higher tumor stage and grade (HR: 1.25, 95% CI = 1.12–1.39; and HR: 1.07, 95% CI = 1.01–1.14; respectively) [65]. LVI occurs during the early metastatic phase by invasion of tumor cells to the lymphatic/vascular channels. It represents the dynamic state of the disease. High SII is an indicator of pro-tumor inflammatory response and a weak anti-tumor immune state (as implied by high neutrophil and platelet and low lymphocyte count) [95].

5.4. Surgical Margins

Positive surgical margin, following RNU, is associated with a higher chance of metastases (5-year metastasis-free survival (MFS) of 51.6% vs. 79.3%) [96]. A positive margin was found to be associated with lower MFS [97]. Pooled analysis of 37984 patients from eight comparative trials revealed that robot-assisted RNU was associated with significantly lower positive surgical margins, compared to open RNU (OR 0.33, 95% CI 0.12, 0.92; $p = 0.03$) [98].

5.5. Lymph Node Status

Poor overall survival comes with nodal metastasis [99]. A study on 306 node-positive patients indicated that the number of removed or positive lymph nodes was not associated with survival indices. Meanwhile, positive lymph node density (best cutoff = 27%) was associated with lower OS and CSS (HR: 1.62, $p = 0.036$, and HR: 1.75, $p = 0.014$, respectively). The 5-year OS rate for patients with density < 27% was 18.7%, compared to 34.2% for those with density $\geq$ 27% ($p < 0.05$) [100].

5.6. Mutational Landscape

UTUC has distinct genetic characteristics. Various mutations are common in UTUC including FGFR3, KMT2D, KMT2a, TP53, and MDM2. A recent robust study proposed a mutational classification flow chart for UTUC, composed of 5 subgroups: the hyper-, TP53/MDM2-, RAS-, FGFR3-, and triple-negative-mutated subtypes. These subgroups differ in prognosis. The triple-negative-subtype shares a similar prognosis to the TP53/MDM2-mutated subtype, which exhibits the most aggressive clinical course. On the contrary, low-grade histology and higher survival rates are seen in the FGFR3-mutated subtype. The

RAS-mutated subtype is characterized by high-grade tumors and squamous cell differentiation [101,102].

By performing unsupervised hierarchical clustering, Su et al. identified two DNA methylation-based epi-clusters. Frequent hyper-methylation was witnessed in the EpiC-C1 cluster, which was more frequently associated with muscle-invasive UTUC, and shorter OS. The Epic-C2 was hypo-methylated, enriched in FGFR3 mutation, and associated with non-muscle invasive disease [103].

5.7. Other Factors

A meta-analysis of 14,368 patients revealed the significant association of sessile tumor architecture with disease recurrence and CSM (pooled HR: 1.454, and 1.416, respectively) [104]. In a study on 811 patients, sessile architecture was an independent predictor of muscle-invasive disease at RNU ($p < 0.0001$) [47]. In another study on 1214 patients who underwent RNU, sessile architecture was significantly associated with muscle-invasive or node-positive disease (OR: 2.31, 95% CI 1.58–3.36, $p < 0.001$) [49]. Papillary configuration was associated with a higher risk of IVR (RR: 3.244 $p < 0.0001$) [77].

Concomitant carcinoma in situ is associated with worse CSS and RFS (HR: 1.25; $p = 0.004$, and HR: 1.24; $p = 0.006$, respectively) [105]. Urothelial bladder cancer occurring at the same time (synchronous) or a different time (metachronous) with UTUC is a predictor of worse PFS (HR: 3.326 CI 95% 1.474–7.503, $p = 0.004$), but not OS [94].

Histological variants of UTUC are associated with the presence of adverse pathological features including higher stage and grade, tumor necrosis, positive surgical margins, and lymph node invasion. The micropapillary variant is associated with worse recurrence, and the sarcomatoid variant is linked to worse CSM. However, variant histology was not associated with survival outcomes in multivariate analyses [106,107].

A recent study assessed the tumor-stroma ratio according to histologic sections. It indicated an association between high-stroma tumors, poorer survival outcomes, and inferior responsiveness to chemotherapy. In addition, a correlation was shown between high-stroma tumors and immuno-evasive microenvironment with exhausted $CD8^+$ T-cells [107].

6. Pre-Operative Predictive Tools

Due to the imperfection of imaging, endoscopy, and biopsy, it is still difficult to achieve precise preoperative characterization of UTUC in terms of grading, staging, and prognosis. Mori et al. indicated a huge discordance between pre-operative clinical and post-operative pathological staging and grading. URS biopsy underestimated the stage in 59.5% of patients. Final pathology of 89.6% of patients with clinical $\leq$ cT1 disease, indicated muscle-invasion. Concordance between clinical and pathological grading occurred in 54.2% of patients [48]. Despite these, CT urography and URS biopsy are still the main sources of pre-operative information, and several predictive models are designed by employing data obtained from these modalities and combining them with other prognosticators. Table 2 summarizes the features of 10 multivariable models that predict muscle-invasive/NOC disease.

Table 2. Pre-operative predictive tools for muscle-invasive, NOC, or node positive UTUC.

First Author	Year	Prediction Form	Number of Patients	Prognosticators	Prediction of	Accuracy	Validation
Brien [108]	2010	Risk group stratification	172	Hydronephrosis, biopsy grade and urinary cytology	NOC UTUC Muscle Invasive	PPV 73 NPV 100 PPV 89 NPV 100	
Margulis [109]	2010	Nomogram	659	Tumor architecture, tumor grade and tumor location	NOC UTUC	76.6	Internal
Favaretto [91]	2012	Risk group stratification	274	Ureteroscopic grade, tumor location, Hydronephrosis and invasion on imaging	NOC Muscle Invasive	70 71	
Chen [110]	2013	Nomogram	693	Gender, architecture, multifocality, tumor location, grade and Hydronephrosis	NOC Muscle Invasive	79 79	Internal

Table 2. *Cont.*

First Author	Year	Prediction Form	Number of Patients	Prognosticators	Prediction of	Accuracy	Validation
Petros [92]	2018	Nomogram	566	Ureteroscopic grade, Architecture, Hemoglobin, Clinical stage	NOC UTUC	82 Development 77 Validation	Internal & External
Yoshida [111]	2020	Nomogram	1101	NLR, CKD, Tumor location, Hydronephrosis, Local invasion on imaging	NOC UTUC	77	Internal & External
Foerster [49]	2021	Nomogram	1214	Previous RC, architecture, multifocality, invasion on imaging, tumor size, Preoperative hydronephrosis, Cytology, Biopsy staging, biopsy grading, sex, age	≥pT2/N+	75 (bias corrected)	Internal
Marcq [47]	2022	Risk group stratification	1214	≥cT3, sessile architecture, hydronephrosis, High grade cytology, high grade biopsy, age at Dx	≥pT2	77	
Venkat [46]	2022	Nomogram	6143	Age, architecture, urine cytology, biopsy grade, LVI, Tumor size, cN	≥pT2	80	Internal
Venkat [46]	2022	Nomogram	6143	LVI, cN, Biopsy grade, tumor size	Positive Node	87.8	Internal

NOC: Non-organ confined; PPV: Positive predictive value; NPV: Negative predictive value; NLR: Neutrophil to lymphocyte ratio; CKD: Chronic kidney disease; RC: Radical cystectomy; Dx: Diagnosis; cN: clinical Node-positive.

Brien et al. used the data of 172 patients from five centers in the US and developed a pre-operative risk group stratification combining ureteroscopic biopsy grade, hydronephrosis, and urine cytology. Their model yielded 100% negative predictive value (NPV), when all three factors were negative, and positive predictive value (PPV) of 73% and 89% for NOC and muscle-invasive disease, respectively [108]. Using data from 274 patients from a single center in the US, Favaretto et al. proposed a risk group stratification model composed of ureteroscopic grade, tumor location, hydronephrosis, and invasion on imaging. Their model had an accuracy of 70% and 71% NOC and muscle-invasive disease, respectively [91]. These two models were not validated by the authors.

Margulis et al. studied 659 patients across 13 centers, mostly in the US and Europe, and developed an internally validated model for NOC prediction with 76.6% accuracy. Their nomogram comprised ureteroscopic tumor architecture, grade and location [109]. Chen et al. developed a nomogram using data from 693 Chinese patients from a single center. Gender, tumor architecture, multifocality, location, grade, and hydronephrosis were predictive factors of this internally validated model with 79% accuracy for NOC and muscle-invasive disease prediction [110]. Singla et al. compared predictive factors of NOC in UTUC patients from the US and China. They indicated that in the US cohort, clinical T3 stage and high-grade pathology on ureteroscopic biopsy were significant NOC disease predictors. Significant predictors of NOC in the Chinese cohort were male gender, tumor location and size on imaging, NLR, and pre-operative estimated glomerular filtration rate (eGFR). They further applied Margulis et al. and Chen et al. models to their study cohorts and found that the Western model (i.e., Margulis et al.) has an accuracy of 75% and 67% in the US and Chinese cohorts, respectively. The Chinese model (i.e., Chen et al.), was 76.3% and 82.8% accurate for US and Chinese populations, respectively [112]. Their results, somehow externally validated these models, and proposed that population-based differences should be considered during the clinical application of predictive models.

Petros et al. developed a nomogram for NOC disease prediction, using data from 566 patients from three centers in the US. The predictive factors used are ureteroscopic grade, tumor architecture, clinical stage, and pre-operative serum hemoglobin. An accuracy of 82% was achieved in the development cohort. Internal and external validation was performed and the model showed 77% accuracy in the test cohort. They further suggested an easily-remembered cut-off point ≥ 0.49 for high-risk disease on their nomogram [92]. Yoshida et al. used two independent Japanese databases to develop and validate a nomogram for NOC disease prediction. Their nomogram composed of NLR, chronic kidney disease (CKD), tumor location, hydronephrosis, and local invasion on imaging, achieved 77% accuracy [111]. URS data are not implemented in the Yoshida et al. nomogram, hence its applicability in patients whose UTUC is detected in imaging upon initial evaluation. These two models can be effectively applied to select patients for pre-operative systemic therapy.

Foerster et al. performed an international multi-institutional study and analyzed data of 1214 patients from 21 centers across North America, Europe, and Eastern Asia. Multivariate logistic regression analysis revealed invasion on imaging, biopsy cT1+ staging, sessile architecture, high-grade biopsy, hydronephrosis, tumor size, and age (OR: 5.10, 3.23, 2.31, 1.81, 1.37, 1.09, 1.02, respectively), were significantly associated with ≥pT2/N+ disease. In addition to these factors, they employed four other factors (previous radical cystectomy, multifocality, cytology, and sex) to develop an internally validated nomogram with a resultant bias-corrected accuracy of 75%. The additional clinical net reduction of 4 per 100 patients over the EAU model, is a superiority. This means using this model in a probability threshold of 20–40%, prevents up to 4 additional patients per 100 from unnecessary RNU, meaning they can benefit from kidney-sparing surgeries. They emphasized the robust role of biopsy staging and tumor architecture in NOC disease prediction, as two factors not used in the EAU risk stratification model [49]. An odds ratio (OR) of 9 was reported for the clinical T stage of 1+ in the prediction of muscle-invasive disease [113]. Foerster et al. indicated that Applying tumor architecture is the advantage of the NCCN model over the EAU model [49].

In their 2022 study, Marcq et al. strived to find predictors of muscle-invasive disease. Non–organ-confined disease on preoperative imaging, sessile architecture, hydronephrosis, high-grade cytology or biopsy, and higher age at diagnosis were found significant in the multivariable analysis of data from 1214 patients from 21 centers. They proposed a new trichotomous classification in contrast to the dichotomous risk categories of EAU guidelines, categorizing UTUC patients as low- intermediate- and high-risk. Due to limitations imposed by tumor size on endoscopic management, Marcq et al. kept this factor along with other significant predictors found on multivariate analysis, as indicators of high-risk disease. Previous radical cystectomy and tumor multifocality are used to divide non-high-risk patients into low and intermediate groups. In comparison to the low-risk group, the odds ratios for muscle invasion were 5.5 (95% CI: 1.3–24.0; $p = 0.023$) and 12.7 (95% CI: 3.0–54.5; $p = 0.0006$) for intermediate- and high-risk groups, respectively. Their model's area under the curve was 77% [47].

Venkat et al. identified 6143 patients from the National Cancer Database, who underwent extirpative surgery and lymph node dissection. LVI, ureteroscopic grade, positive clinical lymph node status, tumor size, and patient age were predictors of muscle-invasive disease. Node-positive disease predictors were positive clinical lymph node status, LVI, ureteroscopic grade, and tumor size. They developed two nomograms for the prediction of muscle-invasive disease, particularly to decide on administering neo-adjuvant systemic therapy, and node-positive disease, to guide the extent of lymph-node dissection. One advantage of their nomograms is that they offer and unknown/indeterminate option for LVI, tumor grade, and clinical lymph node status. This will allow the physician to estimate the probability of muscle-invasive or lymph-node-positive disease despite the lack of data on those factors. Their internally validated nomograms have an accuracy of 80%, and 87.8% for muscle-invasive, and positive-node disease prediction, respectively [46].

Besides nomograms for the prediction of muscle-invasive or NOC disease, studies were carried out to develop nomograms predicting pathologic grade and renal insufficiency following RNU. Ma et al. indicated that ureteroscopic biopsy high-grade, positive urinary cytology, sessile architecture, and age (ORs: 10.85, 6.87, 3.86, and 1.03, respectively; all p-values < 0.05) were pre-operative predictors of pathological high-grade following RNU. The corresponding nomogram, which was developed based on data from 245 patients from one center in China, achieved an Area under the ROC Curve (AUC) of 78%. This nomogram helps reduce the likelihood of undergrading by URS biopsy [114].

A study by Fang et al. on 606 Chinese patients showed that older age, tumors with smaller size, or located in the renal pelvis, lower preoperative eGFR, and the absence of hydronephrosis or multifocality were significant predictors of decreased renal function after RNU. They developed two nomograms for predicting ineligibility for full-dose and reduced-dose adjuvant chemotherapy with accuracies of 75.7% and 83.6%, respectively. Furthermore, they showed postoperative renal function did not have any correlation with patients' survival [115]. Analyzing data from 226 patients from 17 institutions worldwide, Wu et al. developed a nomogram incorporating age, pre-operative eGFR, hydroureteronephrosis, and body mass index (BMI) to predict renal function <50 mL/min/1.73 m^2 following RNU. They performed external validation on an additional 135 patients, which confirmed the 77% discrimination ability of the nomogram [116].

7. Post-Operative Predictive Tools

Post-operative risk stratification helps physicians decide on administering adjuvant chemotherapy and plan the follow-up strategy. Various post-operative nomograms have been developed to predict oncological outcomes in UTUC patients. A recent systematic review and meta-analysis comprehensively sums up these nomograms up to December 2021 [1]. Twenty-six nomograms were identified, only four of which were externally validated. It was not possible for authors to pool the concordance index (c-index) of each nomogram separately, so they categorized nomograms into four groups and calculated the overall performance of each group. Nomograms predicting OS, CSS, RFS, IVR after surgery, and CSS at the time of IVR were respectively assigned to groups A through E. The c-index for nomograms in groups A, C, and D (Predicting OS, RFS, and IVR following surgery) was >0.6, while this value was >0.7 for group B (predicting CSS). The most reliable negative predictors of OS, and RFS, were pathological tumor stage (pT) 3 or higher, and LVI, respectively. CSS was most reliably predicted by ≥pT2, age, and LVI [1].

This review emphasizes the absence of external validation studies and data limitations regarding clinical utility. It encourages the design and conduct of studies to address these issues, which would yield in the clinical applicability of post-operative nomograms. The authors further provide reference tools to help physicians implement appropriate post-operative nomograms according to their individual needs [1].

Tian et al. developed a nomogram for the prediction of OS in UTUC patients receiving chemotherapy. They extracted data from 1195 from the SEER database and found age, TNM stage, marital status, and surgical methods of the primary site, as significant predictors of OS. The AUC values of 78.9%, 77.2%, and 76.3% show discrimination accuracy of their nomogram for 1-, 3-, and 5-year OS in the development cohort. Their internally validated nomogram showed superior accuracy compared to the American Joint Committee on Cancer (AJCC)-TNM staging system [44].

Recent EAU guideline on UTUC recommends adjuvant platinum-based chemotherapy following RNU to patients with pathologic muscle-invasive or node-positive disease. It also suggests discussing adjuvant nivolumab with patients with NOC disease following RNU, who did not receive neo-adjuvant chemotherapy and refused platinum-based adjuvant chemotherapy, or are not fit for it [6]. Proper therapeutic decision-making and patient counseling require judicious application of post-operative nomograms, for which the mentioned studies would be of greatest help.

8. Future Directions

The current EAU risk-stratification tool for non-metastatic UTUC dichotomizes patients into low- and high-risk groups. If the tumor is unifocal, <2 cm, low-grade on URS biopsy, negative for high-grade cytology, and with no invasion on CT imaging, it is considered low-risk; hence a candidate for KSS. Otherwise, it should undergo RNU.

Overall, with advances in minimally-invasive management and evidence of acceptable oncological outcomes in well-selected patients who underwent conservative surgeries, a revision on the current stratification of non-metastatic UTUC seems a sage act. In this regard, considering proposed stratifications deviating from the classic dichotomizing stratification tool, similar to those of Marcq et al. [47], or Benamran et al. [117] would be helpful.

9. Conclusions

There are various diagnostic tools able to enhance the current techniques used for diagnosing UTUC. Novel proposed pre- and post-operative nomograms can guide the path of management with acceptable accuracy. These new diagnostic and risk stratification tools require further validation by robust prospective studies conducted on an international multi-institutional collaboration basis. Only then, these tools will be applicable to clinical practice, resulting in a greater number of patients benefiting from kidney-sparing procedures.

Author Contributions: M.B.: Conceptualization, Methodology, Validation, Investigation, Resources, Data Curation, Writing—Original Draft Preparation, Writing—Review & Editing, Visualization; M.G.Y.: Methodology, Validation, Investigation, Resources, Data Curation, Writing—Original Draft Preparation; E.A.: Conceptualization, Methodology, Validation, Investigation, Writing—Review & Editing, Supervision, Project Administration. All authors have read and agreed to the published version of the manuscript.

Funding: This research received no external funding.

Conflicts of Interest: The authors declare no conflict of interest.

References

1. Pallauf, M.; König, F.; D'Andrea, D.; Laukhtina, E.; Mostafaei, H.; Sari Motlagh, R.; Quhal, F.; Aydh, A.; Yanagisawa, T.; Kawada, T. A systematic review and meta-analysis of prognostic nomograms after utuc surgery. *Front. Oncol.* **2022**, *12*, 2393. [CrossRef] [PubMed]
2. Luo, Y.; She, D.-L.; Xiong, H.; Fu, S.-J.; Yang, L. Kidney-sparing management versus nephroureterectomy for upper tract urothelial carcinoma: A systematic review and meta-analysis. *Asian Pac. J. Cancer Prev.* **2015**, *16*, 5907–5912. [CrossRef] [PubMed]
3. Zhao, Y.; Deng, F.-M.; Melamed, J.; Huang, W.C.; Huang, H.; Ren, Q. Diagnostic role of urine cytology and ureteroscopic biopsies in detection of high grade upper tract urothelial carcinoma. *Am. J. Clin. Exp. Urol.* **2021**, *9*, 221–228. [PubMed]
4. Messer, J.; Shariat, S.F.; Brien, J.C.; Herman, M.P.; Ng, C.K.; Scherr, D.S.; Scoll, B.; Uzzo, R.G.; Wille, M.; Eggener, S. Urinary cytology has a poor performance for predicting invasive or high-grade upper-tract urothelial carcinoma. *BJU Int.* **2011**, *108*, 701–705. [CrossRef]
5. Malm, C.; Grahn, A.; Jaremko, G.; Tribukait, B.; Brehmer, M. Diagnostic accuracy of upper tract urothelial carcinoma: How samples are collected matters. *Scand. J. Urol.* **2017**, *51*, 137–145. [CrossRef]
6. Rouprêt, M.; Seisen, T.; Birtle, A.J.; Capoun, O.; Compérat, E.M.; Dominguez-Escrig, J.L.; Gürses Andersson, I.; Liedberg, F.; Mariappan, P.; Hugh Mostafid, A.; et al. European association of urology guidelines on upper urinary tract urothelial carcinoma: 2023 update. *Eur. Urol.* **2023**, *84*, 49–64. [CrossRef]
7. Nowak, Ł.; Krajewski, W.; Chorbińska, J.; Kiełb, P.; Sut, M.; Moschini, M.; Teoh, J.Y.-C.; Mori, K.; Del Giudice, F.; Laukhtina, E. The impact of diagnostic ureteroscopy prior to radical nephroureterectomy on oncological outcomes in patients with upper tract urothelial carcinoma: A comprehensive systematic review and meta-analysis. *J. Clin. Med.* **2021**, *10*, 4197. [CrossRef]
8. Liedberg, F.; Hagberg, O.; Häggström, C.; Aljabery, F.; Gårdmark, T.; Hosseini, A.; Jahnson, S.; Jerlström, T.; Ströck, V.; Söderkvist, K.; et al. Preoperative upper tract invasive diagnostic modalities are associated with intravesical recurrence following surgery for upper tract urothelial carcinoma: A population-based study. *PLoS ONE* **2023**, *18*, e0281304. [CrossRef]
9. Luo, Z.; Jiao, B.; Su, C.; Zhao, H.; Yan, Y.; Pan, Y.; Ren, J.; Zhang, G.; Ding, Z. Correlation between the timing of diagnostic ureteroscopy for upper tract urothelial cancer and intravesical recurrence after radical nephroureterectomy. *Front. Oncol.* **2023**, *13*, 1122877. [CrossRef]
10. Anbarasan, T.; Nissar, S.; Turbitt, J.; Walls, K.; McLuckie, S.; Clark, C.; Bourdon, J.C.; Tracey, J.; Bray, S.; Shamsuddin, A.; et al. Urinary bladder recurrences following ureteroscopic biopsies of upper tract urothelial cancers: A multi-centre observational study with genomic assessment for clonality. *Scott. Med. J.* **2023**, *68*, 4–13. [CrossRef]
11. Douglawi, A.; Ghoreifi, A.; Lee, R.; Yip, W.; Seyedian, S.S.L.; Ahmadi, H.; Cai, J.; Miranda, G.; Yu, W.; Bhanvadia, S.; et al. Bladder recurrence following diagnostic ureteroscopy in patients undergoing nephroureterectomy for upper tract urothelial cancer: Is ureteral access sheath protective? *Urology* **2022**, *160*, 142–146. [CrossRef]
12. Ha, J.S.; Jeon, J.; Ko, J.C.; Lee, H.S.; Yang, J.; Kim, D.; Kim, J.S.; Ham, W.S.; Choi, Y.D.; Cho, K.S. Intravesical recurrence after radical nephroureterectomy in patients with upper tract urothelial carcinoma is associated with flexible diagnostic ureteroscopy, but not with rigid diagnostic ureteroscopy. *Cancers* **2022**, *14*, 5629. [CrossRef] [PubMed]
13. Sharma, V.; Miest, T.S.; Juvet, T.S.; Toussi, A.; Packiam, V.; Chamie, K.; Matin, S.F.; Boorjian, S.A.; Thompson, R.H.; Frank, I.; et al. The impact of upper tract urothelial carcinoma diagnostic modality on intravesical recurrence after radical nephroureterectomy: A single institution series and updated meta-analysis. *J. Urol.* **2021**, *206*, 558–567. [CrossRef] [PubMed]
14. İzol, V.; Deger, M.; Ozden, E.; Bolat, D.; Argun, B.; Baltaci, S.; Celik, O.; Akgul, H.M.; Tinay, İ.; Bayazit, Y. The effect of diagnostic ureterorenoscopy on intravesical recurrence in patients undergoing nephroureterectomy for primary upper tract urinary carcinoma. *Urol. Int.* **2021**, *105*, 291–297. [CrossRef]

15. Shsm, H.; Bright, E.; Mantle, M.; Munro, N.; Fahmy, O. Diagnostic ureteroscopy in ct urography-diagnosed upper tract urothelial carcinoma: Delay in definitive treatment and increased intravesical recurrence. *Cureus* **2021**, *13*, e15775. [CrossRef]
16. Chung, Y.; Lee, D.H.; Lee, M.; Kim, H.; Lee, S.; Hong, S.K.; Byun, S.S.; Lee, S.E.; Oh, J.J. Impact of diagnostic ureteroscopy before radical nephroureterectomy on intravesical recurrence in patients with upper tract urothelial cancer. *Investig. Clin. Urol.* **2020**, *61*, 158–165. [CrossRef]
17. Baboudjian, M.; Al-Balushi, K.; Michel, F.; Lannes, F.; Akiki, A.; Gaillet, S.; Delaporte, V.; Ragni, E.; Toledano, H.; Karsenty, G.; et al. Diagnostic ureteroscopy prior to nephroureterectomy for urothelial carcinoma is associated with a high risk of bladder recurrence despite technical precautions to avoid tumor spillage. *World J. Urol.* **2020**, *38*, 159–165. [CrossRef] [PubMed]
18. Lee, H.Y.; Yeh, H.C.; Wu, W.J.; He, J.S.; Huang, C.N.; Ke, H.L.; Li, W.M.; Li, C.F.; Li, C.C. The diagnostic ureteroscopy before radical nephroureterectomy in upper urinary tract urothelial carcinoma is not associated with higher intravesical recurrence. *World J. Surg. Oncol.* **2018**, *16*, 135. [CrossRef]
19. Sankin, A.; Tin, A.L.; Mano, R.; Chevinsky, M.; Jakubowski, C.; Sfakianos, J.P.; Cha, E.K.; Yee, A.; Friedman, F.M.; Sjoberg, D.D.; et al. Impact of ureteroscopy before nephroureterectomy for upper tract urothelial carcinoma on oncologic outcomes. *Urology* **2016**, *94*, 148–153. [CrossRef]
20. Liu, P.; Su, X.H.; Xiong, G.Y.; Li, X.S.; Zhou, L.Q. Diagnostic ureteroscopy for upper tract urothelial carcinoma is independently associated with intravesical recurrence after radical nephroureterectomy. *Int. Braz. J. Urol.* **2016**, *42*, 1129–1135. [CrossRef]
21. Sung, H.H.; Jeon, H.G.; Han, D.H.; Jeong, B.C.; Seo, S.I.; Lee, H.M.; Choi, H.Y.; Jeon, S.S. Diagnostic ureterorenoscopy is associated with increased intravesical recurrence following radical nephroureterectomy in upper tract urothelial carcinoma. *PLoS ONE* **2015**, *10*, e0139976. [CrossRef]
22. Ishikawa, S.; Abe, T.; Shinohara, N.; Harabayashi, T.; Sazawa, A.; Maruyama, S.; Kubota, K.; Matsuno, Y.; Osawa, T.; Shinno, Y.; et al. Impact of diagnostic ureteroscopy on intravesical recurrence and survival in patients with urothelial carcinoma of the upper urinary tract. *J. Urol.* **2010**, *184*, 883–887. [CrossRef] [PubMed]
23. Yonese, I.; Ito, M.; Waseda, Y.; Kobayashi, S.; Toide, M.; Takazawa, R.; Koga, F. Adverse prognostic impact of diagnostic ureterorenoscopy in a subset of patients with high-risk upper tract urothelial carcinoma treated with radical nephroureterectomy. *Cancers* **2022**, *14*, 3962. [CrossRef] [PubMed]
24. Fukuhara, H.; Kurabayashi, A.; Furihata, M.; Setuda, S.; Takahashi, K.; Murakami, K.; Tanaka, T.; Inoue, K. 5-aminolevulinic acid-mediated photodynamic diagnosis using fluorescence ureterorenoscopy for urinary upper tract urothelial carcinoma~Preliminary prospective single centre trial~. *Photodiagnosis Photodyn. Ther.* **2020**, *29*, 101617. [CrossRef]
25. Osman, E.; Alnaib, Z.; Kumar, N. Photodynamic diagnosis in upper urinary tract urothelial carcinoma: A systematic review. *Arab. J. Urol.* **2017**, *15*, 100–109. [CrossRef] [PubMed]
26. Wada, K.; Araki, M.; Tanimoto, R.; Sadahira, T.; Watari, S.; Maruyama, Y.; Mitsui, Y.; Nakajima, H.; Acosta, H.; Katayama, S.; et al. Photodynamic diagnostic ureteroscopy using the visera elite video system for diagnosis of upper-urinary tract urothelial carcinoma: A prospective cohort pilot study. *BMC Urol.* **2021**, *21*, 45. [CrossRef]
27. Traxer, O.; Geavlete, B.; de Medina, S.G.; Sibony, M.; Al-Qahtani, S.M. Narrow-band imaging digital flexible ureteroscopy in detection of upper urinary tract transitional-cell carcinoma: Initial experience. *J. Endourol.* **2011**, *25*, 19–23. [CrossRef]
28. Iordache, V.F.; Geavlete, P.A.; Georgescu, D.A.; Ene, C.V.; Păunescu, M.A.; Niculae, A.; Peride, I.; Neagu, T.P.; Bulai, C.A.; Bălan, G.X.; et al. Nbi-assisted digital flexible ureteroscopy in transitional renal cell carcinoma—An evidence-based assessment "through the looking glass" of the pathological analysis. *Rom. J. Morphol. Embryol.* **2018**, *59*, 1091–1096.
29. Bus, M.T.; Muller, B.G.; de Bruin, D.M.; Faber, D.J.; Kamphuis, G.M.; van Leeuwen, T.G.; de Reijke, T.M.; de la Rosette, J.J. Volumetric In Vivo visualization of upper urinary tract tumors using optical coherence tomography: A pilot study. *J. Urol.* **2013**, *190*, 2236–2242. [CrossRef]
30. Bus, M.T.; de Bruin, D.M.; Faber, D.J.; Kamphuis, G.M.; Zondervan, P.J.; Laguna-Pes, M.P.; van Leeuwen, T.G.; de Reijke, T.M.; de la Rosette, J.J. Optical coherence tomography as a tool for In Vivo staging and grading of upper urinary tract urothelial carcinoma: A study of diagnostic accuracy. *J. Urol.* **2016**, *196*, 1749–1755. [CrossRef] [PubMed]
31. Chen, S.P.; Liao, J.C. Confocal laser endomicroscopy of bladder and upper tract urothelial carcinoma: A new era of optical diagnosis? *Curr. Urol. Rep.* **2014**, *15*, 437. [CrossRef] [PubMed]
32. Bui, D.; Mach, K.E.; Zlatev, D.V.; Rouse, R.V.; Leppert, J.T.; Liao, J.C. A pilot study of in vivo confocal laser endomicroscopy of upper tract urothelial carcinoma. *J. Endourol.* **2015**, *29*, 1418–1423. [CrossRef] [PubMed]
33. Breda, A.; Territo, A.; Guttilla, A.; Sanguedolce, F.; Manfredi, M.; Quaresima, L.; Gaya, J.M.; Algaba, F.; Palou, J.; Villavicencio, H. Correlation between confocal laser endomicroscopy (cellvizio®) and histological grading of upper tract urothelial carcinoma: A step forward for a better selection of patients suitable for conservative management. *Eur. Urol. Focus* **2018**, *4*, 954–959. [CrossRef]
34. Freund, J.E.; Liem, E.; Savci-Heijink, C.D.; Baard, J.; Kamphuis, G.M.; de la Rosette, J.; de Bruin, D.M. Confocal laser endomicroscopy for upper tract urothelial carcinoma: Validation of the proposed criteria and proposal of a scoring system for real-time tumor grading. *World J. Urol.* **2019**, *37*, 2155–2164. [CrossRef] [PubMed]
35. Lama, D.J.; Safiullah, S.; Patel, R.M.; Lee, T.K.; Balani, J.P.; Zhang, L.; Okhunov, Z.; Margulis, V.; Savage, S.J.; Uchio, E.J.U. Multi-institutional evaluation of upper urinary tract biopsy using backloaded cup biopsy forceps, a nitinol basket, and standard cup biopsy forceps. *Urology* **2018**, *117*, 89–94. [CrossRef]
36. Breda, A.; Territo, A.; Sanguedolce, F.; Basile, G.; Subiela, J.D.; Reyes, H.V.; Ferrer, O.M.; Gaya, J.M.; Palou, J. Comparison of biopsy devices in upper tract urothelial carcinoma. *World J. Urol.* **2019**, *37*, 1899–1905. [CrossRef]

37. Verges, D.P.; Lallas, C.D.; Hubosky, S.G.; Bagley, D.H., Jr. Endoscopic treatment of upper tract urothelial carcinoma. *Curr. Urol Rep.* **2017**, *18*, 31. [CrossRef]
38. Klein, J.T.; John, A.; Bohnert, L.; Enderle, M.D.; Linzenbold, W.; Bolenz, C. Improving the quality of human upper urinary tract specimens by cryobiopsy. *Front. Oncol.* **2022**, *12*, 810367. [CrossRef]
39. Klett, D.E.; Alom, M.; Wymer, K.; Potretzke, A.J. A novel upper tract ureteroscopic biopsy technique: The "form tackle". *Int. Braz J Urol* **2022**, *48*, 367–368. [CrossRef]
40. Huang, S.Y.; Ahrar, K.; Gupta, S.; Wallace, M.J.; Ensor, J.E.; Krishnamurthy, S.; Matin, S.F. Safety and diagnostic accuracy of percutaneous biopsy in upper tract urothelial carcinoma. *BJU Int.* **2015**, *115*, 625–632. [CrossRef]
41. Joseph, J.P.; Potretzke, T.A.; Packiam, V.; Sharma, V.; Toussi, A.; Miest, T.S.; Juvet, T.; Boorjian, S.A.; Thompson, R.H.; Welle, C.L. et al. Percutaneous image-guided core needle biopsy for upper tract urothelial carcinoma. *Urology* **2020**, *135*, 95–100. [CrossRef]
42. Kim, H.S.; Jeong, C.W.; Kwak, C.; Kim, H.H.; Ku, J.H. Association between demographic factors and prognosis in urothelial carcinoma of the upper urinary tract: A systematic review and meta-analysis. *Oncotarget* **2017**, *8*, 7464–7476. [CrossRef] [PubMed]
43. Qi, F.; Wei, X.; Zheng, Y.; Sha, Y.; Lu, Y.; Li, X. Nomograms to predict overall and cancer-specific survival in patients with upper tract urothelial carcinoma: A large population-based study. *Transl. Androl. Urol.* **2020**, *9*, 1177. [CrossRef] [PubMed]
44. Tian, C.; Liu, J.; An, L.; Hong, Y.; Xu, Q. Prognostic nomogram for overall survival in upper urinary tract urothelial carcinoma (utuc) patients treated with chemotherapy: A seer-based retrospective cohort study. *BMC Urol.* **2023**, *23*, 2.
45. Martinez-Salamanca, J.I.; Shariat, S.F.; Rodriguez, J.C.; Chromecki, T.F.; Ficarra, V.; Fritsche, H.M.; Kassouf, W.; Matsumoto, K.; Cabello, L.O.; Seitz, C.; et al. Prognostic role of ecog performance status in patients with urothelial carcinoma of the upper urinary tract: An international study. *BJU Int.* **2012**, *109*, 1155–1161. [CrossRef] [PubMed]
46. Venkat, S.; Khan, A.I.; Lewicki, P.J.; Borregales, L.; Scherr, D.S. Novel nomograms to predict muscle invasion and lymph node metastasis in upper tract urothelial carcinoma. In *Urologic Oncology: Seminars and Original Investigations*; Elsevier: Amsterdam, The Netherlands, 2022; pp. 108.e111–108.e117.
47. Marcq, G.; Foerster, B.; Abufaraj, M.; Matin, S.F.; Azizi, M.; Gupta, M.; Li, W.-M.; Seisen, T.; Clinton, T.; Xylinas, E. Novel classification for upper tract urothelial carcinoma to better risk-stratify patients eligible for kidney-sparing strategies: An international collaborative study. *Eur. Urol. Focus* **2022**, *8*, 491–497. [CrossRef] [PubMed]
48. Mori, K.; Katayama, S.; Laukhtina, E.; Schuettfort, V.M.; Pradere, B.; Quhal, F.; Motlagh, R.S.; Mostafaei, H.; Grossmann, N.C.; Rajwa, P. Discordance between clinical and pathological staging and grading in upper tract urothelial carcinoma. *Clin. Genitourin. Cancer* **2022**, *20*, 95.e91–95.e96. [CrossRef]
49. Foerster, B.; Abufaraj, M.; Matin, S.F.; Azizi, M.; Gupta, M.; Li, W.-M.; Seisen, T.; Clinton, T.; Xylinas, E.; Mir, M. Pretreatment risk stratification for endoscopic kidney-sparing surgery in upper tract urothelial carcinoma: An international collaborative study. *Eur. Urol.* **2021**, *80*, 507–515. [CrossRef]
50. Mori, K.; Mostafaei, H.; Enikeev, D.V.; Lysenko, I.; Quhal, F.; Kimura, S.; Karakiewicz, P.I.; Egawa, S.; Shariat, S.F. Differential effect of sex on outcomes after radical surgery for upper tract and bladder urothelial carcinoma: A systematic review and meta-analysis. *J. Urol.* **2020**, *204*, 58–62. [CrossRef]
51. Singla, N.; Fang, D.; Su, X.; Bao, Z.; Cao, Z.; Jafri, S.M.; Xiong, G.; Zhang, L.; Hutchinson, R.; Sagalowsky, A. A multi-institutional comparison of clinicopathological characteristics and oncologic outcomes of upper tract urothelial carcinoma in china and the United States. *J. Urol.* **2017**, *197*, 1208–1213. [CrossRef]
52. Collà Ruvolo, C.; Wenzel, M.; Nocera, L.; Würnschimmel, C.; Tian, Z.; Shariat, S.F.; Saad, F.; Longo, N.; Imbimbo, C.; Briganti, A.; et al. The effect of race on stage at presentation and survival in upper tract urothelial carcinoma. *Urol. Oncol.* **2021**, *39*, 788.e7–788.e13. [CrossRef]
53. Raman, J.D.; Messer, J.; Sielatycki, J.A.; Hollenbeak, C. Incidence and survival of patients with carcinoma of the ureter and renal pelvis in the USA, 1973–2005. *BJU Int.* **2011**, *107*, 1059–1064. [CrossRef]
54. Rink, M.; Xylinas, E.; Margulis, V.; Cha, E.K.; Ehdaie, B.; Raman, J.D.; Chun, F.K.; Matsumoto, K.; Lotan, Y.; Furberg, H. Impact of smoking on oncologic outcomes of upper tract urothelial carcinoma after radical nephroureterectomy. *Eur. Urol.* **2013**, *63*, 1082–1090. [CrossRef] [PubMed]
55. Xylinas, E.; Kluth, L.A.; Rieken, M.; Lee, R.K.; Elghouayel, M.; Ficarra, V.; Margulis, V.; Lotan, Y.; Rouprêt, M.; Martinez-Salamanca, J. Impact of smoking status and cumulative exposure on intravesical recurrence of upper tract urothelial carcinoma after radical nephroureterectomy. *BJU Int.* **2014**, *114*, 56–61. [CrossRef]
56. van Osch, F.H.; Jochems, S.H.; van Schooten, F.J.; Bryan, R.T.; Zeegers, M. Significant role of lifetime cigarette smoking in worsening bladder cancer and upper tract urothelial carcinoma prognosis: A meta-analysis. *J. Urol.* **2016**, *195*, 872–879. [CrossRef] [PubMed]
57. Xia, L.; Taylor, B.L.; Pulido, J.E.; Guzzo, T.J. Impact of surgical waiting time on survival in patients with upper tract urothelial carcinoma: A national cancer database study. In *Urologic Oncology: Seminars and Original Investigations*; Elsevier: Amsterdam, The Netherlands, 2018; pp. 10.e15–10.e22.
58. Sundi, D.; Svatek, R.S.; Margulis, V.; Wood, C.G.; Matin, S.F.; Dinney, C.P.; Kamat, A.M. Upper tract urothelial carcinoma: Impact of time to surgery. *Urol. Oncol. Semin. Orig. Investig.* **2012**, *30*, 266–272. [CrossRef] [PubMed]
59. Surov, A.; Wienke, A. Prevalence of sarcopenia in patients with solid tumors: A meta-analysis based on 81,814 patients. *JPEN J. Parenter. Enter. Nutr.* **2022**, *46*, 1761–1768. [CrossRef]

60. Pickl, C.; Engelmann, S.; Girtner, F.; Gužvić, M.; van Rhijn, B.W.; Hartmann, V.; Holbach, S.; Kälble, S.; Haas, M.; Rosenhammer, B. Body composition as a comorbidity-independent predictor of survival following nephroureterectomy for urothelial cancer of the upper urinary tract. *Cancers* **2023**, *15*, 450. [CrossRef]
61. Liu, J.; Wu, P.; Lai, S.; Song, X.; Wang, M.; Wang, X.; Liu, S.; Hou, H.; Zhang, Y.; Wang, J.J.N.; et al. Clinicopathological and prognostic significance of preoperative prognostic nutritional index in patients with upper urinary tract urothelial carcinoma. *Nutr. Cancer* **2022**, *74*, 2964–2974. [CrossRef]
62. Xue, W.; Tan, P.; Xu, H.; Yang, L.; Wei, Q. Impact of the preoperative prognostic nutritional index on survival outcomes in upper tract urothelial carcinomas. *Cancer Med.* **2019**, *8*, 2971–2978. [CrossRef]
63. Gao, X.; Lin, B.; Lin, Q.; Ye, T.; Zhou, T.; Hu, M.; Zhu, H.; Lu, F.; Chen, W.; Xia, P. A halp score-based prediction model for survival of patients with the upper tract urothelial carcinoma undergoing radical nephroureterectomy. *Bosn. J. Basic. Med. Sci.* **2022**, *22*, 280. [PubMed]
64. Zhao, Z.; Xie, S.; Feng, B.; Zhang, S.; Sun, Y.; Guo, H.; Yang, R. Preoperative risk classification using neutrophil-to-lymphocyte ratio and albumin for upper tract urothelial carcinoma treated with radical nephroureterectomy. *Cancer Manag. Res.* **2020**, *12*, 9023–9032. [CrossRef]
65. Li, X.; Ma, X.; Tang, L.; Wang, B.; Chen, L.; Zhang, F.; Zhang, X. Prognostic value of neutrophil-to-lymphocyte ratio in urothelial carcinoma of the upper urinary tract and bladder: A systematic review and meta-analysis. *Oncotarget* **2017**, *8*, 62681–62692. [CrossRef]
66. Xu, H.; Ai, J.Z.; Tan, P.; Lin, T.H.; Jin, X.; Gong, L.N.; Lei, H.R.; Yang, L.; Wei, Q. Pretreatment elevated fibrinogen level predicts worse oncologic outcomes in upper tract urothelial carcinoma. *Asian J. Androl.* **2020**, *22*, 177–183. [PubMed]
67. Egger, V.; Hutterer, G.C.; Mischinger, J.; Seles, M.; Pichler, R.; Mannweiler, S.; Huber, K.; Balihodzic, A.; Spiegelberg, J.; Bauernhofer, T.; et al. Preoperative fibrinogen/crp score predicts survival in upper urothelial tract carcinoma patients undergoing radical curative surgery. *World J. Urol.* **2023**, *41*, 1359–1364. [CrossRef]
68. Liao, C.-I.; Fang, H.-C.; Lee, P.-T.; Hsu, C.-Y.; Chen, C.-L.; Huang, C.-W.; Chen, X.-Y.; Ou, S.-H.; Tsai, C.-T.; Chou, K.-J. Trends in the incidence of urothelial carcinoma in taiwan after the ban on aristolochic acid-containing chinese herbal preparations, 2001–2018: A national population-based cohort study. *J. Cancer Res. Clin. Oncol.* **2023**, *149*, 8201–8211. [CrossRef]
69. Pfau, W.; Schmeiser, H.H.; Wiessler, M.J.C. 32p-postlabelling analysis of the DNA adducts formed by aristolochic acid i and ii. *Carcinogenesis* **1990**, *11*, 1627–1633. [CrossRef]
70. Nortier, J.L.; Martinez, M.-C.M.; Schmeiser, H.H.; Arlt, V.M.; Bieler, C.A.; Petein, M.; Depierreux, M.F.; De Pauw, L.; Abramowicz, D.; Vereerstraeten, P. Urothelial carcinoma associated with the use of a chinese herb (*Aristolochia fangchi*). *N. Engl. J. Med.* **2000**, *342*, 1686–1692. [CrossRef]
71. Dickman, K.G.; Chen, C.-H.; Grollman, A.P.; Pu, Y.-S. Aristolochic acid-containing chinese herbal medicine and upper urinary tract urothelial carcinoma in taiwan: A narrative review. *World J. Urol.* **2023**, *41*, 899–907. [CrossRef] [PubMed]
72. Chen, C.-H.; Dickman, K.G.; Moriya, M.; Zavadil, J.; Sidorenko, V.S.; Edwards, K.L.; Gnatenko, D.V.; Wu, L.; Turesky, R.J.; Wu, X.-R. Aristolochic acid-associated urothelial cancer in Taiwan. *Proc. Natl. Acad. Sci. USA* **2012**, *109*, 8241–8246. [CrossRef]
73. Chen, C.H.; Dickman, K.G.; Huang, C.Y.; Moriya, M.; Shun, C.T.; Tai, H.C.; Huang, K.H.; Wang, S.M.; Lee, Y.J.; Grollman, A. Aristolochic acid-induced upper tract urothelial carcinoma in Taiwan: Clinical characteristics and outcomes. *Int. J. Cancer* **2013**, *133*, 14–20. [CrossRef] [PubMed]
74. Mbeutcha, A.; Rouprêt, M.; Kamat, A.M.; Karakiewicz, P.I.; Lawrentschuk, N.; Novara, G.; Raman, J.D.; Seitz, C.; Xylinas, E.; Shariat, S. Prognostic factors and predictive tools for upper tract urothelial carcinoma: A systematic review. *World J. Urol.* **2017**, *35*, 337–353. [CrossRef] [PubMed]
75. Margulis, V.; Shariat, S.F.; Matin, S.F.; Kamat, A.M.; Zigeuner, R.; Kikuchi, E.; Lotan, Y.; Weizer, A.; Raman, J.D.; Wood, C. Outcomes of radical nephroureterectomy: A series from the upper tract urothelial carcinoma collaboration. *Cancer* **2009**, *115*, 1224–1233. [CrossRef] [PubMed]
76. van Doeveren, T.; van der Mark, M.; van Leeuwen, P.J.; Boormans, J.L.; Aben, K.K.H. Rising incidence rates and unaltered survival rates for primary upper urinary tract urothelial carcinoma: A dutch population-based study from 1993 to 2017. *BJU Int.* **2021**, *128*, 343–351. [CrossRef] [PubMed]
77. Huang, W.W.; Huang, H.Y.; Liao, A.C.; Shiue, Y.L.; Tai, H.L.; Lin, C.M.; Wang, Y.H.; Lin, C.N.; Shen, K.H.; Li, C.F. Primary urothelial carcinoma of the upper tract: Important clinicopathological factors predicting bladder recurrence after surgical resection. *Pathol. Int.* **2009**, *59*, 642–649. [CrossRef]
78. Katayama, S.; Mori, K.; Schuettfort, V.M.; Pradere, B.; Mostafaei, H.; Quhal, F.; Rajwa, P.; Motlagh, R.S.; Laukhtina, E.; Moschini, M. Accuracy and clinical utility of a tumor grade-and stage-based predictive model in localized upper tract urothelial carcinoma. *Eur. Urol. Focus* **2022**, *8*, 761–768. [CrossRef]
79. Sun, K.N.; Wu, J.H.; Chen, Z.H.; He, Y.J.; Chen, Y.L.; Hu, J.Z.; Sheng, L. Predictive value of flank pain and gross hematuria on long-term survival in patients with upper tract urothelial carcinoma treated by radical nephroureterectomy. *Clin. Med. Insights Oncol.* **2023**, *17*, 11795549221147993. [CrossRef]
80. Yeh, H.-C.; Chang, C.-H.; Fang, J.-K.; Chen, I.-H.A.; Lin, J.-T.; Hong, J.-H.; Huang, C.-Y.; Wang, S.-S.; Chen, C.-S.; Lo, C.-W. The value of preoperative local symptoms in prognosis of upper tract urothelial carcinoma after radical nephroureterectomy: A retrospective, multicenter cohort study. *Front. Oncol.* **2022**, *12*, 872849. [CrossRef]

81. Messer, J.C.; Terrell, J.D.; Herman, M.P.; Ng, C.K.; Scherr, D.S.; Scoll, B.; Boorjian, S.A.; Uzzo, R.G.; Wille, M.; Eggener, S.E.; et al. Multi-institutional validation of the ability of preoperative hydronephrosis to predict advanced pathologic tumor stage in upper-tract urothelial carcinoma. *Urol. Oncol.* **2013**, *31*, 904–908. [CrossRef]
82. Ito, Y.; Kikuchi, E.; Tanaka, N.; Miyajima, A.; Mikami, S.; Jinzaki, M.; Oya, M. Preoperative hydronephrosis grade independently predicts worse pathological outcomes in patients undergoing nephroureterectomy for upper tract urothelial carcinoma. *J. Urol.* **2011**, *185*, 1621–1626. [CrossRef]
83. Kaczmarek, K.; Lemiński, A.; Gołąb, A.; Słojewski, M. Survival differences of patients with ureteral versus pelvicalyceal tumours: A systematic review and meta-analysis. *Arch. Med. Sci. AMS* **2021**, *17*, 603–612. [CrossRef] [PubMed]
84. Lwin, A.A.; Hsu, C.H.; Chipollini, J. Urothelial carcinoma of the renal pelvis and ureter: Does location make a difference? *Clin. Genitourin. Cancer* **2020**, *18*, 45–49.e41. [CrossRef] [PubMed]
85. Miyake, M.; Hori, S.; Owari, T.; Oda, Y.; Tatsumi, Y.; Nakai, Y.; Fujii, T.; Fujimoto, K. Clinical impact of tumor-infiltrating lymphocytes and pd-l1-positive cells as prognostic and predictive biomarkers in urological malignancies and retroperitoneal sarcoma. *Cancers* **2020**, *12*, 3153. [CrossRef] [PubMed]
86. Miyake, M.; Iida, K.; Nishimura, N.; Inoue, T.; Matsumoto, H.; Matsuyama, H.; Fujiwara, Y.; Komura, K.; Inamoto, T.; Azuma, H. Site-specific risk stratification models for postoperative recurrence and survival prediction in patients with upper tract urothelial carcinoma undergoing radical nephroureterectomy: Better stratification for adjuvant therapy. *Eur. Urol. Open Sci.* **2022**, *41*, 95–104. [CrossRef] [PubMed]
87. Shibing, Y.; Liangren, L.; Qiang, W.; Hong, L.; Turun, S.; Junhao, L.; Lu, Y.; Zhengyong, Y.; Yonghao, J.; Guangqing, F. Impact of tumour size on prognosis of upper urinary tract urothelial carcinoma after radical nephroureterectomy: A multi-institutional analysis of 795 cases. *BJU Int.* **2016**, *118*, 902–910. [CrossRef]
88. Simone, G.; Papalia, R.; Loreto, A.; Leonardo, C.; Sentinelli, S.; Gallucci, M. Independent prognostic value of tumour diameter and tumour necrosis in upper urinary tract urothelial carcinoma. *BJU Int.* **2009**, *103*, 1052–1057. [CrossRef]
89. Ma, R.; Liu, Z.; Cheng, Y.; Zhou, P.; Pan, Y.; Bi, H.; Tao, L.; Yang, B.; Xia, H.; Zhu, X. Prognostic value of tumor size in patients with upper tract urothelial carcinoma: A systematic review and meta-analysis. *Eur. Urol. Open Sci.* **2022**, *42*, 19–29. [CrossRef]
90. Foerster, B.; Abufaraj, M.; Mari, A.; Seisen, T.; Bandini, M.; Schweitzer, D.; Czech, A.K.; Moschini, M.; D'Andrea, D.; Bianchi, M. The performance of tumor size as risk stratification parameter in upper tract urothelial carcinoma (utuc). *Clin. Genitourin. Cancer* **2021**, *19*, 272.e271–272.e277. [CrossRef]
91. Favaretto, R.L.; Shariat, S.F.; Savage, C.; Godoy, G.; Chade, D.C.; Kaag, M.; Bochner, B.H.; Coleman, J.; Dalbagni, G. Combining imaging and ureteroscopy variables in a preoperative multivariable model for prediction of muscle-invasive and non-organ confined disease in patients with upper tract urothelial carcinoma. *BJU Int.* **2012**, *109*, 77–82. [CrossRef]
92. Petros, F.G.; Qiao, W.; Singla, N.; Clinton, T.N.; Robyak, H.; Raman, J.D.; Margulis, V.; Matin, S.F. Preoperative multiplex nomogram for prediction of high-risk nonorgan-confined upper-tract urothelial carcinoma. In *Urologic Oncology: Seminars and Original Investigations*; Elsevier: Amsterdam, The Netherlands, 2019; pp. 292.e291–292.e299.
93. Stangl-Kremser, J.; Muto, G.; Grosso, A.A.; Briganti, A.; Comperat, E.; Di Maida, F.; Montironi, R.; Remzi, M.; Pradere, B.; Soria, F.; et al. The impact of lymphovascular invasion in patients treated with radical nephroureterectomy for upper tract urothelial carcinoma: An extensive updated systematic review and meta-analysis. *Urol. Oncol. Semin. Orig. Investig.* **2022**, *40*, 243–261. [CrossRef]
94. Meireles, S.; Dias, N.; Martins, D.; Dias, C.; Gonçalves, M.; Silva, J.; Silva, C.M.; Oliveira, P.D.; Soares, P.; Lopes, J.M. Prognostic value of bladder involvement in the outcome of upper tract urothelial carcinoma. *Diagnostics* **2023**, *13*, 153. [CrossRef] [PubMed]
95. Jan, H.-C.; Wu, K.-Y.; Tai, T.-Y.; Weng, H.-Y.; Yang, W.-H.; Ou, C.-H.; Hu, C.-Y. The systemic immune-inflammation index (sii) increases the prognostic significance of lymphovascular invasion in upper tract urothelial carcinoma after radical nephroureterectomy. *Cancer Manag. Res.* **2022**, *14*, 3139–3149. [CrossRef] [PubMed]
96. Colin, P.; Ouzzane, A.; Yates, D.R.; Audenet, F.; Pignot, G.; Arvin-Berod, A.; Merigot de Treigny, O.; Laurent, G.; Valeri, A.; Irani, J.; et al. Influence of positive surgical margin status after radical nephroureterectomy on upper urinary tract urothelial carcinoma survival. *Ann. Surg. Oncol.* **2012**, *19*, 3613–3620. [CrossRef] [PubMed]
97. Hurel, S.; Rouprêt, M.; Ouzzane, A.; Rozet, F.; Xylinas, E.; Zerbib, M.; Berod, A.A.; Ruffion, A.; Adam, E.; Cussenot, O.; et al. Impact of lymphovascular invasion on oncological outcomes in patients with upper tract urothelial carcinoma after radical nephroureterectomy. *BJU Int.* **2013**, *111*, 1199–1207. [CrossRef]
98. Li, K.P.; Chen, S.Y.; Wang, C.Y.; Wan, S.; Yang, L. Comparison between robot-assisted versus open nephroureterectomy for upper tract urothelial carcinoma: Outcomes from a pooled analysis. *J. Robot. Surg.* **2023**, *17*, 1227–1238. [CrossRef]
99. Pelcovits, A.; Mueller-Leonhard, C.; Mega, A.; Amin, A.; Kim, S.P.; Golijanin, D.; Gershman, B. Outcomes of upper tract urothelial carcinoma with isolated lymph node involvement following surgical resection: Implications for multi-modal management. *World J. Urol.* **2020**, *38*, 1243–1252. [CrossRef]
100. Xia, H.R.; Li, S.G.; Zhai, X.Q.; Liu, M.; Guo, X.X.; Wang, J.Y. The value of lymph node dissection in patients with node-positive upper urinary tract urothelial cancer: A retrospective cohort study. *Front. Oncol.* **2022**, *12*, 889144. [CrossRef]
101. Fujii, Y.; Sato, Y.; Suzuki, H.; Kakiuchi, N.; Yoshizato, T.; Lenis, A.T.; Maekawa, S.; Yokoyama, A.; Takeuchi, Y.; Inoue, Y. Molecular classification and diagnostics of upper urinary tract urothelial carcinoma. *Cancer Cell* **2021**, *39*, 793–809.e798. [CrossRef]

102. Evmorfopoulos, K.; Mitrakas, L.; Karathanasis, A.; Zachos, I.; Tzortzis, V.; Vlachostergios, P. Upper tract urothelial carcinoma: A rare malignancy with distinct immuno-genomic features in the era of precision-based therapies. *Biomedicines* **2023**, *11*, 1775. [CrossRef]
103. Su, X.; Lu, X.; Bazai, S.K.; Compérat, E.; Mouawad, R.; Yao, H.; Rouprêt, M.; Spano, J.-P.; Khayat, D.; Davidson, I.; et al. Comprehensive integrative profiling of upper tract urothelial carcinomas. *Genome Biol.* **2021**, *22*, 7. [CrossRef]
104. Fan, B.; Hu, B.; Yuan, Q.; Wen, S.; Liu, T.; Bai, S.; Qi, X.; Wang, X.; Yang, D.; Sun, X.; et al. Impact of tumor architecture on disease recurrence and cancer-specific mortality of upper tract urothelial carcinoma treated with radical nephroureterectomy. *Tumour Biol. J. Int. Soc. Oncodev. Biol. Med.* **2017**, *39*, 1010428317710822. [CrossRef]
105. Gao, X.; Ma, Y.; Chen, G.; Chen, J.; Li, H.; Li, H.; Wei, X.; Wang, K. Concomitant carcinoma in situ as a prognostic factor in the upper tract urothelial carcinoma after radical nephroureterectomy: A systematic review and meta-analysis. *Urol. Oncol.* **2020**, *38*, 574–581. [CrossRef] [PubMed]
106. Zamboni, S.; Foerster, B.; Abufaraj, M.; Seisen, T.; Roupret, M.; Colin, P.; De la Taille, A.; Di Bona, C.; Peyronnet, B.; Bensalah, K.; et al. Incidence and survival outcomes in patients with upper urinary tract urothelial carcinoma diagnosed with variant histology and treated with nephroureterectomy. *BJU Int.* **2019**, *124*, 738–745. [CrossRef]
107. Xu, L.; Zhong, W.; Li, C.; Hong, P.; Xia, K.; Lin, R.; Cheng, S.; Wang, B.; Yang, M.; Chen, J.; et al. The tumour-associated stroma correlates with poor clinical outcomes and immunoevasive contexture in patients with upper tract urothelial carcinoma: Results from a multicenter real-world study (tsu-01 study). *Br. J. Cancer* **2023**, *128*, 310–320. [CrossRef]
108. Brien, J.C.; Shariat, S.F.; Herman, M.P.; Ng, C.K.; Scherr, D.S.; Scoll, B.; Uzzo, R.G.; Wille, M.; Eggener, S.E.; Terrell, J. Preoperative hydronephrosis, ureteroscopic biopsy grade and urinary cytology can improve prediction of advanced upper tract urothelial carcinoma. *J. Urol.* **2010**, *184*, 69–73. [CrossRef] [PubMed]
109. Margulis, V.; Youssef, R.F.; Karakiewicz, P.I.; Lotan, Y.; Wood, C.G.; Zigeuner, R.; Kikuchi, E.; Weizer, A.; Raman, J.D.; Remzi, M. Preoperative multivariable prognostic model for prediction of nonorgan confined urothelial carcinoma of the upper urinary tract. *J. Urol.* **2010**, *184*, 453–458. [CrossRef]
110. Chen, X.P.; Xiong, G.Y.; Li, X.S.; Matin, S.F.; Garcia, M.; Fang, D.; Wang, T.Y.; Yu, W.; Gong, K.; Song, Y.; et al. Predictive factors for worse pathological outcomes of upper tract urothelial carcinoma: Experience from a nationwide high-volume centre in china. *BJU Int.* **2013**, *112*, 917–924. [CrossRef] [PubMed]
111. Yoshida, T.; Kobayashi, T.; Kawaura, T.; Miyake, M.; Ito, K.; Okuno, H.; Murota, T.; Makita, N.; Kawakita, M.; Kawa, G. Development and external validation of a preoperative nomogram for predicting pathological locally advanced disease of clinically localized upper urinary tract carcinoma. *Cancer Med.* **2020**, *9*, 3733–3741. [CrossRef] [PubMed]
112. Singla, N.; Fang, D.; Su, X.; Bao, Z.; Cao, Z.; Robyak, H.; Xiong, G.; Zhang, L.; Woldu, S.; Hutchinson, R. Preoperative predictors of nonorgan-confined disease in upper-tract urothelial carcinoma differ between china and the United States. In *Urologic Oncology: Seminars and Original Investigations*; Elsevier: Amsterdam, The Netherlands, 2018; pp. 88.e11–88.e18.
113. Margolin, E.J.; Matulay, J.T.; Li, G.; Meng, X.; Chao, B.; Vijay, V.; Silver, H.; Clinton, T.N.; Krabbe, L.-M.; Woldu, S. Discordance between ureteroscopic biopsy and final pathology for upper tract urothelial carcinoma. *J. Urol.* **2018**, *199*, 1440–1445. [CrossRef] [PubMed]
114. Ma, R.; Xia, H.; Qiu, M.; Tao, L.; Lu, M.; Huang, R.; Lu, J.; Ma, L. A diagnostic nomogram of pathologic grade for preoperative risk stratification in upper tract urothelial carcinoma. *Clin. Med. Insights Oncol.* **2020**, *14*, 1179554920927662. [CrossRef]
115. Fang, D.; Zhang, Q.; Li, X.; Qian, C.; Xiong, G.; Zhang, L.; Chen, X.; Zhang, X.; Yu, W.; He, Z. Nomogram predicting renal insufficiency after nephroureterectomy for upper tract urothelial carcinoma in the chinese population: Exclusion of ineligible candidates for adjuvant chemotherapy. *BioMed Res. Int.* **2014**, *2014*, 529186. [CrossRef] [PubMed]
116. Wu, Z.; Chen, Q.; Djaladat, H.; Minervini, A.; Uzzo, R.G.; Sundaram, C.P.; Rha, K.H.; Gonzalgo, M.L.; Mehrazin, R.; Mazzone, E. A preoperative nomogram to predict renal function insufficiency for cisplatin-based adjuvant chemotherapy following minimally invasive radical nephroureterectomy (robuust collaborative group). *Eur. Urol. Focus* **2022**, *8*, 173–181. [CrossRef] [PubMed]
117. Benamran, D.; Seisen, T.; Naoum, E.; Vaessen, C.; Parra, J.; Mozer, P.; Shariat, S.F.; Rouprêt, M. Risk stratification for upper tract urinary carcinoma. *Transl. Androl. Urol.* **2020**, *9*, 1799. [CrossRef] [PubMed]

cancers

MDPI

Review

Overview, Diagnosis, and Perioperative Systemic Therapy of Upper Tract Urothelial Carcinoma

Adam Kolawa [1], Anishka D'Souza [2,*] and Varsha Tulpule [2]

[1] IRD 620, Department of Internal Medicine, University of Southern California, 2020 Zonal Avenue, Los Angeles, CA 90033, USA; adam.kolawa@med.usc.edu

[2] USC Norris Comprehensive Cancer Center, 1441 Eastlake Ave, Los Angeles, CA 90033, USA; varsha.tulpule@med.usc.edu

* Correspondence: anishkad@med.usc.edu; Tel.: +1-323-865-3903; Fax: +1-323-865-0061

Simple Summary: As upper tract urothelial carcinoma is a relatively rare disease, much of clinical practice has been extrapolated from urothelial carcinoma data. Here we summarize data, current guidelines, and future directions in the management of upper tract urothelial carcinoma with a particular focus on systemic therapy.

Abstract: Upper tract urothelial carcinoma comprises 5–10% of all urothelial carcinoma cases. This disease tends to have a more aggressive course than its lower urinary tract counterpart, with 60% of patients presenting with invasive disease and 30% of patients presenting with metastatic disease at diagnosis. The diagnostic workup of UTUC involves imaging with CT urogram, urine cytology, and direct visualization and biopsy of suspected lesions via ureteroscopy. Standard treatment of high-grade UTUC involves radical nephroureterectomy (RNU) and excision of the ipsilateral bladder cuff. Both the NCCN and EAU Guidelines include neoadjuvant chemotherapy as a treatment option for select patients with UTUC; however, there are no strict guidelines. Much of the rationale for neoadjuvant chemotherapy is based on extrapolation from data from muscle-invasive bladder cancer, which has demonstrated a 5-year OS benefit of 5–8%. Retrospective studies evaluating the use of NACT in urothelial carcinoma have yielded pathologic objective response rates of 48% in UTUC cohorts. The randomized Phase III POUT study noted a DFS advantage with adjuvant platinum-based chemotherapy, compared with surveillance in UTUC, of 70% vs. 51% at 2 years. Though not the standard of care, multiple studies have explored the use of perioperative immunotherapy or chemoimmunotherapy in the management of invasive urothelial carcinoma. The PURE-02 study explored the use of neoadjuvant pembrolizumab in patients with high-risk UTUC. A small study of 10 patients, it showed no significant signals of activity with neoadjuvant pembrolizumab. Another Phase II study of neoadjuvant ipilimumab and nivolumab in cisplatin-ineligible UTUC yielded more promising findings, with 3/9 patients attaining a pathologic CR and the remaining six pathologically downstaged. The ABACUS trial found a 31% pathologic complete response rate amongst cisplatin-ineligible MIBC patients treated with neoadjuvant atezolizumab. The use of adjuvant immunotherapy has been explored over three phase III trials. The CheckMate-274 trial found a DFS benefit with the addition of one year of adjuvant nivolumab in patients with high-risk urothelial carcinoma. The IMvigor-010 study of adjuvant atezolizumab was a negative study. The AMBASSADOR trial of adjuvant pembrolizumab is pending results. With the FDA approval of erdafitinib in metastatic urothelial carcinoma, similar targets have been explored for use in perioperative use in invasive urothelial carcinoma, as with adjuvant infigratinib in the PROOF-302 trial. As the treatment paradigm for urothelial carcinoma evolves, further prospective studies are needed to expand the perioperative treatment landscape of UTUC.

Keywords: upper tract urothelial; perioperative; immunotherapy

1. Introduction

Urothelial cell carcinoma (UCC), also known as transitional cell carcinoma, is the predominant histological subtype of urinary tract cancer. It is the sixth most common tumor entity in developed countries [1]. The majority of these cases, approximately 90–95%, occur within the bladder. The remaining 5–10% originate in the upper urinary tract, which encompasses the renal pelvis, renal calyx, and the ureter [1]. This form is referred to as upper tract urothelial carcinoma (UTUC).

Although UTUC constitutes a minority of urothelial carcinomas, it is of particular interest due to its relatively aggressive biological behavior and higher mortality rate compared to other genitourinary tract malignancies. UTUC has a tendency to present at an advanced stage; at the time of diagnosis, around 60% of patients have invasive disease, and 30% present with metastatic disease [2]. This is in stark comparison to bladder cancer, where only 25% of patients present with invasive pathology [3]. Consequently, the overall 5-year disease specific survival is less favorable than lower tract UCC, ranging between 57 to 73% [4].

Global incidence of UTUC exhibits geographic variation. Western countries report a rate of 1–2 cases per 100,000 individuals annually, whereas in certain regions, such as Taiwan, UTUC comprises nearly a quarter of all urothelial carcinomas due to specific endemic factors [5]. Several risk factors for UTUC have been identified, including exposure to specific chemicals and drugs, tobacco smoking, prior pelvic radiation therapy, and inherited conditions such as Lynch syndrome. For instance, UTUC incidence is 2–3 times greater in individuals with a history of tobacco use, which is implicated in approximately 50% of cases in males and 33% in females [6]. Moreover, analgesic misuse and exposure to carcinogenic chemicals are associated with a fourfold and sixfold increase in risk, respectively. Furthermore, pathological risk factors significantly influence general outcomes in UTUC [6]. The European Association of Urology defines high-risk upper tract urothelial carcinoma as: high-grade cytology, high-grade-ureteroscopic biopsy, local invasion on CT, tumor size > 2 cm, multifocal disease, variant histology, and previous radical cystectomy for high-grade BC [7].

Despite advancements in diagnostic methodologies and therapeutic strategies, there has been limited improvement in the 5-year survival rate of UTUC over the preceding decades, underscoring the critical necessity for ongoing research. The advent of genomic sequencing techniques has facilitated the identification of a significant amount of genetic and epigenetic alterations within UTUC, thus providing a richer understanding of its pathogenesis and revealing novel potential therapeutic targets. The following sections will delve deeper into the intricacies of urothelial carcinoma of the upper urinary tract, shedding light on its diagnostic modalities, therapeutic approaches, and future directions in research. By doing so, we hope to provide a comprehensive understanding that may guide healthcare providers in delivering optimal care and contribute to the ongoing quest to improve outcomes for patients afflicted with UTUC.

2. Diagnosis

Upper tract urothelial carcinoma (UTUC) often elicits diagnostic consideration upon the manifestation of clinical symptoms such as hematuria and flank pain. Hematuria is particularly notable, present in an estimated 75% of UTUC cases (albeit non-exclusive to this malignancy, which consequently may contribute to diagnostic delay) [8]. Other common presenting symptoms are flank pain and presence of a lumbar mass occurring in 20–40% and 10–20% of cases, respectively [9]. The initial clinical suspicion is then followed by employment of imaging modalities which are integral to the detection and diagnosis of UTUC. Computed tomography urography (CTU) typically boasts high sensitivity and specificity, with respective rates ranging from 67–100% and 93–99% [8]. However, it is important to note that the sensitivity decreases to 89% for lesions less than 5 mm and 40% for lesions less than 3 mm, thereby presenting a potential limitation in diagnostic precision [10]. Alternative imaging modalities, such as magnetic resonance urography (MRU), offer similar rates of sensitivity and specificity to CTU.

Parallel to imaging, urine cytology adds another dimension to the diagnostic paradigm. Despite its high specificity of 94–98%, the sensitivity of cytology is quite variable, particularly for low-grade tumors, with sensitivity rates of 20–50%, increasing to 60–80% for high-grade tumors [11]. In an attempt to augment the sensitivity of UTUC detection, emerging research is directed towards the application of novel biomarkers, such as nuclear matrix protein 22 (NMP22) and fibroblast growth factor receptor 3 (FGFR3) mutation assays. Preliminary studies indicate encouraging results, with NMP22 demonstrating sensitivity and specificity rates up to 85% and 77% respectively [12].

The diagnostic paradigm for UTUC also incorporates the direct visualization and biopsy of suspected lesions via ureteroscopy. Biopsies in UTUC can be challenging due to difficulties accessing the upper urinary tract anatomy. Reported rates of nondiagnostic biopsies range from 10–20% [13]. Sampling error is a concern as UTUCs can be heterogeneous and solitary biopsies may miss higher grade components in up to 42% of cases [13]. There is also a small risk of tumor-seeding along the instrument tract during biopsy, estimated at <1% with proper technique [14]. Specimen interpretation is complicated by artifacts like crush and cautery effect, making it difficult to differentiate non-invasive from invasive disease in a significant number of samples. Furthermore, given the complexities of the procedure, the anatomy and the malignancy itself, upstaging from pT1 can occur in 61% of cases and upgrading from low to high grade can occur in 30% of cases [15]. There is no clear guideline on when a biopsy is absolutely needed versus proceeding directly to resection for suspected UTUC. Overall, issues with access, sampling, seeding risk, artifacts, and lack of consensus guidelines pose difficulties for biopsies in UTUC that require careful technique and interpretation.

The diagnosis of UTUC constitutes a complex, multifaceted process, encompassing aspects of clinical symptomatology, imaging, urine cytology, and endoscopic biopsy. Nonetheless, inherent limitations within each of these modalities underscore the imperative for continued advancement in diagnostic technologies and strategies. As research progresses, the future may see enhancements in imaging techniques, the introduction of novel biomarkers, and potentially novel diagnostic methodologies, all culminating in earlier and more accurate diagnoses of UTUC.

3. Treatment:

3.1. Perioperative Chemotherapy

Treatment of high-grade upper tract urothelial carcinoma (UTUC) with radical nephroureterectomy (RNU) and excision of the ipsilateral bladder cuff is standard for tumors of the renal pelvis. Endoscopic ablation and segmental ureterectomy can be considered for low-risk tumors, as is further discussed in subsequent chapters of this manuscript [2,16]. National Cancer Center Network (NCCN) and European Association of Urology (EAU) Guidelines do mention consideration of neoadjuvant chemotherapy in select patients with UTUC, though there are no strict guidelines [7]. The rationale for neoadjuvant chemotherapy (NAC), platinum-based, for UTUC is extrapolated from data in localized muscle-invasive bladder cancer (MIBC) to treat micro-metastatic disease, and downstage the tumor burden in those with optimal renal function [17]. Specifically, NAC prior to radical cystectomy in localized MIBC has shown a 5–8% improvement in OS at 5 years [18–20].

Unfortunately, the accurate staging of UTUC is much more challenging than in bladder cancer given the limitations and feasibility of biopsies [21–23]. Clinicians rely on radiologic imaging to clinically stage patients, though restaging is not often performed post-NAC and prior to RNU [24,25]. Despite these challenges, the multi-centric retrospective analysis by D'Andrea et al. showed similar outcomes of downstaging with use of NAC in both MIBC and UTUC [26,27]. In this study, a retrospective analysis was performed on 1830 patients treated with NAC, which was subsequently followed by radical cystectomy or RNU. Patients with metastatic disease were excluded from the trial. Results showed a pathological complete response in 19.2% of patients with urothelial carcinoma of the bladder (UCB) and 8.3% in patients with UTUC. A pathological objective response was seen in 40.3% of UCB patients and 48.2% in UTUC patients. In addition, Leow et al. also conducted a systematic review and meta-analysis that examined the efficacy of NAC and AC for non-metastatic UTUC. For NAC, pooled analysis of 14 studies (n = 811 patients) demonstrated an 11% pathologic complete response rate (defined as ≤ypT0N0M0) and 43% partial response rate (defined as ≤ypT1N0M0). Pathologic downstaging from the clinical tumor stage occurred in 33% across six studies. In comparative studies, NAC was associated with improved overall survival (OS) (hazard ratio [HR] 0.44, $p < 0.001$) and cancer-specific survival (CSS) (HR 0.38, $p < 0.001$) versus radical nephroureterectomy (RNU) alone. For AC, pooled analysis of 14 studies (n = 7983 patients) revealed an OS benefit (HR 0.77, $p = 0.004$), while 18 studies (n = 5659 patients) showed improved CSS (HR 0.79, $p = 0.001$) and 4 studies (n = 602 patients) demonstrated superior disease-free survival (HR 0.52, $p < 0.001$) with AC compared to RNU alone [28]. Overall, there have been many retrospective and prospective studies supporting peri-operative systemic therapy in the treatment of UTUC by benefiting improvement in OS and DSS, some of which we will outline in this review [29–32].

Neoadjuvant cisplatin-based therapy is the clinicians' preference, rather than adjuvant platinum-based therapy, given the possible decline in renal function post-RNU which may render a patient ineligible for cisplatin-based therapy. One prospective study of neoadjuvant split-dose gemcitabine and cisplatin of 53 patients showed a CR of 19%, downstaging to ypT1 or less in 60% of patients, 2-year PFS of 76% [33]. Adjuvant cisplatin-based chemotherapy does also have a benefit in DFS as noted in the POUT study, a prospective, randomized phase III trial which showed DFS improvement at 2 years by 70% vs. 51% with the use of adjuvant platinum-based chemotherapy. Non-cisplatin-based therapies, including gemcitabine-based regimens, did not have an impact on mortality. The POUT trial arm of adjuvant carboplatin and gemcitabine for those with insufficient renal function noted that the DFS benefit at 3 years was upheld, though lacked improvement in OS [34]. Similarly, as in the treatment of MIBC, carboplatin-based regimens are not standard in either the neoadjuvant or adjuvant setting for patients who are cisplatin-eligible. However, carboplatin and gemcitabine can be considered adjuvantly in cisplatin-ineligible patients with high-risk upper tract disease.

Adibi et al. conducted a retrospective study between 2004–2017 of 126 patients with high-risk UTUC who were treated with NAC prior to RNU. NAC regimens did differ, as 62 received ddMVAC (methotrexate, vinblastine, Adriamycin, and cisplatin), 28 received cisplatin with or without gemcitabine, and 19 were treated with gemcitabine, paclitaxel, and doxorubicin. Seventeen patients received multiple different regimens or non-platinum-based therapy due to decreased renal function. Median OS was 107 months (95% CI 86–125), 14.3% achieved a pathologic complete response, while 60% were downstaged to ypT0-1N0. Estimated 5- and 10-year DSS rates were 89.8% (95% CI 0.836–0.965) and 80.6% (95% CI 0.691–0.94), respectively. Five- and 10-year metastasis free survival rates were 81% (95% CI 74–88.6) and 75.4% (95% CI 65.3–87), respectively, and 5- and 10-year OS were 73.7% (95% CI 65.3–83.1) and 35.9% (95% CI 23.9–54). Median time to recurrence was 15.5 months, with 24 metastatic recurrences documented, 50% to retroperitoneal, pelvic, of supraclavicular lymph nodes and 25% in the lung. This study supported the benefit of NAC prior to RNU with a durable 5-and 10-year OS and DSS [35]. Margulis et al. conducted a prospective multicenter phase II study consisting of 30 patients with high-grade UTUC receiving neoadjuvant accelerated MVAC (aMVAC) prior to nephroureterectomy. The pathologic complete response rate was 14% (4/29, 90% CI 4.9–28.8%). Overall, 62% achieved ≤pT1 at surgery. At a median 21 months follow-up, the 2-year recurrence-free and cancer-specific survival rates were 67% and 91%, respectively. Grade 3–4 toxicity occurred in 23% with aMVAC. While median creatinine clearance remained stable after chemotherapy (82 to 75 mL/min), it declined substantially to 48 mL/min after surgery, with 59% of patients becoming cisplatin-ineligible [29]. This study demonstrated neoadjuvant aMVAC appears safe and active for eligible patients with high-grade upper tract urothelial carcinoma, supporting further evaluation of this approach. Cisplatin ineligibility frequently develops after surgery, further highlighting the potential benefit of preoperative systemic therapy.

3.2. Perioperative Immunotherapy

There is limited data on the use of perioperative immunotherapy in the management of UTUC. The PURE-02 study was a feasibility study evaluating the use of three cycles of neoadjuvant pembrolizumab in patients with high-risk UTUC [36]. Despite the small sample size of 10 patients, there were no significant signals of activity with neoadjuvant pembrolizumab. Only one patient was characterized as a major responder, with a radiographic complete response to therapy. The remaining patients were defined as either nonresponders or with uncertain responses to therapy. A phase II study evaluated the use of neoadjuvant nivolumab and ipilimumab in patients with cisplatin-ineligible, high-grade UTUC [37]. The Stage I portion of the study enrolled nine patients, three of whom attained a pathologic CR (pCR); the remaining six patients were pathologically downstaged (<pT2pN0). Next-generation sequencing was performed on the pre-treatment tumor specimens. Interestingly, three patients were found to have germline variants in mismatch repair genes; one attained a pCR and the other two ypTaN0. The ABACUS trial was a single-arm, phase II study evaluating two cycles of neoadjuvant atezolizumab prior to cystectomy in 95 cisplatin-ineligible muscle-invasive bladder cancer patients. At a median follow-up of 25 months, the 2-year disease-free and overall survival rates were 68% (95% CI 58–76%) and 77% (95% CI 68–85%), respectively. In the 31% of patients achieving a pathologic complete response, the 2-year disease-free survival rate was 85% (95% CI 65–94%). High baseline stromal CD8+ T cells and negative baseline circulating tumor DNA status correlated with improved relapse-free survival, while post-treatment fibroblast activation protein positivity was associated with worse outcomes. Serial circulating tumor DNA analysis demonstrated conversion to negative status after neoadjuvant therapy in some baseline-positive patients and was highly prognostic for relapse when positive post-cystectomy [38]. In summary, atezolizumab showed promising preliminary efficacy in patients with MIBC. Further research is warranted to confirm these findings and determine if similar efficacy and safety of neoadjuvant atezolizumab can be reproduced in patients with UTUC prior to radical nephroureterectomy.

Gao et al. further evaluated the efficacy of PD-L1 plus CTLA-4 blockade in the neoadjuvant setting. In this open-label, single-arm pilot study, 28 cisplatin-ineligible patients with high-risk muscle-invasive urothelial carcinoma received neoadjuvant durvalumab plus tremelimumab every 4 weeks for two doses. The pathologic complete response (pCR) rate was 38% (9/24 patients, 95% CI 19–59%) among those completing cystectomy. In 12 patients with T3/T4 disease, the pCR rate was 42% (5/12 patients). The overall downstaging rate to $\leq$pT1N0 was 58% (14/24 patients, 95% CI 36–77%). At a median follow-up of 19 months, the 1-year overall survival rate was 89% (95% CI 70–96%) and 1-year relapse-free survival rate was 83% (95% CI 61–93%). Grade $\geq$ 3 treatment-related adverse events occurred in 21% (6/28 patients) of patients. High baseline tertiary lymphoid structure density was significantly associated with improved survival. [39] In summary, neoadjuvant durvalumab plus tremelimumab showed encouraging antitumor activity and manageable toxicity in high-risk cisplatin-ineligible muscle-invasive bladder cancer. Two ongoing trials are evaluating the use of neoadjuvant durvalumab combined with chemotherapy for patients with high-risk UTUC [40,41].

Several Phase III studies have explored the use of adjuvant immunotherapy in patients with high-risk muscle-invasive urothelial carcinoma. The CheckMate-274 trial, which randomized patients to receive one-year of adjuvant nivolumab or placebo, found a disease-free survival benefit with the addition of adjuvant nivolumab; overall survival results are not mature. Of the 709 patients in the intention-to-treat population, 149 had upper tract disease [42]. On subgroup analysis, there was no benefit of the addition of nivolumab for upper tract disease (HR [renal pelvis] 1.23, 95% CI 0.67–2.23; HR [ureter] 1.56 95% CI 0.70–3.48); however, the study was not powered to specifically evaluate this. The IMvigor-010 study evaluated the use of adjuvant atezolizumab in patients with locally advanced or metastatic UTUC who had previously received platinum-based chemotherapy. This was a negative trial with no disease-free survival benefit in the intention-to-treat population (HR 0.89, 95% CI 0.74–1.08; $p = 0.24$) [43]. On the horizon is the AMBASSADOR trial, which is a phase III randomized, double-blind, placebo-controlled clinical trial evaluating the use of adjuvant pembrolizumab after nephroureterectomy in patients with high-risk UTUC. The trial aimed to enroll 360 patients who underwent radical nephroureterectomy for high-risk, non-metastatic UTUC. Patients were randomized 1:1 to receive either adjuvant pembrolizumab every 3 weeks or placebo for up to eighteen cycles. The primary endpoint is overall survival and disease-free survival. Key eligibility criteria include: high-grade UTUC (either high-grade papillary cancer or invasive urothelial carcinoma), pT2-T4 or pTany with positive lymph nodes, and no neoadjuvant chemotherapy. The results from this trial have the potential to establish adjuvant pembrolizumab as a new standard of care for high-risk UTUC patients after nephroureterectomy. The trial is expected to be completed in 2025 [44].

4. Future Directions

In recent years, advancements in the genomic understanding of UTUC have delineated the potential therapeutic promise of the Fibroblast Growth Factor Receptor (FGFR) pathway. Comprising a group of receptor tyrosine kinases, FGFR is instrumental in the regulation of critical cellular processes, including proliferation, differentiation, and survival. The dysregulation of FGFR signaling pathways, predominantly due to gene mutations or fusions, is implicated in the tumorigenesis of a wide range of cancers, UTUC included. The prevalence of FGFR mutations or fusions in UTUC is relatively high, with genetic alterations involving FGFR reported in an estimated 20% of patients with advanced urothelial cell cancer [45]. This revelation has sparked substantial interest in the development of FGFR-targeted therapies, resulting in several clinical trials examining the potential benefits of FGFR inhibitors, such as erdafitinib and infigratinib, for UTUC.

Erdafitinib, an FGFR1-4 inhibitor, has been tested in the clinical setting for patients with UTUC and other urothelial carcinomas. It was granted accelerated approval by the FDA based primarily on the results of a multicenter, open-label, single-arm study conducted by Loriot et al. In this open-label phase 2 trial, 99 patients with metastatic or unresectable urothelial carcinoma harboring FGFR alterations received the pan-FGFR inhibitor erdafitinib continuously at 8 mg or 9 mg daily doses. The confirmed objective response rate was 40% (95% CI 31–50%). Among FGFR mutation patients, the response rate was 49%. Median progression-free survival was 5.5 months and median overall survival was 13.8 months. The 12-month overall survival rate was 55%. Grade ≥ 3 treatment-related adverse events occurred in 46% of patients, most commonly hyponatremia, stomatitis and asthenia [46]. Erdafitinib showed promising antitumor activity and manageable toxicity in this patient population who had progressed on prior chemotherapy and/or immunotherapy.

Infigratinib, a selective FGFR1-3 inhibitor, has also shown promise in FGFR-altered urothelial cancer, including UTUC. Lyou et al. conducted an open-label multicenter phase 1b study, where 13 patients received the FGFR1-3 inhibitor infigratinib early-line before platinum chemotherapy for metastatic urothelial carcinoma, while 54 received it after $\geq$1 prior therapies. The confirmed objective response rate was 31% (4/13 patients, 95% CI 9.1–61.4%) with early-line and 24% (13/54 patients, 95% CI 13.5–37.6%) with later-line infigratinib. Disease control rates were 46% (6/13 patients, 95% CI 19.2–74.9%) and 69% (37/54 patients, 95% CI 54.4–80.5%) in the early-line and salvage settings, respectively. Median progression-free survival was 12.0 months versus 5.6 months, and median overall survival was 13.8 months versus 12.9 months in the early-line compared to later-line groups [47]. Infigratinib demonstrated clinically meaningful antitumor activity regardless of treatment line in metastatic urothelial carcinoma, supporting further evaluation across different settings.

Notwithstanding the encouraging preliminary results of FGFR-targeted therapies, multiple challenges endure. These include the emergence of resistance to FGFR inhibitors, the management of therapy-associated side effects, and the necessity for reliable biomarkers to guide patient selection. Moreover, the definitive impact of FGFR inhibitors on overall survival remains under investigation. These studies represent important strides in the treatment of UTUC and other urothelial carcinomas. They underscore the importance of genomic profiling in urothelial cancer to identify patients who might benefit from these targeted treatments. As further studies are conducted, the role of FGFR inhibitors in the treatment paradigm of UTUC is likely to become better defined.

In addition to immunotherapy and chemotherapy, there is significant interest in the role of radiation therapy in the adjuvant space. A systematic review by Iwata et al. evaluated the role of adjuvant radiotherapy (ART) after surgery for bladder cancer and UTUC. For bladder cancer, the review included three randomized controlled trials comprising 456 patients and 11 retrospective studies comprising 7571 patients [48]. Some studies found ART improved recurrence-free survival (5-year rates of 49% vs. 25% in one RCT) and local recurrence-free survival (5-year rates of 87% vs. 50% in one RCT), but most studies found no statistically significant impact on metastasis-free or overall survival [48]. For UTUC, 14 retrospective studies comprising 6047 patients were included. Most studies did not find a survival advantage for ART, except two studies that showed improved overall survival in locally advanced UTUC (29.9 vs. 11.4 months in one study) [48]. Toxicity from ART is decreasing with improved radiotherapy techniques, with recent studies showing lower rates of severe gastrointestinal toxicity and bowel obstruction compared to older studies [48]. The quality and quantity of data on ART in bladder cancer and UTUC was found to be limited. The combination of ART and chemotherapy may be beneficial for locally advanced tumors. The authors concluded there is currently no clear evidence for the survival benefit of ART after surgery for bladder cancer or UTUC, and future efforts should focus on multimodal therapy with ART plus chemotherapy or immunotherapy.

5. Conclusions

Further prospective, randomized clinical trials of peri-operative chemo- and immunotherapy in the treatment of UTUC are needed to answer efficacy questions and establish a new standard of care.

Author Contributions: Conceptualization, A.K., V.T. and A.D.; validation, A.K., V.T. and A.D.; formal analysis, A.K., V.T. and A.D.; investigation, A.K., V.T. and A.D.; resources A.K., V.T. and A.D.; data curation, A.K., V.T. and A.D.; writing—original draft preparation, A.K., V.T. and A.D.; writing—review and editing, A.K., V.T. and A.D.; visualization, A.K., V.T. and A.D.; supervision, V.T. and A.D.; project administration, V.T. and A.D.; funding acquisition, V.T. and A.D. All authors have read and agreed to the published version of the manuscript.

Funding: This research received no external funding.

Conflicts of Interest: The authors declare no conflict of interest.

Appendix A

Table A1 and Figure A1 show a basic frame work of working up UTUC.

Table A1. Trial Summaries of the key clinical trials investigating the role of neoadjuvant, adjuvant, and systemic therapies in the management of UTUC. DFS = Disease Free Survival, ORR = Objective Response Rate, PRR = Pathological Response Rate, PCR = Pathologic Complete Response, OS = Overall Survival.

Name of Trial or Study Drug	NCT Identifier	Trial Setting	Clinical Setting	Number of Study Subjects/UTUC Patients	Primary Measure	Treatment Efficacy	Treatment
POUT	NCT01993979	Phase 3	Adjuvant	261 total/ 261 UTUC patients	Disease-free Survival	3-year DFS: 77% vs. 46% (Treatment vs. Surveillance)	Chemotherapy (Cisplatin or Carboplatin) vs. Surveillance
PURE-02	NCT02736266	Phase 2	Neoadjuvant	10 total/ 10 UTUC	Pathological Response	Not Reported	Pembrolizumab
Checkmate 274	NCT02632409	Phase 3	Adjuvant	709 total/ 149 UTUC patients	Disease-free Survival	DFS: 21.2 months vs. 20.8 months (Nivolumab vs. Placebo)	Nivolumab vs. Placebo
Imvigor-210	NCT02108652	Phase 2	Advanced	119 total/ 33 UTUC patients	Objective Response Rate	Not Reported	Atezolizumab
AMBASSADOR	NCT03244384	Phase 3	Adjuvant	739 total	Overall Survival, Disease-free Survival	DFS: 16.9 months vs. 8.3 months (Pembrolizumab vs. Surveillance)	Pembrolizumab vs. Surveillance
Infigratanib (Lyou et al. [47])	NCT01004224	Phase 1b	Advanced	67 total/8 UTUC patients	Objective Response Rate	ORR: 31%	Infigratanib
Erdafitinib (Loriot et al. [46])	NCT02365597	Phase 2	Advanced	99 total/ 99 UTUC patients	Objective Response Rate	ORR: 40%	Erdafitinib
Gemcitabine and Cisplatin (Coleman et al. [33])	NCT01261728	Phase 2	Neoadjuvant	57 total/ 57 UTUC patients	Pathological Response Rate	PRR: 63%	Gemcitabine and Cisplatin
aMVAC vs. GCa (Margulis et al. [29])	NCT02412670	Phase 2	Neoadjuvant	30 total/ 30 UTUC patients	Pathologic Complete Response	PCR: 14% (aMVAC arm)	Accelerated Methotrexate, Vinblastine, Doxorubicin, Cisplatin vs. Gemcitabine and Carboplatin
Nivolumab plus Ipilimumab (Teo M. et al. [37])	NCT03520491	Phase 2	Neoadjuvant	45 total	Pathologic Complete Response	Not Reported	Nivolumab vs. Nivolumab + Ipilimumab
ABACUS	NCT02662309	Phase 2	Neoadjuvant	96 total	Pathologic Complete Response	PCR: 31%	Atezolizumab
DANUBE	NCT02516241	Phase 3	Advanced	1032 total	Overall Survival	OS: 15.1 months vs. 12.1 months (Treatment vs. Standard of Care)	Durvalumab + Tremelimumab vs. SOC
iNDUCT	NCT04617756	Phase 2	Neoadjuvant	50 total	Pathologic Complete Response	Not Reported	Durvalumab + Gemcitabine/(Cisplatin or Carboplatin)

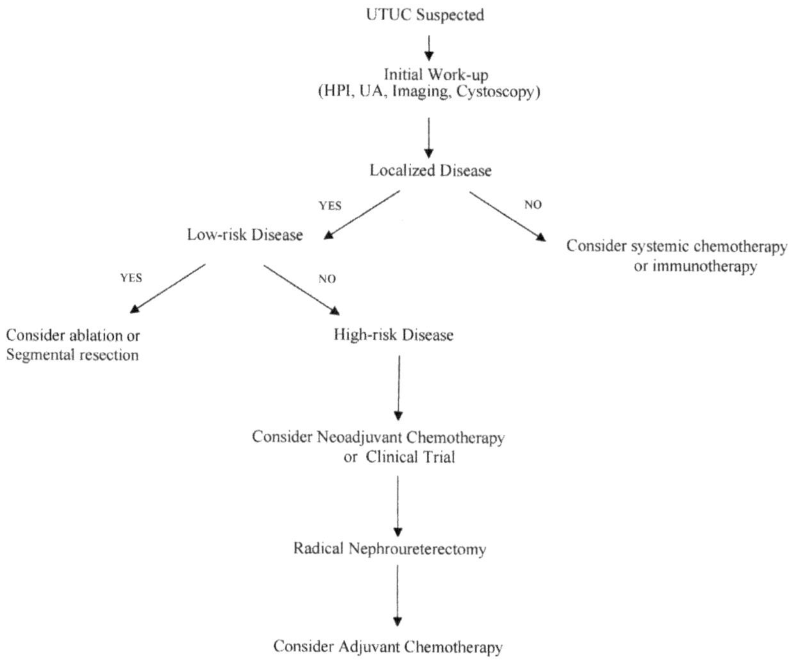

Figure A1. UTUC Work-up Flowsheet: a proposed work-up and approach to the management of UTUC. Low-risk UTUC refers to localized, low-grade tumors with small volume, papillary architecture, limited depth of invasion (non-invasive or lamina propria only), and lack of aggressive features like carcinoma in situ, lymphovascular invasion, lymph node metastases, or radiographic evidence of advanced disease. High-risk UTUC refers to tumors with aggressive features like high-grade disease (G3), carcinoma in situ (CIS), large size (>2 cm), infiltrative architecture, multifocality, advanced local extent on imaging, muscularis propria invasion or beyond (≥pT2), lymphovascular invasion (LVI), lymph node involvement or metastases (pN1–3 or M1), or high volume even if low stage/grade.

References

1. Siegel, R.L.; Miller, K.D.; Fuchs, H.E.; Jemal, A. Cancer Statistics, 2021. *CA Cancer J. Clin.* **2021**, *71*, 7–33. [CrossRef] [PubMed]
2. Margulis, V.; Shariat, S.F.; Matin, S.F.; Kamat, A.M.; Zigeuner, R.; Kikuchi, E.; Lotan, Y.; Weizer, A.; Raman, J.D.; Wood, C.G.; et al. Outcomes of radical nephroureterectomy: A series from the Upper Tract Urothelial Carcinoma Collaboration. *Cancer* **2009**, *115*, 1224–1233. [CrossRef] [PubMed]
3. Comperat, E.; Larre, S.; Roupret, M.; Neuzillet, Y.; Pignot, G.; Quintens, H.; Houede, N.; Roy, C.; Durand, X.; Varinot, J.; et al. Clinicopathological characteristics of urothelial bladder cancer in patients less than 40 years old. *Virchows Arch.* **2015**, *466*, 589–594. [CrossRef]
4. Oswald, D.; Pallauf, M.; Deininger, S.; Torzsok, P.; Sieberer, M.; Eiben, C. Neoadjuvant Chemotherapy before Nephroureterectomy in High-Risk Upper Tract Urothelial Cancer: A Systematic Review and Meta-Analysis. *Cancers* **2022**, *14*, 4841. [CrossRef]
5. Wu, J.; Chen, S.; Wu, X.; Mao, W.; Wang, Y.; Xu, B.; Zheng, D.; Chen, M. Trends of incidence and prognosis of upper tract urothelial carcinoma. *Bosn. J. Basic. Med. Sci.* **2021**, *21*, 607–619. [CrossRef]
6. Ng, K.L. The Etiology of Renal Cell Carcinoma and Upper Tract Urothelial Carcinoma. In *Urologic Cancers*; Barber, N., Ali, A., Eds.; Exon Publications: Brisbane, Australia, 2022.
7. Roupret, M.; Babjuk, M.; Burger, M.; Capoun, O.; Cohen, D.; Comperat, E.M.; Cowan, N.C.; Dominguez-Escrig, J.L.; Gontero, P.; Hugh Mostafid, A.; et al. European Association of Urology Guidelines on Upper Urinary Tract Urothelial Carcinoma: 2020 Update. *Eur. Urol.* **2021**, *79*, 62–79.
8. Cowan, N.C. CT urography for hematuria. *Nat. Rev. Urol.* **2012**, *9*, 218–226. [CrossRef]
9. Fiuk, J.V.; Schwartz, B.F. Upper tract urothelial carcinoma: Paradigm shift towards nephron sparing management. *World J. Nephrol.* **2016**, *5*, 158–165. [CrossRef]

10. Baard, J.; de Bruin, D.M.; Zondervan, P.J.; Kamphuis, G.; de la Rosette, J.; Laguna, M.P. Diagnostic dilemmas in patients with upper tract urothelial carcinoma. *Nat. Rev. Urol.* **2017**, *14*, 181–191. [CrossRef]
11. Zhao, Y.; Deng, F.M.; Melamed, J.; Huang, W.C.; Huang, H.; Ren, Q. Diagnostic role of urine cytology and ureteroscopic biopsies in detection of high grade upper tract urothelial carcinoma. *Am. J. Clin. Exp. Urol.* **2021**, *9*, 221–228.
12. Dogan, C.; Pelit, E.S.; Yildirim, A.; Zemheri, I.E.; Canakci, C.; Basok, E.K.; Caskurlu, T. The value of the NMP22 test for superficial bladder cancer diagnosis and follow-up. *Turk. J. Urol.* **2013**, *39*, 137–142. [CrossRef] [PubMed]
13. Freund, J.E.; Liem, E.; Savci-Heijink, C.D.; Baard, J.; Kamphuis, G.M.; de la Rosette, J.; de Bruin, D.M. Confocal laser endomicroscopy for upper tract urothelial carcinoma: Validation of the proposed criteria and proposal of a scoring system for real-time tumor grading. *World J. Urol.* **2019**, *37*, 2155–2164. [CrossRef] [PubMed]
14. Cutress, M.L.; Stewart, G.D.; Zakikhani, P.; Phipps, S.; Thomas, B.G.; Tolley, D.A. Ureteroscopic and percutaneous management of upper tract urothelial carcinoma (UTUC): Systematic review. *BJU Int.* **2012**, *110*, 614–628. [CrossRef]
15. Koll, F.J.; Meisenzahl, E.; Haller, B.; Maisch, P.; Kirchhoff, F.; Horn, T.; Gschwend, J.E.; Schmid, S.C. Evaluation of Pre-operative Biopsy, Surgical Procedures and Oncologic Outcomes in Upper Tract Urothelial Carcinoma (UTUC). *Front. Surg.* **2021**, *8*, 790738. [CrossRef] [PubMed]
16. Raman, J.D.; Scherr, D.S. Management of patients with upper urinary tract transitional cell carcinoma. *Nat. Clin. Pract. Urol.* **2007**, *4*, 432–443. [CrossRef]
17. Audenet, F.; Yates, D.R.; Cussenot, O.; Roupret, M. The role of chemotherapy in the treatment of urothelial cell carcinoma of the upper urinary tract (UUT-UCC). *Urol. Oncol.* **2013**, *31*, 407–413. [CrossRef] [PubMed]
18. Witjes, J.A.; Bruins, H.M.; Cathomas, R.; Comperat, E.M.; Cowan, N.C.; Gakis, G.; Hernandez, V.; Linares Espinos, E.; Lorch, A.; Neuzillet, Y.; et al. European Association of Urology Guidelines on Muscle-invasive and Metastatic Bladder Cancer: Summary of the 2020 Guidelines. *Eur. Urol.* **2021**, *79*, 82–104. [CrossRef]
19. Grossman, H.B.; Natale, R.B.; Tangen, C.M.; Speights, V.O.; Vogelzang, N.J.; Trump, D.L.; de Vere White, R.W.; Sarosdy, M.F.; Wood, D.P., Jr.; Raghavan, D.; et al. Neoadjuvant chemotherapy plus cystectomy compared with cystectomy alone for locally advanced bladder cancer. *N. Engl. J. Med.* **2003**, *349*, 859–866. [CrossRef]
20. Advanced Bladder Cancer Meta-analysis, C. Neoadjuvant chemotherapy in invasive bladder cancer: Update of a systematic review and meta-analysis of individual patient data advanced bladder cancer (ABC) meta-analysis collaboration. *Eur. Urol.* **2005**, *48*, 202–205, discussion 205–206.
21. Clements, T.; Messer, J.C.; Terrell, J.D.; Herman, M.P.; Ng, C.K.; Scherr, D.S.; Scoll, B.; Boorjian, S.A.; Uzzo, R.G.; Wille, M.; et al. High-grade ureteroscopic biopsy is associated with advanced pathology of upper-tract urothelial carcinoma tumors at definitive surgical resection. *J. Endourol.* **2012**, *26*, 398–402. [CrossRef]
22. Rojas, C.P.; Castle, S.M.; Llanos, C.A.; Santos Cortes, J.A.; Bird, V.; Rodriguez, S.; Reis, I.M.; Zhao, W.; Gomez-Fernandez, C.; Leveillee, R.J.; et al. Low biopsy volume in ureteroscopy does not affect tumor biopsy grading in upper tract urothelial carcinoma. *Urol. Oncol.* **2013**, *31*, 1696–1700. [CrossRef] [PubMed]
23. Brown, G.A.; Matin, S.F.; Busby, J.E.; Dinney, C.P.; Grossman, H.B.; Pettaway, C.A.; Munsell, M.F.; Kamat, A.M. Ability of clinical grade to predict final pathologic stage in upper urinary tract transitional cell carcinoma: Implications for therapy. *Urology* **2007**, *70*, 252–256. [CrossRef] [PubMed]
24. Seisen, T.; Colin, P.; Roupret, M. Risk-adapted strategy for the kidney-sparing management of upper tract tumours. *Nat. Rev. Urol.* **2015**, *12*, 155–166. [CrossRef]
25. Honda, Y.; Nakamura, Y.; Teishima, J.; Goto, K.; Higaki, T.; Narita, K.; Akagi, M.; Terada, H.; Kaichi, Y.; Fujii, S.; et al. Clinical staging of upper urinary tract urothelial carcinoma for T staging: Review and pictorial essay. *Int. J. Urol.* **2019**, *26*, 1024–1032. [CrossRef]
26. D'Andrea, D.; Matin, S.; Black, P.C.; Petros, F.G.; Zargar, H.; Dinney, C.P.; Cookson, M.S.; Kassouf, W.; Dall'Era, M.A.; McGrath, J.S.; et al. Comparative effectiveness of neoadjuvant chemotherapy in bladder and upper urinary tract urothelial carcinoma. *BJU Int.* **2021**, *127*, 528–537. [CrossRef]
27. Siefker-Radtke, A.O.; Dinney, C.P.; Shen, Y.; Williams, D.L.; Kamat, A.M.; Grossman, H.B.; Millikan, R.E. A phase 2 clinical trial of sequential neoadjuvant chemotherapy with ifosfamide, doxorubicin, and gemcitabine followed by cisplatin, gemcitabine, and ifosfamide in locally advanced urothelial cancer: Final results. *Cancer* **2013**, *119*, 540–547. [CrossRef]
28. Leow, J.J.; Chong, Y.L.; Chang, S.L.; Valderrama, B.P.; Powles, T.; Bellmunt, J. Neoadjuvant and Adjuvant Chemotherapy for Upper Tract Urothelial Carcinoma: A 2020 Systematic Review and Meta-analysis, and Future Perspectives on Systemic Therapy. *Eur. Urol.* **2021**, *79*, 635–654. [CrossRef]
29. Margulis, V.; Puligandla, M.; Trabulsi, E.J.; Plimack, E.R.; Kessler, E.R.; Matin, S.F.; Godoy, G.; Alva, A.; Hahn, N.M.; Carducci, M.A.; et al. Phase II Trial of Neoadjuvant Systemic Chemotherapy Followed by Extirpative Surgery in Patients with High Grade Upper Tract Urothelial Carcinoma. *J. Urol.* **2020**, *203*, 690–698. [CrossRef]
30. McConkey, D.J.; Choi, W.; Shen, Y.; Lee, I.L.; Porten, S.; Matin, S.F.; Kamat, A.M.; Corn, P.; Millikan, R.E.; Dinney, C.; et al. A Prognostic Gene Expression Signature in the Molecular Classification of Chemotherapy-naive Urothelial Cancer is Predictive of Clinical Outcomes from Neoadjuvant Chemotherapy: A Phase 2 Trial of Dose-dense Methotrexate, Vinblastine, Doxorubicin, and Cisplatin with Bevacizumab in Urothelial Cancer. *Eur. Urol.* **2016**, *69*, 855–862.

31. Youssef, R.F.; Shariat, S.F.; Lotan, Y.; Wood, C.G.; Sagalowsky, A.I.; Zigeuner, R.; Kikuchi, E.; Weizer, A.; Raman, J.D.; Remzi, M.; et al. Upper urinary tract urothelial carcinoma with loco-regional nodal metastases: Insights from the Upper Tract Urothelial Carcinoma Collaboration. *BJU Int.* **2011**, *108*, 1286–1291. [CrossRef]
32. Meng, X.; Chao, B.; Vijay, V.; Silver, H.; Margolin, E.J.; Balar, A.; Taneja, S.S.; Shah, O.; Bjurlin, M.A.; Anderson, C.B.; et al. High Response Rates to Neoadjuvant Chemotherapy in High-Grade Upper Tract Urothelial Carcinoma. *Urology* **2019**, *129*, 146–152. [CrossRef] [PubMed]
33. Coleman, J.A.; Yip, W.; Wong, N.C.; Sjoberg, D.D.; Bochner, B.H.; Dalbagni, G.; Donat, S.M.; Herr, H.W.; Cha, E.K.; Donahue, T.F.; et al. Multicenter Phase II Clinical Trial of Gemcitabine and Cisplatin as Neoadjuvant Chemotherapy for Patients With High-Grade Upper Tract Urothelial Carcinoma. *J. Clin. Oncol.* **2023**, *41*, 1618–1625. [CrossRef] [PubMed]
34. Birtle, A.; Johnson, M.; Chester, J.; Jones, R.; Dolling, D.; Bryan, R.T.; Harris, C.; Winterbottom, A.; Blacker, A.; Catto, J.W.F.; et al. Adjuvant chemotherapy in upper tract urothelial carcinoma (the POUT trial): A phase 3, open-label, randomised controlled trial. *Lancet* **2020**, *395*, 1268–1277. [CrossRef]
35. Adibi, M.; McCormick, B.; Economides, M.P.; Petros, F.; Xiao, L.; Guo, C.; Shah, A.; Kamat, A.M.; Dinney, C.; Navai, N.; et al. Five and Ten-Year Outcomes of Neoadjuvant Chemotherapy and Surgery for High-Risk Upper Tract Urothelial Carcinoma. *Clin. Genitourin. Cancer* **2022**, *20*, 176–182. [CrossRef] [PubMed]
36. Necchi, A.; Martini, A.; Raggi, D.; Cucchiara, V.; Colecchia, M.; Luciano, R.; Villa, L.; Mazzone, E.; Basile, G.; Scuderi, S.; et al. A feasibility study of preoperative pembrolizumab before radical nephroureterectomy in patients with high-risk, upper tract urothelial carcinoma: PURE-02. *Urol. Oncol.* **2022**, *40*, 10.e11–10.e16. [CrossRef] [PubMed]
37. Teo, M.; Guercio, B.; Pietzak, E.J. Neoadjuvant nivolumab (N) + ipilimumab (I) in cisplatin-ineligible patients with upper tract urothelial cancer (UTUC). *J. Clin. Oncol.* **2023**, *41*, 511. [CrossRef]
38. Szabados, B.; Kockx, M.; Assaf, Z.J.; van Dam, P.J.; Rodriguez-Vida, A.; Duran, I.; Crabb, S.J.; Van Der Heijden, M.S.; Pous, A.F.; Gravis, G.; et al. Final Results of Neoadjuvant Atezolizumab in Cisplatin-ineligible Patients with Muscle-invasive Urothelial Cancer of the Bladder. *Eur. Urol.* **2022**, *82*, 212–222. [CrossRef]
39. Gao, J.; Navai, N.; Alhalabi, O.; Siefker-Radtke, A.; Campbell, M.T.; Tidwell, R.S.; Guo, C.C.; Kamat, A.M.; Matin, S.F.; Araujo, J.C.; et al. Neoadjuvant PD-L1 plus CTLA-4 blockade in patients with cisplatin-ineligible operable high-risk urothelial carcinoma. *Nat. Med.* **2020**, *26*, 1845–1851. [CrossRef]
40. National Cancer Institute. Testing the Addition of MEDI4736 (Durvalumab) to Chemotherapy Before Surgery for Patients with High-Grade Upper Urinary Tract Cancer. ClinicalTrials.gov Identifier: NCT04628767. Available online: https://classic.clinicaltrials.gov/ct2/show/NCT04628767 (accessed on 26 June 2023).
41. Centre Hospitalier Universitaire de Nîmes. Safety & Efficacy of Durvalumab+Neoadjuvant Chemotherapy for High-Risk Urothelial Carcinoma of the Upper Urinary Tract (iNDUCT). ClinicalTrials.gov Identifier: NCT04617756. Available online: https://classic.clinicaltrials.gov/ct2/show/NCT04617756 (accessed on 25 June 2023).
42. Bajorin, D.F.; Witjes, J.A.; Gschwend, J.E.; Schenker, M.; Valderrama, B.P.; Tomita, Y.; Bamias, A.; Lebret, T.; Shariat, S.F.; Park, S.H.; et al. Adjuvant Nivolumab versus Placebo in Muscle-Invasive Urothelial Carcinoma. *N. Engl. J. Med.* **2021**, *384*, 2102–2114. [CrossRef]
43. Bellmunt, J.; Hussain, M.; Gschwend, J.E.; Albers, P.; Oudard, S.; Castellano, D.; Daneshmand, S.; Nishiyama, H.; Majchrowicz, M.; Degaonkar, V.; et al. Adjuvant atezolizumab versus observation in muscle-invasive urothelial carcinoma (IMvigor010): A multicentre, open-label, randomised, phase 3 trial. *Lancet Oncol.* **2021**, *22*, 525–537. [CrossRef]
44. Apolo, A.B. ASCO GU 2019: Pembrolizumab in Muscle-Invasive and Locally Advanced Urothelial Carcinoma—AMBASSADOR versus Observation. 2019. Available online: urotoday.com (accessed on 5 August 2023).
45. Knowles, M.A.; Hurst, C.D. Molecular biology of bladder cancer: New insights into pathogenesis and clinical diversity. *Nat. Rev. Cancer* **2015**, *15*, 25–41. [CrossRef] [PubMed]
46. Loriot, Y.; Necchi, A.; Park, S.H.; Garcia-Donas, J.; Huddart, R.; Burgess, E.; Fleming, M.; Rezazadeh, A.; Mellado, B.; Varlamov, S.; et al. Erdafitinib in Locally Advanced or Metastatic Urothelial Carcinoma. *N. Engl. J. Med.* **2019**, *381*, 338–348. [CrossRef] [PubMed]
47. Lyou, Y.; Rosenberg, J.E.; Hoffman-Censits, J.; Quinn, D.I.; Petrylak, D.; Galsky, M.; Vaishampayan, U.; De Giorgi, U.; Gupta, S.; Burris, H.; et al. Infigratinib in Early-Line and Salvage Therapy for FGFR3-Altered Metastatic Urothelial Carcinoma. *Clin. Genitourin. Cancer* **2022**, *20*, 35–42. [CrossRef]
48. Iwata, T.; Kimura, S.; Abufaraj, M.; Janisch, F.; Karakiewicz, P.I.; Seebacher, V.; Roupret, M.; Nasu, Y.; Shariat, S.F. The role of adjuvant radiotherapy after surgery for upper and lower urinary tract urothelial carcinoma: A systematic review. *Urol. Oncol.* **2019**, *37*, 659–671. [CrossRef]

cancers

MDPI

Review

Intravesical Therapy for Upper Urinary Tract Urothelial Carcinoma: A Comprehensive Review

Zheng Wang [1,†], Haoqing Shi [1,†], Yifan Xu [1], Yu Fang [1], Jiaao Song [1], Wentao Jiang [1], Demeng Xia [2], Zhenjie Wu [1,*] and Linhui Wang [1,*]

1 Department of Urology, Changhai Hospital, Naval Medical University, Shanghai 200433, China; wangzheng@smmu.edu.cn (Z.W.); shihaoqing2007@163.com (H.S.); xuyifan@smmu.edu.cn (Y.X.); 13916943129@163.com (Y.F.); songjiaao@smmu.edu.cn (J.S.); jiangwentao@smmu.edu.cn (W.J.)

2 Department of Pharmacy, Seventh People's Hospital of Shanghai University of Traditional Chinese Medicine, Shanghai 200137, China; demengxia@smmu.edu.cn

* Correspondence: wuzhenjie17@163.com (Z.W.); wanglinhui@smmu.edu.cn (L.W.)

† These authors contributed equally to this work.

Simple Summary: This comprehensive review discusses the current status and future prospects of intravesical therapy for upper urinary tract urothelial carcinoma (UTUC). It emphasizes the need to understand its role in UTUC management and the importance of personalized strategies for drug selection, dosage, timing and frequency to optimize treatment outcomes and reduce intravesical recurrence. By summarizing historical development, clinical trials, guideline recommendations, and clinical applications, this review provides valuable insights. We aim to guide future studies and impact the research in UTUC, advancing the understanding and utilization of intravesical therapy for UTUC.

Abstract: Upper tract urothelial carcinoma (UTUC) poses unique challenges in diagnosis and treatment. This comprehensive review focuses on prophylactic intravesical therapy for UTUC, summarizing key aspects of intravesical therapy in various clinical scenarios, including concurrent with or following radical nephroureterectomy, kidney-sparing surgery, ureteroscopy-guided biopsy. The incidence of intravesical recurrence in UTUC after surgical treatment is significant, necessitating effective preventive measures. Intravesical therapy plays a vital role in reducing the risk of bladder recurrence following UTUC surgery. Tailoring timing, drug selection, dosage, and frequency is vital in optimizing treatment outcomes and reducing intravesical recurrence risk in UTUC. This review provides a comprehensive summary of the history, clinical trials, guideline recommendations, and clinical applications of intravesical therapy for UTUC. It also discusses the future directions based on current clinical needs and ongoing trials. Future directions entail optimizing dosage, treatment duration, and drug selection, as well as exploring novel agents and combination therapies. Intravesical therapy holds tremendous potential in improving outcomes for UTUC patients and reducing the risk of bladder recurrence. Although advancements have been made in UTUC treatment research, further refinements are necessary to enhance efficacy and safety.

Keywords: upper urinary tract urothelial carcinoma; intravesical recurrence; intravesical therapy; bladder instillation; chemotherapy; ureteroscopy; radical nephroureterectomy; UGN-101; mitomycin C; Bacillus Calmette–Guerin

1. Introduction

Upper tract urothelial carcinoma (UTUC) is a rare and challenging malignancy that primarily affects the inner urothelial lining of the renal pelvis, calyces, and ureters. It accounts for approximately 5–10% of all urothelial carcinoma (UC) and presents unique diagnostic and therapeutic considerations [1].

The incidence of UTUC is on the rise, with an estimated annual incidence of 1–2 cases per 100,000 individuals. Moreover, there is an observable trend of UTUC affecting patients at older ages, as reflected by the increasing mean age at diagnosis from 71.5 to 73.4 years. Encouragingly, advancements in treatment strategies have contributed to improved prognoses for UTUC patients, as demonstrated by an upward trend in the five-year cancer-specific survival rate from 57.4% to 65.4% [2,3].

After treatment, the intravesical recurrence (IVR) of UTUC is observed in 22–47% of patients, with the rate varying based on the initial tumor grade [4–7]. IVR of UTUC is believed to occur through a dual-stage process known as the "seeding" and "field" hypothesis [8–11]. In this theory, short-term recurrences primarily occur due to the dissemination of tumor cells, while long-term recurrences are associated with the field effect, indicating the presence of a molecularly altered urothelium that is prone to tumor development. A shorter interval between IVR and UTUC is considered indicative of a poorer prognosis [12]. Moreover, the period of 2–2.5 years post-surgery is considered a high-risk phase for IVR, highlighting the importance of implementing adjuvant therapies in conjunction with surgery to reduce IVR [13–17]. This aspect not only warrants significant attention but also necessitates further research and investigation.

Although UTUC and bladder carcinomas share common pathogenic mechanisms and exhibit similar tumor characteristics, leading to the adoption of bladder cancer treatment strategies as a reference point for UTUC management [18,19], it is, however, important to note that UTUC and BC also have distinct differences, leading to variations in treatment approaches [20]. While significant progress has been made in UTUC treatment research, further advancements and refinements are still needed in comparison to the advancements made in non-muscle-invasive bladder cancer (NMIBC) [21].

Based on the American Urological Association (AUA) guidelines, it is strongly recommended that UTUC patients meeting the eligibility criteria should undergo a postoperative intravesical therapy to decrease the risk of IVR (Grade A evidence level) [8]. Currently, research on intravesical therapy for UTUC primarily focuses on postoperative bladder instillation. If a concurrent bladder tumor is present at the time of UTUC diagnosis or if there is bladder tumor recurrence after nephroureterectomy (RNU), treatment strategies for NMIBC can be considered as a reference.

Thus, the primary focus of this review is to comprehensively summarize and discuss the key elements pertaining to postoperative intravesical therapy for UTUC. These elements encompass strategy development, optimal timing and duration of therapy, drug selection, and emerging therapeutic agents. Through an in-depth analysis, this review aims to provide valuable insights into the field of intravesical therapy for UTUC in order to enhance the prevention of bladder recurrence and improve patient outcomes.

2. Definition of Intravesical Therapy

Intravesical therapy, also commonly referred to as bladder instillation, involves the administration of drugs or solutions directly into the bladder. This therapeutic approach aims to prevent or treat tumor recurrence within the bladder following UTUC surgery. By delivering medications directly to the bladder lining, intravesical therapy targets residual cancer cells and inhibits their growth, leading to improved treatment outcomes. It is an important adjunctive treatment option that requires careful monitoring and individualized selection of chemotherapy agents, immunotherapies, or other medications [6]. According to Hwang et al., a single-dose intravesical chemotherapy instillation significantly reduces bladder cancer recurrence risk compared to no instillation. During a 12-month follow-up period, prophylactic intravesical instillation could potentially lead to a significant reduction of 127 bladder cancer recurrences per 1000 participants [22].

The risk stratification influences the choice of treatment strategies for bladder management, and different surgical approaches are recommended for individuals with different risk categories. For patients with low-risk tumors, kidney-sparing management is offered as a preferred treatment option. In contrast, radical nephroureterectomy (RNU) (both open and minimally invasive), along with complete bladder cuff excision (BCE), is considered the standard surgical approach for localized high-risk UTUC [23–27]. Therefore, it can be concluded that patients undergoing different surgical procedures based on their risk profile would require distinct postoperative intravesical instillation treatment plans (Figure 1).

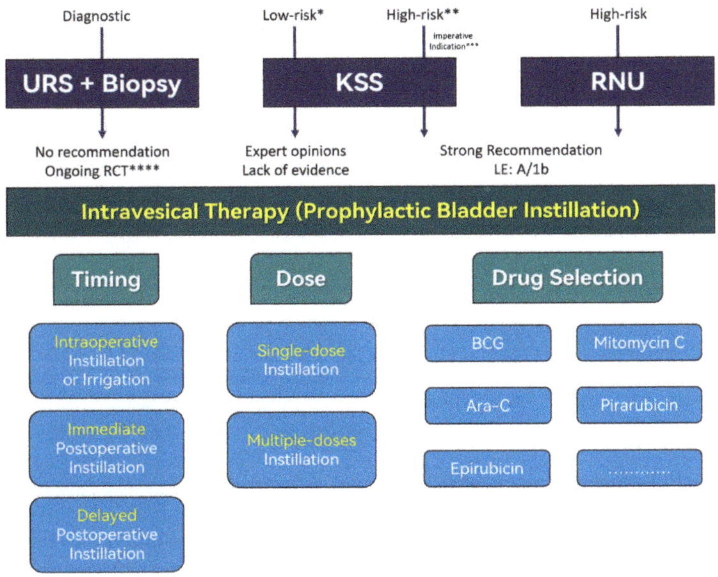

Figure 1. This diagram illustrates recommendations for postoperative prophylactic intravesical therapy based on clinical evidence in different clinical scenarios, as well as the timing (intraoperative instillation [28,29] or irrigation [30], immediate postoperative instillation [31] and delayed postoperative instillation [32,33]), dosage (single-dose instillation [31,33] and multiple-doses instillation [32,34]), and choice of medications for intravesical therapy. * "Low-risk" requires meeting the following conditions simultaneously: unifocal disease, tumor size < 2 cm, negative for high-grade cytology, low-grade ureteroscopy biopsy, and no invasive aspect on CT. ** "High-risk" can be satisfied by meeting any of the following criteria: multifocal disease, tumor size ≥ 2 cm, high-grade cytology, local invasion on CT, hydronephrosis, previous radical cystectomy for high-grade bladder cancer, or histological subtype. *** "Imperative indication" refers to cases involving patients with a solitary kidney, bilateral UTUC, chronic kidney disease, or patients who are medically ineligible or unwilling to undergo RNU. **** NCT05810623. URS: ureteroscopy; KSS: kidney-sparing surgery; RNU: radical nephroureterectomy; RCT: randomized controlled trial; LE: level of evidence; BCG: Bacillus Calmette–Guerin; Ara-C: cytosine arabinoside.

3. Search Strategy

A comprehensive literature search was conducted using the following databases: Pubmed, Web of Science, Medline, Embase, Cochrane controlled trials databases, and clinicaltrials.gov (accessed on 30 July 2023). Additionally, guidelines and abstracts from relevant associations and conferences, including the European Association of Urology (EAU), American Urological Association (AUA) and American Society of Clinical Oncology (ASCO), among others, were also reviewed. The search strategy employed the following keywords:

Intravesical therapy, intravesical treatment, intravesical instillation, bladder instillation, local therapy, adjuvant therapy, intravesical chemotherapy, upper urinary tract urothelial carcinoma, upper tract urothelial carcinoma, renal pelvis carcinoma, ureteral carcinoma, bladder recurrence.

The search strategy aimed to identify studies and the literature related to intravesical therapy for upper urinary tract urothelial carcinoma. The databases were searched for articles published up until the date of the literature search.

The search results were imported into reference management software (Endnote) for initial screening. Titles and abstracts were screened to identify potentially relevant articles. Full texts of the selected articles were retrieved and reviewed for eligibility based on predefined inclusion and exclusion criteria. Inclusion criteria encompassed studies that examined intravesical therapy for upper urinary tract urothelial carcinoma, including clinical trials, observational studies, and systematic reviews. Studies that merely focused on non-urothelial malignancies were excluded.

Data extraction was performed on the included studies, capturing relevant information such as study design, patient characteristics, intervention details, outcomes assessed, and key findings. The extracted data were synthesized and presented in a narrative format, highlighting the main findings, trends, and limitations of the included studies.

The quality of the included studies was assessed using appropriate tools based on the study design. For randomized controlled trials, the Cochrane Collaboration's risk of bias tool was used, while observational studies were evaluated using relevant quality assessment tools.

The limitations of this review include potential publication bias and the exclusion of non-English articles, which may introduce a language bias. Efforts were made to minimize bias by conducting a comprehensive search across multiple databases and including diverse sources of evidence.

Overall, the search strategy outlined above aimed to identify relevant studies on intravesical therapy for upper urinary tract urothelial carcinoma from a variety of databases and sources. Clinical studies related to intravesical therapy are listed in Table 1, including completed trials, studies currently recruiting patients, trials about to commence recruitment, as well as clinical trials with an unknown status. The findings from this comprehensive review will contribute to a thorough understanding of the topic and provide valuable insights for clinical practice and future research.

Table 1. Summary of clinical trials on intravesical therapy for prevention of intravesical recurrence after treatment for UTUC.

ID	Abbreviation	Author + Year	Status	Drugs	Dose and Timing	Follow-Up
/	/	Sakamoto 2001	Completed	MMC 20 mg and Ara-C 200 mg	A total of 28 instillations were given over 2 years.	45 months
/	/	Wu 2010	Completed	Epirubicin 20 mg or MMC 10 mg	6 to 8 times after RNU	55.6 months
ISRCTN 36343644	ODMIT-C	O'Brien 2011	Completed	MMC 40 mg	Single dose at least 1 week after RNU	12 months
/	THP Monotherapy	Ito 2012	Completed	THP 30 mg	Single dose within 48 h after RNU	24 months
UMIN000009682	/	Yamamoto 2013	Unknown status	THP	Single dose after RNU	/
NCT02438865	/	Osman 2015	Completed	Epirubicin 50 mg	Single dose with 48 h or maintenance therapy after RNU	24 months
NCT02923557	/	Li 2015	Unknown status	THP 40 mg	Single dose within 24 h after RNU	
NCT02740426	/	Li 2017	Unknown status	THP 40 mg	Single dose within 24 h after diagnostic URS	36 months
NCT03062059	/	Seo 2017	Recruiting	Gemcitabine 2000 mg	During RNU	72 months
NCT03209206	/	Ku 2017	Unknown status	Docetaxel 75 mg	Single dose within 48 h after RNU	24 months
NCT03030157	/	Huang 2019	Recruiting	THP 30 mg	Single dose within 72–168 h postoperatively plus 1 year long-term after RNU	12 months
/	REBACARE	Van Doeveren 2018	Completed	MMC 40 mg	Single dose immediately (within 3 h) before RNU or KSS	24 months
UMIN000024267	JCOG1403	Miyamoto 2018	Completed	THP 30 mg	Single dose within 24 h after RNU	36 months
NCT03658304	/	Crispen 2018	Not yet recruiting	MMC 40 mg	Single dose during RNU	36 months
NCT04398368	GEMINI	Boorjian 2020	Terminated	Gemcitabine	Single dose at least 1 h at the time of RNU	24 months
NCT05810623	MINERVA	D'Andrea 2023	Not yet recruiting	/	Single dose within 24 h after diagnostic URS	24 months
NCT05731622	SINCERE	Baard, 2023	Not yet recruiting	MMC	Single dose after URS	24 months

UTUC: upper tract urothelial carcinoma; URS: ureteroscopy; KSS: kidney-sparing surgery; RNU: radical nephroureterectomy; MMC: Mitomycin C; Ara-C: cytosine arabinoside;
THP: tetrahydropyranyldoxorubicin.

4. Intraoperative Bladder Instillation and Irrigation

Intraoperative intravesical therapy primarily involves two approaches. One approach is the administration of medication directly during the surgical procedure, aiming to maximize therapeutic efficacy by avoiding delays caused by drug absorption through the mucosa. The other approach involves continuous bladder irrigation with saline or distilled water to prevent the potential dissemination of tumor cells from the surgical site to the bladder.

Continuous irrigation, predominantly utilizing non-medicated solutions such as distilled water or saline, serves as a mechanism to perpetually flush the bladder. This approach is grounded in the rationale that dislodged tumor cells are effectively eliminated. In this study investigating the effect of intraoperative irrigation, a total of 109 UTUC patients with a median follow-up of 26.1 months were included [30]. Among them, 48 patients received bladder irrigation with either normal saline or distilled water intraoperatively. In the irrigation group, the recurrence rate was significantly lower compared to the non-irrigation group, with rates of 25.0% vs. 52.5%, respectively ($p = 0.0066$).

The instillation of chemotherapeutic agents presents a more assertive strategy. Direct administration into the bladder is designed to annihilate free-floating tumor cells on contact. MMC (Mitomycin C) is a potent chemotherapeutic drug widely employed in the management of various malignancies [35]. When used in bladder instillation, MMC plays a crucial role in targeting and treating bladder cancer, thereby minimizing the risk of recurrence and enhancing overall patient prognosis. In a retrospective analysis, 30 patients who received intraoperative (IO) instillation of MMC during RNU were compared with 21 patients who received postoperative (PO) instillation for UTUC. The estimated probability of 1-year bladder tumor recurrence rates was 16% in the IO group and 33% in the PO group ($p = 0.09$). Cox analysis revealed a significantly lower rate of recurrence rate in the first year postoperatively in the IO group (HR = 0.113, 95% CI = 0.28–0.63, $p = 0.01$) [36]. However, this approach introduces challenges related to timing. Given the variability in surgical duration, determining the optimal drug retention period becomes critical. Late conclusion of surgery might necessitate reconsideration of drug retention to mitigate potential toxicities, as opposed to adhering to a standardized duration.

In the study conducted by Nadler et al., MMC (40 mg MMC in 40 mL 0.9% saline) was instilled in 47 patients after BCE and retained for a maximum duration of one hour during RNU [28]. The safety and feasibility of instillation during the surgical procedure have been confirmed, as no complications were observed. However, due to limited sample size and trial design, the efficacy of MMC in suppressing bladder recurrence has not been adequately validated.

Immunotherapy, with agents like Bacillus Calmette–Guerin (BCG), offers an alternative therapeutic mechanism. Rather than direct cytotoxicity, the goal is to harness the body's immune response to target and obliterate tumor cells. The enduring effect of this method, even post-agent removal, underscores its potential. Yet, the administration's timing, be it preoperative for enhanced immune activation or postoperative to capitalize on the surgical milieu, remains a pivotal consideration. Notably, previous studies suggest that recurrent tumor cells might not respond to BCG as robustly as they do in NMIBC [20,37]. The efficacy of intraoperative or preoperative BCG administration remains an area warranting further exploration.

The procedure of bladder cuff excision (BCE) introduces additional intricacies. Drug spillage during BCE is a genuine concern. The primary concern is drug spillage due to incomplete healing of the excision site, risking leakage into the abdominal cavity. The technical skill in suturing the BCE site is crucial. Using normal saline or distilled water minimizes leakage risks. Using normal saline or distilled water can reduce the adverse reactions associated with drug spillage into the abdominal cavity. However, this approach may concurrently elevate the risk of disseminating tumor cells, potentially leading to implantation within the peritoneal cavity. If leakage occurs, the patient, under anesthesia, may require additional sutures for reinforcement.

Given these considerations, it is clear that a singular approach may not suffice. Personalizing the strategy and factoring in patient-specific attributes, tumor pathology, and surgical specifics are of utmost importance. Advancements in this realm will undoubtedly be driven by rigorous clinical trials and a profound understanding of tumor biology, setting the stage for enhanced intraoperative bladder management following RNU.

Intraoperative instillations offer a more feasible and potentially higher utilization option [29]. As for intraoperative irrigation, while not currently a prominent area of research, it continues to be a viable strategy to reduce bladder recurrence.

5. Intravesical Therapy Following Radical Nephroureterectomy

Given the increased propensity for recurrence in high-risk UTUC, the standard treatment approach involves radical nephroureterectomy (RNU). Extensive investigation has been undertaken to explore the role of perioperative bladder instillation in RNU, considering both the optimal timing and frequency of instillations. This section aims to delve into the specific aspects of bladder instillation during the perioperative period of RNU, with particular emphasis on addressing these crucial questions.

5.1. Immediate Postoperative Single Instillation

Immediate single instillation involves administering intravesical chemotherapy directly after surgical procedures, typically within 24–48 h or even sooner [38]. Due to the multifocality and potential dissemination of tumors, residual tumor cells may still exist in the bladder after RNU surgery [9,39]. Immediate single instillation is a focused approach that specifically targets and addresses residual disease and disseminated tumor cells within the bladder, minimizing the opportunity for tumor growth [40].

It has been found in non-muscle-invasive bladder cancer that immediate single instillation following transurethral resection of bladder tumors (TURBT) helps to reduce recurrence [41]. This strategy takes advantage of the active state of tumor cells during the early postoperative period, optimizing the effectiveness of treatment [42].

Among all the studies on immediate postoperative single-dose bladder instillation, the prospective, randomized, phase II study conducted by Ito et al. holds significant representative value. Their findings demonstrated that administering a single dose of intravesical pirarubicin (THP) within 48 h after surgery significantly reduced bladder recurrence rates in UTUC patients [31]. Pirarubicin is an anthracycline anticancer drug commonly used in the treatment of various cancers. In this systematic review, two multicenter randomized clinical trials (RCT) were included. The evidence suggested that single-dose intravesical chemotherapy for UTUC patients who had undergone RNU may significantly lower the risk of bladder cancer recurrence compared to no instillation, as indicated by a hazard ratio of 0.51 (95% CI: 0.32 to 0.82, low-certainty evidence) [22]. Another meta-analysis [43], involving 532 patients from three multicenter randomized controlled trials and one large retrospective study, showed a significant reduction in bladder recurrence with an overall hazard ratio of 0.54 (95% CI: 0.38–0.76) for patients receiving intravesical instillation.

These results support the use of intravesical therapy as an effective approach to prevent bladder recurrence after RNU. Now, both EAU and AUA guidelines strongly recommend delivering postoperative bladder instillation to reduce the rate of bladder recurrence.

5.2. Delayed Postoperative Single Instillation

Delayed single instillation involves administering intravesical chemotherapy at a later time point after surgery, usually within one or two weeks. The delayed approach allows for proper healing of the surgical site and potentially reduces the risk of complications associated with immediate instillation, such as extravasation, the risk of which mainly depends on the suture of the bladder wall [31]. In the event of drug extravasation, it not only increases patient discomfort but also poses an increased risk of implantation [44].

In 2001, an RCT was launched to investigate the efficacy of prophylactic intravesical therapy (1 to 2 weeks after RNU) of MMC and cytosine arabinoside (Ara-C) on bladder recurrence of UTUC. In the bladder instillation group, the bladder recurrence rate was slightly lower compared to the non-instillation group, indicating a trend but not statistical significance. It should be noted that this study is relatively early, and the drug regimen and dosage are still being explored. Additionally, the sample size was small (instillation group n = 13 vs. non-instillation group n = 12), limiting the generalizability of the findings [32].

The ODMIT-C trial, which spanned six years and recruited 284 patients, demonstrated that administering intravesical mitomycin C (MMC) instillation at least one week after surgery significantly reduced the risk of bladder recurrence within one year while maintaining a low risk of complications [33]. However, Goel et al. pointed out that delaying MMC instillation for at least one week after surgery may have an impact on treatment efficacy [45].

Based on the currently available clinical evidence, the advantages of delayed instillation compared to immediate instillation are not clearly demonstrated. Furthermore, the optimal timing for delayed instillation is still under investigation and may vary depending on factors such as the specific chemotherapy agent used and individual patient characteristics.

5.3. Multiple Bladder Instillations

The optimal instillation regimen, whether single or multiple doses, remains a focus of investigation in the field of intravesical instillation.

In 2010, Wu et al. published a retrospective study regarding 196 UTUC patients receiving 20 mg epirubicin or 10 mg MMC six to eight times for intravesical instillation after RNU, respectively. In comparison to patients who do not undergo bladder instillation, those receiving either epirubicin or MMC exhibit reduced rates of bladder recurrence, prolonged time to bladder recurrence, and enhanced recurrence-free survival rates [22]. However, since this study did not compare single instillation with multiple instillations, no conclusion can be drawn regarding the superior efficacy of either approach.

Harraz initiated an RCT with the primary objective of comparing the effects of one-year maintenance intravesical chemotherapy (MIC) to a single intravesical instillation (SIC) in terms of reducing bladder recurrence following RNU for UTUC patients. Both groups received epirubicin 50 mg. In the MIC group, the treatment regimen involved weekly instillations for 6 weeks followed by monthly instillations for 1 year. The rates of bladder recurrence-free survival at 3, 6, and 12 months were similar between the two groups, indicating that multiple instillations of intravesical chemotherapy did not lead to a significant reduction in bladder recurrence rates [34].

For patients with in situ (CIS) bladder tumors, intravesical BCG instillation after TURBT is considered the standard treatment [46]. UTUC patients with IVR after RNU exhibited a worse prognosis compared to the primary NMIBC group, especially regarding the occurrence of secondary IVR. The results emphasize the complexities involved in managing recurrent bladder tumors in patients who have undergone RNU for UTUC [44].

Undoubtedly, multiple bladder instillations pose a greater burden to patients and exacerbate side effects. Hence, unless multiple bladder instillations exhibit compelling benefits, their widespread adoption may be challenging. As for the unsatisfying aforementioned results, current guidelines do not provide explicit recommendations for administering multiple bladder instillations in patients after RNU.

5.4. Bladder Instillations and Neoadjuvant Chemotherapy

Neoadjuvant chemotherapy (NAC) has become a cornerstone in managing UTUC, offering significant improvements in overall survival (OS) and progression-free survival (PFS) [47–50]. Given before surgery, NAC aims to shrink tumors and clear potential micrometastases, enhancing surgical success [51]. Recent research underscores NAC's value, highlighting its role in reducing intravesical recurrence after nephroureterectomy for UTUC, especially in advanced cases [52].

Alongside NAC, bladder instillation acts as another adjuvant treatment, specifically targeting post-surgical bladder recurrence. While their methods differ, both therapies share a goal: improving patient outcomes and reducing disease return. NAC, given preoperatively in RNU for UTUC, exerts systemic therapeutic effects that may limit the dissemination of tumor cells. On the other hand, bladder instillation is usually applied intraoperatively or postoperatively, delivering therapeutic agents directly to the bladder, aiming to eradicate any residual tumor cells and prevent recurrence. Given the distinct administration timelines of NAC (preoperatively) and bladder instillation (intra- or postoperatively), there is minimal overlap in their therapeutic windows, ensuring that one does not impede the other's efficacy. This temporal separation also offers a strategic advantage, potentially providing a prolonged period of therapeutic intervention against tumor cells. However, the combined strategy's true potential remains to be fully elucidated. Future research should focus on determining the optimal sequencing of these treatments, their combined safety profile, and their overall impact on patient outcomes in UTUC. Such studies will be instrumental in refining treatment protocols and maximizing therapeutic benefits for UTUC patients.

6. Intravesical Therapy following Kidney-Sparing Management

Kidney-sparing surgery (KSS) is a valuable approach for managing UTUC and preserving renal function. Approaches considered for KSS were segmental ureterectomy (SU), ureteroscopy (URS), percutaneous management (PC), and chemo-ablation [53–55]. Different from intravesical instillation, which involves injecting chemotherapeutic agents into the bladder to prevent tumor recurrence, chemo-ablation in UTUC is a kidney-sparing technique where the chemotherapeutic agents are directly applied to the tumor site in the upper urinary tract, aiming to destroy tumor cells. The selection of the most appropriate approach depends on factors such as tumor characteristics, location, and patient-specific considerations and should be made in consultation with a multidisciplinary team of urologists and oncologists.

A systematic review and meta-analysis found no differences in oncological outcomes among different drug administration methods for UTUC or CIS of the upper urinary tract treated with KSS and adjuvant endocavitary treatment [56]. However, the efficacy of these interventions in localized low-risk UTUC had only been validated in a small-scale population for localized low-risk UTUC, as the recurrence rates following adjuvant instillations were similar to those observed in untreated patients [57]. Therefore, European Association of Urology (EAU) guidelines do not recommend postoperative bladder instillation for low-risk UTUC. According to AUA guidelines, clinicians may consider adjuvant pelvicalyceal chemotherapy and intravesical chemotherapy following UTUC ablation if no bladder or UT perforation is observed to reduce the risk of implantation metastasis (Expert Opinion) [58].

KSS can be considered for high-risk patients with imperative indications such as a solitary kidney, bilateral UTUC, chronic kidney disease, or those who are medically ineligible or unwilling to undergo RNU. However, KSS for high-risk patients may carry a higher risk of progression and reduced OS [54]. In such cases, postoperative prophylactic medication instillation is vital, and a single dose of intravesical chemotherapy is recommended to prevent recurrence [59].

Therefore, for high-risk UTUC patients who have undergone KSS and face a heightened risk of postoperative intravesical recurrence, prophylactic intravesical therapy may be considered an urgent treatment option.

7. Intravesical Therapy Following Ureteroscopy-Guided Biopsy

Performing pre-RNU URS biopsy aids in accurate UTUC staging and classification. This preoperative evaluation helps in surgical planning, guiding the choice between KSS and RNU [60,61]. Additionally, it serves as an effective means of screening and monitoring high-risk individuals, further emphasizing its significance in managing this patient population [62]. However, it is important to note that recent evidence suggests that URS prior to RNU has been associated with a higher risk of IVR [63].

In the first meta-analysis investigating preoperative URS prior to RNU (16 studies, n = 5489), patients who underwent URS had a significantly higher rate of bladder recurrence post-RNU compared to those without URS. However, long-term survival outcomes were comparable between the groups [64]. The findings of other meta-analyses were consistent with the aforementioned results [65,66]. Sharma et al. provided additional evidence supporting the association between preoperative URS with biopsy and increased risk of IVR after RNU, while percutaneous biopsy showed no such association [63].

These findings, along with other related studies, highlighted the need for careful consideration and close monitoring of patients who undergo URS before RNU, as it has emerged as a risk factor for postoperative IVR [67–69]. The increased risk of tumor dissemination during the URS procedure may account for the higher rate of bladder recurrence observed. However, URS plays a valuable role in providing accurate staging and histological diagnosis, aiding in the formulation of surgical strategies [70–72]. Performing preoperative URS before RNU while effectively controlling IVR incidence remains a challenge. Therefore, considering the previous discussion, postoperative bladder instillation appears to be highly effective in targeting disseminated tumor cells. The follow-up is crucial for patients who undergo both URS and RNU consecutively, as it plays a vital role in promptly diagnosing and guiding treatment for any recurrence. Timely treatment following detection is key to improving the prognosis.

Regrettably, at present, there is a lack of consensus regarding the optimal management strategy for URS prior to RNU, and a definitive standard recommendation is yet to be established. The discussion on the necessity of immediate instillation after URS has become increasingly heated, highlighting the importance of a high-quality clinical study specifically investigating the use of immediate instillation following URS procedures. There is an ongoing clinical trial (NCT05810623), but recruitment has not yet commenced.

In addition to ureteroscopy, any diagnostic interventions focused on the upper urinary tract hold the potential to elevate the incidence of post-RNU IVR. Notably, procedures such as ureteral catheterization could contribute to an increased likelihood of IVR occurrences following RNU [73].

8. Limitations

This comprehensive review of intravesical therapy for UTUC has certain inherent limitations that should be acknowledged. The scope of our coverage, although extensive, may not encompass all facets of intravesical therapy. This limitation is attributable to the specificity of our search keywords and criteria. We acknowledge that certain therapies from other medical domains, repurposed for UTUC treatment, might have been overlooked. Additionally, some outdated therapies that lack clinical relevance or translational potential may not be featured in this review. It is essential to recognize that even in a comprehensive review, the ever-evolving landscape of medical research can introduce new developments, making it challenging to capture every relevant aspect comprehensively. Moreover, our primary focus on clinical aspects, such as efficacy, safety, and guideline adherence, has limited the examination of crucial factors like patient preferences and economic considerations, which can significantly impact treatment decisions but are not comprehensively addressed herein. Furthermore, the interrelatedness of various components of intravesical therapy, including tumor grade and follow-up protocols, could not be exhaustively discussed due to space constraints and the need for focused analysis. Lastly, as with any review, the potential for publication bias exists, where studies with significant or positive outcomes are more likely to be published. Despite our efforts to mitigate this bias through stringent search and inclusion criteria, it is important to acknowledge this inherent limitation. As observed in the provided data, many clinical trials remain incomplete or do not publish their clinical data. Consequently, our review is limited to focusing on reported clinical trials. This inherent limitation may introduce a potential bias, as unreported or incomplete trials may yield different results. Therefore, readers should interpret our findings with an awareness of these limitations and remain vigilant for updates and emerging research in this continually evolving field.

9. Future Directions

Compared to the current advancements in NMIBC intravesical therapy, the field of intravesical therapy for UTUC still holds vast potential for exploration and research. It is anticipated that there will be an increased focus on optimizing the dosage, dwell time, treatment duration, and drug selection for UTUC intravesical therapy. Each component will surely be supported by a wealth of high-quality clinical evidence. Further exploration into the mechanisms (especially by identifying suitable biomarkers) might guide us in selecting the most appropriate drug regimens for UTUC patients [74,75].

The future research directions for intravesical therapy primarily focus on (1) novel instillation agents (NCT03617003 and NCT02793128) or repurposing systemic and local therapy drugs for intravesical therapy after RNU (NCT04398368 and NCT01606345); (2) combination approaches with other systemic treatments (NCT03504163); (3) standard instillation protocols following ureteroscopy with biopsy prior to RNU (NCT05810623 and NCT05731622); and so on.

Based on the current advancements, UGN-101 (MitoGel™) has shown promising results as an endocavitary administered gel-based formulation containing MMC, providing targeted treatment for urothelial carcinoma [76,77]. The OLYMPUS trial demonstrated its efficacy in treating low-grade upper tract urothelial carcinoma, with notable complete response rates and durability of response [78,79]. Moreover, UGN-101 holds the potential as a kidney-sparing treatment option for high-grade UTUC patients [80–82]. The efficacy of UGN-101 in treating UTUC through kidney-sparing surgery hints at its potential for future prophylactic applications against the recurrence of UTUC. An initial study aimed at its role in recurrent UTUC of the renal pelvis and ureter (NCT04006691) was withdrawn due to insufficient participant enrollment. However, just as with the original intent of this study, further research was warranted to explore its role in preventing recurrence in different parts of the urinary tract, especially intravesical recurrence.

10. Conclusions

In the treatment of UTUC, intravesical therapy has emerged as an important therapeutic approach, demonstrating significant progress and research outcomes. By delivering medications directly into the bladder, it reduces the risk of IVR and improves patient survival rates. Various drugs and treatment regimens have been utilized for intravesical instillation. Additionally, there is ongoing research exploring novel agents and combination therapies. However, the current clinical evidence is still relatively limited, necessitating further studies to assess and refine the efficacy and safety of intravesical therapy.

Bladder instillation for UTUC should not be viewed in isolation but rather as part of a comprehensive approach that integrates diagnosis, surgical treatment, adjuvant therapy, and follow-up. It is crucial to thoroughly study the role of intravesical therapy in specific clinical contexts. This includes the use of intraoperative bladder instillation and irrigation, which involves the administration of therapeutic agents directly into the bladder during surgery to minimize the risk of recurrence. Another significant scenario is the intravesical therapy following radical nephroureterectomy, where both single-dose and multiple-dose regimens are employed post-surgery to reduce the chances of tumor recurrence and provide sustained therapeutic effects. Furthermore, in situations where kidney preservation is prioritized, intravesical therapy post kidney-sparing procedures becomes instrumental in both managing the existing condition and thwarting the disease's progression. It is also noteworthy that URS elevates the risk of IVR, underscoring the heightened significance of intravesical therapy in such contexts. By examining these specific scenarios, we can assess the overall impact of intravesical therapy and work towards the development of new comprehensive treatment strategies.

Author Contributions: Conceptualization, Z.W. (Zhenjie Wu) and L.W.; data collection, Z.W. (Zheng Wang), D.X., J.S. and W.J.; writing—original draft preparation, Z.W. (Zheng Wang) and H.S.; writing—reviewing and editing, Y.X., Y.F., Z.W. (Zhenjie Wu) and L.W. All authors have read and agreed to the published version of the manuscript.

Funding: This work was supported by the National Natural Science Foundation of China (82072825 and 81874093 to Zhenjie Wu; 81730073 and 81872074 to Linhui Wang), a grant from the Program of Shanghai Municipal Health Bureau (Hospital New Star Program of Shanghai, YYXX to Zhenjie Wu), the Shuguang Program of Shanghai Education Development Foundation and Shanghai Municipal Education Commission (22SG35 to Zhenjie Wu), and the Excellent Ph. D. Talents Program of Changhai Hospital (to Zhenjie Wu).

Institutional Review Board Statement: This article is a review and did not require ethical approval.

Informed Consent Statement: Not applicable, as this review article did not involve new studies of human or animal subjects performed by any of the authors.

Data Availability Statement: The data supporting this review are from previously reported studies and datasets, which have been cited.

Conflicts of Interest: The authors declare no conflict of interest.

References

1. Siegel, R.L.; Miller, K.D.; Fuchs, H.E.; Jemal, A. Cancer Statistics, 2021. *CA Cancer J. Clin.* **2021**, *71*, 7–33. [CrossRef] [PubMed]
2. Almas, B.; Halvorsen, O.J.; Johannesen, T.B.; Beisland, C. Higher than expected and significantly increasing incidence of upper tract urothelial carcinoma. A population based study. *World J. Urol.* **2021**, *39*, 3385–3391. [CrossRef] [PubMed]
3. Soria, F.; Shariat, S.F.; Lerner, S.P.; Fritsche, H.M.; Rink, M.; Kassouf, W.; Spiess, P.E.; Lotan, Y.; Ye, D.; Fernandez, M.I.; et al. Epidemiology, diagnosis, preoperative evaluation and prognostic assessment of upper-tract urothelial carcinoma (UTUC). *World J. Urol.* **2017**, *35*, 379–387. [CrossRef]
4. Kates, M.; Badalato, G.M.; Gupta, M.; McKiernan, J.M. Secondary bladder cancer after upper tract urothelial carcinoma in the US population. *BJU Int.* **2012**, *110*, 1325–1329. [CrossRef] [PubMed]
5. Sato, G.; Yoshida, T.; Yanishi, M.; Saito, R.; Murota, T.; Kawa, G.; Kinoshita, H.; Matsuda, T. Preoperative Pyuria Predicts for Intravesical Recurrence in Patients with Urothelial Carcinoma of the Upper Urinary Tract After Radical Nephroureterectomy Without a History of Bladder Cancer. *Clin. Genitourin. Cancer* **2020**, *18*, e167–e173. [CrossRef]
6. Seisen, T.; Granger, B.; Colin, P.; Leon, P.; Utard, G.; Renard-Penna, R.; Comperat, E.; Mozer, P.; Cussenot, O.; Shariat, S.F.; et al. A Systematic Review and Meta-analysis of Clinicopathologic Factors Linked to Intravesical Recurrence After Radical Nephroureterectomy to Treat Upper Tract Urothelial Carcinoma. *Eur. Urol.* **2015**, *67*, 1122–1133. [CrossRef] [PubMed]
7. Xylinas, E.; Rink, M.; Margulis, V.; Karakiewicz, P.; Novara, G.; Shariat, S.F.; Upper Tract Urothelial Carcinoma, C. Multifocal carcinoma in situ of the upper tract is associated with high risk of bladder cancer recurrence. *Eur. Urol.* **2012**, *61*, 1069–1070. [CrossRef]
8. Habuchi, T.; Takahashi, R.; Yamada, H.; Kakehi, Y.; Sugiyama, T.; Yoshida, O. Metachronous multifocal development of urothelial cancers by intraluminal seeding. *Lancet* **1993**, *342*, 1087–1088. [CrossRef]
9. Hafner, C.; Knuechel, R.; Stoehr, R.; Hartmann, A. Clonality of multifocal urothelial carcinomas: 10 years of molecular genetic studies. *Int. J. Cancer* **2002**, *101*, 1–6. [CrossRef]
10. Harris, A.L.; Neal, D.E. Bladder cancer—Field versus clonal origin. *N. Engl. J. Med.* **1992**, *326*, 759–761. [CrossRef]
11. Jones, T.D.; Wang, M.; Eble, J.N.; MacLennan, G.T.; Lopez-Beltran, A.; Zhang, S.; Cocco, A.; Cheng, L. Molecular evidence supporting field effect in urothelial carcinogenesis. *Clin. Cancer Res.* **2005**, *11*, 6512–6519. [CrossRef] [PubMed]
12. Zeng, S.; Ying, Y.; Yu, X.; Wang, L.; Zhang, Z.; Xu, C. Impact of previous, simultaneous or intravesical recurrence bladder cancer on prognosis of upper tract urothelial carcinoma after nephroureterectomy: A large population-based study. *Transl. Androl. Urol.* **2021**, *10*, 4365–4375. [CrossRef]
13. Azawi, N.H.; Naeraa, S.H.; Subhi, Y.; Vasquez, J.L.; Norus, T.; Dahl, C.; Thind, P.; Jensen, J.B. Oncological outcomes of radical nephroureterectomy for upper urinary tract urothelial neoplasia in Denmark. *Scand. J. Urol.* **2020**, *54*, 58–64. [CrossRef]
14. Krogh, J.; Kvist, E.; Rye, B. Transitional cell carcinoma of the upper urinary tract: Prognostic variables and post-operative recurrences. *Br. J. Urol.* **1991**, *67*, 32–36. [CrossRef] [PubMed]
15. Sakamoto, N.; Naito, S.; Kotoh, S.; Nakashima, M.; Nakamura, M.; Ueda, T.; Kumazawa, J. Recurrence of bladder tumors following surgery for transitional cell carcinoma of the upper urinary tract. *Eur. Urol.* **1991**, *20*, 136–139. [CrossRef]
16. Takaoka, E.; Hinotsu, S.; Joraku, A.; Oikawa, T.; Sekido, N.; Miyanaga, N.; Kawai, K.; Shimazui, T.; Akaza, H. Pattern of intravesical recurrence after surgical treatment for urothelial cancer of the upper urinary tract: A single institutional retrospective long-term follow-up study. *Int. J. Urol.* **2010**, *17*, 623–628. [CrossRef] [PubMed]

17. Yamashita, S.; Ito, A.; Mitsuzuka, K.; Tochigi, T.; Namima, T.; Soma, F.; Aizawa, M.; Ioritani, N.; Kaiho, Y.; Arai, Y. Clinical implications of intravesical recurrence after radical nephroureterectomy for upper urinary tract urothelial carcinoma. *Int. J. Urol.* **2016**, *23*, 378–384. [CrossRef]
18. Jain, R.K.; Ross, J.S.; Necchi, A.; Spiess, P.E. Should Upper-tract Urothelial Carcinoma and Bladder Carcinoma Be Treated the Same or Different? *Eur. Urol. Oncol.* **2021**, *4*, 180–181. [CrossRef]
19. Kobayashi, T. Understanding the biology of urothelial cancer metastasis. *Asian J. Urol.* **2016**, *3*, 211–222. [CrossRef]
20. Miyake, M.; Tatsumi, Y.; Matsumoto, H.; Nagao, K.; Matsuyama, H.; Inamoto, T.; Azuma, H.; Yasumoto, H.; Shiina, H.; Fujimoto, K.; et al. Outcomes of subsequent non-muscle-invasive bladder cancer treated with intravesical Bacillus Calmette-Guerin after radical nephroureterectomy for upper urinary tract urothelial carcinoma. *BJU Int.* **2018**, *121*, 764–773. [CrossRef]
21. Sfakianos, J.P.; Gul, Z.; Shariat, S.F.; Matin, S.F.; Daneshmand, S.; Plimack, E.; Lerner, S.; Roupret, M.; Pal, S. Genetic Differences Between Bladder and Upper Urinary Tract Carcinoma: Implications for Therapy. *Eur. Urol. Oncol.* **2021**, *4*, 170–179. [CrossRef] [PubMed]
22. Hwang, E.C.; Sathianathen, N.J.; Jung, J.H.; Kim, M.H.; Dahm, P.; Risk, M.C. Single-dose intravesical chemotherapy after nephroureterectomy for upper tract urothelial carcinoma. *Cochrane Database Syst. Rev.* **2019**, *5*, CD013160. [CrossRef] [PubMed]
23. Margulis, V.; Shariat, S.F.; Matin, S.F.; Kamat, A.M.; Zigeuner, R.; Kikuchi, E.; Lotan, Y.; Weizer, A.; Raman, J.D.; Wood, C.G.; et al. Outcomes of radical nephroureterectomy: A series from the Upper Tract Urothelial Carcinoma Collaboration. *Cancer* **2009**, *115*, 1224–1233. [CrossRef]
24. Ni, S.; Tao, W.; Chen, Q.; Liu, L.; Jiang, H.; Hu, H.; Han, R.; Wang, C. Laparoscopic versus open nephroureterectomy for the treatment of upper urinary tract urothelial carcinoma: A systematic review and cumulative analysis of comparative studies. *Eur. Urol.* **2012**, *61*, 1142–1153. [CrossRef] [PubMed]
25. Phe, V.; Cussenot, O.; Bitker, M.O.; Roupret, M. Does the surgical technique for management of the distal ureter influence the outcome after nephroureterectomy? *BJU Int.* **2011**, *108*, 130–138. [CrossRef] [PubMed]
26. Roupret, M.; Seisen, T.; Birtle, A.J.; Capoun, O.; Comperat, E.M.; Dominguez-Escrig, J.L.; Gurses Andersson, I.; Liedberg, F.; Mariappan, P.; Hugh Mostafid, A.; et al. European Association of Urology Guidelines on Upper Urinary Tract Urothelial Carcinoma: 2023 Update. *Eur. Urol.* **2023**, *84*, 49–64. [CrossRef] [PubMed]
27. Xylinas, E.; Rink, M.; Cha, E.K.; Clozel, T.; Lee, R.K.; Fajkovic, H.; Comploj, E.; Novara, G.; Margulis, V.; Raman, J.D.; et al. Impact of distal ureter management on oncologic outcomes following radical nephroureterectomy for upper tract urothelial carcinoma. *Eur. Urol.* **2014**, *65*, 210–217. [CrossRef]
28. Nadler, N.; Oedorf, K.; Jensen, J.B.; Azawi, N. Intraoperative Mitomycin C Bladder Instillation During Radical Nephroureterectomy Is Feasible and Safe. *Eur. Urol. Open Sci.* **2021**, *34*, 41–46. [CrossRef]
29. Freifeld, Y.; Ghandour, R.; Singla, N.; Woldu, S.; Bagrodia, A.; Lotan, Y.; Rapoport, L.M.; Gazimiev, M.; Delafuente, K.; Kulangara, R.; et al. Intraoperative prophylactic intravesical chemotherapy to reduce bladder recurrence following radical nephroureterectomy. *Urol. Oncol.* **2020**, *38*, 737.e11–737.e16. [CrossRef]
30. Yamamoto, S.; Sakamoto, S.; Imamura, Y.; Sazuka, T.; Nakamura, K.; Inoue, T.; Chiba, K.; Miyazaki, K.; Inoue, A.; Nagata, M.; et al. Intravesical irrigation might prevent bladder recurrence in patients undergoing radical nephroureterectomy for upper urinary tract urothelial carcinoma. *Int. J. Urol.* **2019**, *26*, 791–796. [CrossRef]
31. Ito, A.; Shintaku, I.; Satoh, M.; Ioritani, N.; Aizawa, M.; Tochigi, T.; Kawamura, S.; Aoki, H.; Numata, I.; Takeda, A.; et al. Prospective randomized phase II trial of a single early intravesical instillation of pirarubicin (THP) in the prevention of bladder recurrence after nephroureterectomy for upper urinary tract urothelial carcinoma: The THP Monotherapy Study Group Trial. *J. Clin. Oncol.* **2013**, *31*, 1422–1427. [CrossRef] [PubMed]
32. Sakamoto, N.; Naito, S.; Kumazawa, J.; Ariyoshi, A.; Osada, Y.; Omoto, T.; Fujisawa, Y.; Morita, I.; Yamashita, H.; Kyushu University Urological Oncology, G. Prophylactic intravesical instillation of mitomycin C and cytosine arabinoside for prevention of recurrent bladder tumors following surgery for upper urinary tract tumors: A prospective randomized study. *Int. J. Urol.* **2001**, *8*, 212–216. [CrossRef] [PubMed]
33. O'Brien, T.; Ray, E.; Singh, R.; Coker, B.; Beard, R.; British Association of Urological Surgeons Section of Oncology. Prevention of bladder tumours after nephroureterectomy for primary upper urinary tract urothelial carcinoma: A prospective, multicentre, randomised clinical trial of a single postoperative intravesical dose of mitomycin C (the ODMIT-C Trial). *Eur. Urol.* **2011**, *60*, 703–710. [CrossRef] [PubMed]
34. Harraz, A.M.; El-Shabrawy, M.; El-Nahas, A.R.; El-Kappany, H.; Osman, Y. Single Versus Maintenance Intravesical Chemotherapy for the Prevention of Bladder Recurrence after Radical Nephroureterectomy for Upper Tract Urothelial Carcinoma: A Randomized Clinical Trial. *Clin. Genitourin. Cancer* **2019**, *17*, e1108–e1115. [CrossRef] [PubMed]
35. Tomasz, M.; Palom, Y. The mitomycin bioreductive antitumor agents: Cross-linking and alkylation of DNA as the molecular basis of their activity. *Pharmacol. Ther.* **1997**, *76*, 73–87. [CrossRef]
36. Noennig, B.; Bozorgmehri, S.; Terry, R.; Otto, B.; Su, L.M.; Crispen, P.L. Evaluation of Intraoperative Versus Postoperative Adjuvant Mitomycin C with Nephroureterectomy for Urothelial Carcinoma of the Upper Urinary Tract. *Bladder Cancer* **2018**, *4*, 389–394. [CrossRef]
37. Yates, D.R.; Catto, J.W. Distinct patterns and behaviour of urothelial carcinoma with respect to anatomical location: How molecular biomarkers can augment clinico-pathological predictors in upper urinary tract tumours. *World J. Urol.* **2013**, *31*, 21–29. [CrossRef]

38. Oosterlinck, W.; Kurth, K.H.; Schroder, F.; Bultinck, J.; Hammond, B.; Sylvester, R. A prospective European Organization for Research and Treatment of Cancer Genitourinary Group randomized trial comparing transurethral resection followed by a single intravesical instillation of epirubicin or water in single stage Ta, T1 papillary carcinoma of the bladder. *J. Urol.* **1993**, *149*, 749–752 [CrossRef]
39. Catto, J.W.; Hartmann, A.; Stoehr, R.; Bolderson, E.; Rehman, I.; Rosario, D.J.; Hamdy, F.C.; Meuth, M. Multifocal urothelial cancers with the mutator phenotype are of monoclonal origin and require panurothelial treatment for tumor clearance. *J. Urol.* **2006**, *175*, 2323–2330. [CrossRef]
40. Sylvester, R.J.; Oosterlinck, W.; Holmang, S.; Sydes, M.R.; Birtle, A.; Gudjonsson, S.; De Nunzio, C.; Okamura, K.; Kaasinen, E.; Solsona, E.; et al. Systematic Review and Individual Patient Data Meta-analysis of Randomized Trials Comparing a Single Immediate Instillation of Chemotherapy After Transurethral Resection with Transurethral Resection Alone in Patients with Stage pTa-pT1 Urothelial Carcinoma of the Bladder: Which Patients Benefit from the Instillation? *Eur. Urol.* **2016**, *69*, 231–244. [CrossRef]
41. Sylvester, R.J.; Oosterlinck, W.; van der Meijden, A.P. A single immediate postoperative instillation of chemotherapy decreases the risk of recurrence in patients with stage Ta T1 bladder cancer: A meta-analysis of published results of randomized clinical trials. *J. Urol.* **2004**, *171*, 2186–2190, quiz 2435. [CrossRef] [PubMed]
42. Hnotsu, S.; Akaza, H.; Ohashi, Y.; Kotake, T. Intravesical chemotherapy for maximum prophylaxis of new early phase superficial bladder carcinoma treated by transurethral resection: A combined analysis of trials by the Japanese Urological Cancer Research Group using smoothed hazard function. *Cancer* **1999**, *86*, 1818–1826. [CrossRef]
43. Yoo, S.H.; Jeong, C.W.; Kwak, C.; Kim, H.H.; Choo, M.S.; Ku, J.H. Intravesical Chemotherapy after Radical Nephroureterectomy for Primary Upper Tract Urothelial Carcinoma: A Systematic Review and Network Meta-Analysis. *J. Clin. Med.* **2019**, *8*, 1059. [CrossRef] [PubMed]
44. Bosschieter, J.; Nieuwenhuijzen, J.A.; van Ginkel, T.; Vis, A.N.; Witte, B.; Newling, D.; Beckers, G.M.A.; van Moorselaar, R.J.A. Value of an Immediate Intravesical Instillation of Mitomycin C in Patients with Non-muscle-invasive Bladder Cancer: A Prospective Multicentre Randomised Study in 2243 patients. *Eur. Urol.* **2018**, *73*, 226–232. [CrossRef]
45. Goel, A.; Paul, S. Re: Tim O'Brien, Eleanor Ray, Rajinder Singh, Bola Coker, Ralph Beard, British Association of Urological Surgeons Section of Oncology. Prevention of bladder tumours after nephroureterectomy for primary upper urinary tract urothelial carcinoma: A prospective, multicentre, randomised clinical trial of a single postoperative intravesical dose of mitomycin C (the ODMIT-C Trial). Eur Urol 2011;60:703-10. *Eur Urol* **2012**, *61*, e14. [CrossRef]
46. Babjuk, M.; Burger, M.; Capoun, O.; Cohen, D.; Comperat, E.M.; Dominguez Escrig, J.L.; Gontero, P.; Liedberg, F.; Masson-Lecomte, A.; Mostafid, A.H.; et al. European Association of Urology Guidelines on Non-muscle-invasive Bladder Cancer (Ta, T1, and Carcinoma in Situ). *Eur. Urol.* **2022**, *81*, 75–94. [CrossRef]
47. Martini, A.; Daza, J.; Poltiyelova, E.; Gul, Z.; Heard, J.R.; Ferket, B.S.; Waingankar, N.; Galsky, M.D.; Sfakianos, J.P. Pathological downstaging as a novel endpoint for the development of neoadjuvant chemotherapy for upper tract urothelial carcinoma. *BJU Int.* **2019**, *124*, 665–671. [CrossRef]
48. Porten, S.; Siefker-Radtke, A.O.; Xiao, L.; Margulis, V.; Kamat, A.M.; Wood, C.G.; Jonasch, E.; Dinney, C.P.; Matin, S.F. Neoadjuvant chemotherapy improves survival of patients with upper tract urothelial carcinoma. *Cancer* **2014**, *120*, 1794–1799. [CrossRef]
49. Hosogoe, S.; Hatakeyama, S.; Kusaka, A.; Hamano, I.; Iwamura, H.; Fujita, N.; Yamamoto, H.; Tobisawa, Y.; Yoneyama, T.; Yoneyama, T.; et al. Platinum-based Neoadjuvant Chemotherapy Improves Oncological Outcomes in Patients with Locally Advanced Upper Tract Urothelial Carcinoma. *Eur. Urol. Focus.* **2018**, *4*, 946–953. [CrossRef]
50. Meng, X.; Chao, B.; Vijay, V.; Silver, H.; Margolin, E.J.; Balar, A.; Taneja, S.S.; Shah, O.; Bjurlin, M.A.; Anderson, C.B.; et al. High Response Rates to Neoadjuvant Chemotherapy in High-Grade Upper Tract Urothelial Carcinoma. *Urology* **2019**, *129*, 146–152. [CrossRef]
51. Massari, F.; Santoni, M.; di Nunno, V.; Cheng, L.; Lopez-Beltran, A.; Cimadamore, A.; Gasparrini, S.; Scarpelli, M.; Battelli, N.; Montironi, R. Adjuvant and neoadjuvant approaches for urothelial cancer: Updated indications and controversies. *Cancer Treat. Rev.* **2018**, *68*, 80–85. [CrossRef] [PubMed]
52. Yamaguchi, N.; Morizane, S.; Yumioka, T.; Shimizu, R.; Teraoka, S.; Iwamoto, H.; Hikita, K.; Honda, M.; Takenaka, A. Effect of Adjuvant Systemic Chemotherapy on Intravesical Recurrence After Radical Nephroureterectomy for Upper Urinary Tract Urothelial Carcinoma. *Anticancer Res.* **2023**, *43*, 1725–1730. [CrossRef] [PubMed]
53. Strijbos, W.E.; van der Heij, B. Percutaneous resection of upper tract urothelial cell carcinoma: When, how, and is it safe? *Asian J. Urol.* **2016**, *3*, 134–141. [CrossRef]
54. Seisen, T.; Peyronnet, B.; Dominguez-Escrig, J.L.; Bruins, H.M.; Yuan, C.Y.; Babjuk, M.; Bohle, A.; Burger, M.; Comperat, E.M.; Cowan, N.C.; et al. Oncologic Outcomes of Kidney-sparing Surgery Versus Radical Nephroureterectomy for Upper Tract Urothelial Carcinoma: A Systematic Review by the EAU Non-muscle Invasive Bladder Cancer Guidelines Panel. *Eur. Urol.* **2016**, *70*, 1052–1068. [CrossRef]
55. Cutress, M.L.; Stewart, G.D.; Zakikhani, P.; Phipps, S.; Thomas, B.G.; Tolley, D.A. Ureteroscopic and percutaneous management of upper tract urothelial carcinoma (UTUC): Systematic review. *BJU Int.* **2012**, *110*, 614–628. [CrossRef] [PubMed]
56. Foerster, B.; D'Andrea, D.; Abufaraj, M.; Broenimann, S.; Karakiewicz, P.I.; Roupret, M.; Gontero, P.; Lerner, S.P.; Shariat, S.F.; Soria, F. Endocavitary treatment for upper tract urothelial carcinoma: A meta-analysis of the current literature. *Urol. Oncol.* **2019**, *37*, 430–436. [CrossRef]

57. Bozzini, G.; Gastaldi, C.; Besana, U.; Calori, A.; Casellato, S.; Parma, P.; Pastore, A.; Macchi, A.; Breda, A.; Gozen, A.; et al. Thulium-laser retrograde intra renal ablation of upper urinary tract transitional cell carcinoma: An ESUT Study. *Minerva Urol. Nephrol.* **2021**, *73*, 114–121. [CrossRef]
58. Coleman, J.A.; Clark, P.E.; Bixler, B.R.; Buckley, D.I.; Chang, S.S.; Chou, R.; Hoffman-Censits, J.; Kulkarni, G.S.; Matin, S.F.; Pierorazio, P.M.; et al. Diagnosis and Management of Non-Metastatic Upper Tract Urothelial Carcinoma: AUA/SUO Guideline. *J. Urol.* **2023**, *209*, 1071–1081. [CrossRef]
59. Proietti, S.; Marchioni, M.; Eisner, B.H.; Luciano, R.; Saitta, G.; Rodriguez-Socarras, M.E.; D'Orta, C.; Bellinzoni, P.; Schips, L.; Gaboardi, F.; et al. Conservative treatment of upper urinary tract carcinoma in patients with imperative indications. *Minerva Urol. Nephrol.* **2021**, *73*, 245–252. [CrossRef]
60. Clements, T.; Messer, J.C.; Terrell, J.D.; Herman, M.P.; Ng, C.K.; Scherr, D.S.; Scoll, B.; Boorjian, S.A.; Uzzo, R.G.; Wille, M.; et al. High-grade ureteroscopic biopsy is associated with advanced pathology of upper-tract urothelial carcinoma tumors at definitive surgical resection. *J. Endourol.* **2012**, *26*, 398–402. [CrossRef]
61. Gravestock, P.; Cullum, D.; Somani, B.; Veeratterapillay, R. Diagnosing upper tract urothelial carcinoma: A review of the role of diagnostic ureteroscopy and novel developments over last two decades. *Asian J. Urol.* **2022**. [CrossRef]
62. Lonati, C.; Simeone, C.; Suardi, N.; Spiess, P.E.; Necchi, A.; Moschini, M. Genitourinary manifestations of Lynch syndrome in the urological practice. *Asian J. Urol.* **2022**, *9*, 443–450. [CrossRef] [PubMed]
63. Sharma, V.; Miest, T.S.; Juvet, T.S.; Toussi, A.; Packiam, V.; Chamie, K.; Matin, S.F.; Boorjian, S.A.; Thompson, R.H.; Frank, I.; et al. The Impact of Upper Tract Urothelial Carcinoma Diagnostic Modality on Intravesical Recurrence after Radical Nephroureterectomy: A Single Institution Series and Updated Meta-Analysis. *J. Urol.* **2021**, *206*, 558–567. [CrossRef]
64. Nowak, L.; Krajewski, W.; Chorbinska, J.; Kielb, P.; Sut, M.; Moschini, M.; Teoh, J.Y.; Mori, K.; Del Giudice, F.; Laukhtina, E.; et al. The Impact of Diagnostic Ureteroscopy Prior to Radical Nephroureterectomy on Oncological Outcomes in Patients with Upper Tract Urothelial Carcinoma: A Comprehensive Systematic Review and Meta-Analysis. *J. Clin. Med.* **2021**, *10*, 4197. [CrossRef] [PubMed]
65. Sankin, A.; Tin, A.L.; Mano, R.; Chevinsky, M.; Jakubowski, C.; Sfakianos, J.P.; Cha, E.K.; Yee, A.; Friedman, F.M.; Sjoberg, D.D.; et al. Impact of Ureteroscopy Before Nephroureterectomy for Upper Tract Urothelial Carcinoma on Oncologic Outcomes. *Urology* **2016**, *94*, 148–153. [CrossRef] [PubMed]
66. Guo, R.Q.; Hong, P.; Xiong, G.Y.; Zhang, L.; Fang, D.; Li, X.S.; Zhang, K.; Zhou, L.Q. Impact of ureteroscopy before radical nephroureterectomy for upper tract urothelial carcinomas on oncological outcomes: A meta-analysis. *BJU Int.* **2018**, *121*, 184–193. [CrossRef]
67. Marchioni, M.; Primiceri, G.; Cindolo, L.; Hampton, L.J.; Grob, M.B.; Guruli, G.; Schips, L.; Shariat, S.F.; Autorino, R. Impact of diagnostic ureteroscopy on intravesical recurrence in patients undergoing radical nephroureterectomy for upper tract urothelial cancer: A systematic review and meta-analysis. *BJU Int.* **2017**, *120*, 313–319. [CrossRef]
68. Luo, H.L.; Kang, C.H.; Chen, Y.T.; Chuang, Y.C.; Lee, W.C.; Cheng, Y.T.; Chiang, P.H. Diagnostic ureteroscopy independently correlates with intravesical recurrence after nephroureterectomy for upper urinary tract urothelial carcinoma. *Ann. Surg. Oncol.* **2013**, *20*, 3121–3126. [CrossRef]
69. Sung, H.H.; Jeon, H.G.; Han, D.H.; Jeong, B.C.; Seo, S.I.; Lee, H.M.; Choi, H.Y.; Jeon, S.S. Diagnostic Ureterorenoscopy Is Associated with Increased Intravesical Recurrence following Radical Nephroureterectomy in Upper Tract Urothelial Carcinoma. *PLoS ONE* **2015**, *10*, e0139976. [CrossRef]
70. Smith, A.K.; Stephenson, A.J.; Lane, B.R.; Larson, B.T.; Thomas, A.A.; Gong, M.C.; Jones, J.S.; Campbell, S.C.; Hansel, D.E. Inadequacy of biopsy for diagnosis of upper tract urothelial carcinoma: Implications for conservative management. *Urology* **2011**, *78*, 82–86. [CrossRef]
71. Rojas, C.P.; Castle, S.M.; Llanos, C.A.; Santos Cortes, J.A.; Bird, V.; Rodriguez, S.; Reis, I.M.; Zhao, W.; Gomez-Fernandez, C.; Leveillee, R.J.; et al. Low biopsy volume in ureteroscopy does not affect tumor biopsy grading in upper tract urothelial carcinoma. *Urol. Oncol.* **2013**, *31*, 1696–1700. [CrossRef] [PubMed]
72. Subiela, J.D.; Territo, A.; Mercade, A.; Balana, J.; Aumatell, J.; Calderon, J.; Gallioli, A.; Gonzalez-Padilla, D.A.; Gaya, J.M.; Palou, J.; et al. Diagnostic accuracy of ureteroscopic biopsy in predicting stage and grade at final pathology in upper tract urothelial carcinoma: Systematic review and meta-analysis. *Eur. J. Surg. Oncol.* **2020**, *46*, 1989–1997. [CrossRef] [PubMed]
73. Yonese, I.; Ito, M.; Waseda, Y.; Kobayashi, S.; Toide, M.; Takazawa, R.; Koga, F. Impact of diagnostic ureteral catheterization on intravesical tumour recurrence following radical nephroureterectomy for upper tract urothelial carcinoma. *World J. Urol.* **2023**, *41*, 1869–1875. [CrossRef] [PubMed]
74. Claps, F.; Mir, M.C.; Zargar, H. Molecular markers of systemic therapy response in urothelial carcinoma. *Asian J. Urol.* **2021**, *8*, 376–390. [CrossRef] [PubMed]
75. Wen, L.; Britton, C.J.; Garje, R.; Darbro, B.W.; Packiam, V.T. The emerging role of somatic tumor sequencing in the treatment of urothelial cancer. *Asian J. Urol.* **2021**, *8*, 391–399. [CrossRef]
76. Rosen, G.H.; Nallani, A.; Muzzey, C.; Murray, K.S. Antegrade Instillation of UGN-101 (Mitomycin for Pyelocalyceal Solution) for Low-Grade Upper Tract Urothelial Carcinoma: Initial Clinical Experience. *J. Urol.* **2022**, *207*, 1302–1311. [CrossRef]
77. Donin, N.M.; Duarte, S.; Lenis, A.T.; Caliliw, R.; Torres, C.; Smithson, A.; Strauss-Ayali, D.; Agmon-Gerstein, Y.; Malchi, N.; Said, J.; et al. Sustained-release Formulation of Mitomycin C to the Upper Urinary Tract Using a Thermosensitive Polymer: A Preclinical Study. *Urology* **2017**, *99*, 270–277. [CrossRef]

78. Kleinmann, N.; Matin, S.F.; Pierorazio, P.M.; Gore, J.L.; Shabsigh, A.; Hu, B.; Chamie, K.; Godoy, G.; Hubosky, S.; Rivera, M.; et al. Primary chemoablation of low-grade upper tract urothelial carcinoma using UGN-101, a mitomycin-containing reverse thermal gel (OLYMPUS): An open-label, single-arm, phase 3 trial. *Lancet Oncol.* **2020**, *21*, 776–785. [CrossRef]
79. Matin, S.F.; Pierorazio, P.M.; Kleinmann, N.; Gore, J.L.; Shabsigh, A.; Hu, B.; Chamie, K.; Godoy, G.; Hubosky, S.G.; Rivera, M.; et al. Durability of Response to Primary Chemoablation of Low-Grade Upper Tract Urothelial Carcinoma Using UGN-101, a Mitomycin-Containing Reverse Thermal Gel: OLYMPUS Trial Final Report. *J. Urol.* **2022**, *207*, 779–788. [CrossRef]
80. Labbate, C.; Woldu, S.; Murray, K.; Rose, K.; Sexton, W.; Tachibana, I.; Kaimakliotis, H.; Jacob, J.; Dickstein, R.; Linehan, J.; et al. Efficacy and Safety of Mitomycin Gel (UGN-101) as an Adjuvant Therapy After Complete Endoscopic Management of Upper Tract Urothelial Carcinoma. *J. Urol.* **2023**, *209*, 872–881. [CrossRef]
81. Linehan, J.; Gottlieb, J.; Woldu, S.L.; Labbate, C.; Rose, K.; Sexton, W.; Kaimakliotis, H.; Jacob, J.; Dickstein, R.; Nieder, A.; et al. Route of Administration for UGN-101 and Impact on Oncological and Safety Outcomes. *Eur. Urol. Focus.* **2023**. [CrossRef] [PubMed]
82. Rose, K.M.; Murray, K.S.; Labbate, C.; Woldu, S.; Linehan, J.; Jacob, J.; Kaimakliotis, H.; Dickstein, R.; Feldman, A.; Matin, S.F.; et al. Mitomycin Gel (UGN-101) as a Kidney-sparing Treatment for Upper Tract Urothelial Carcinoma in Patients with Imperative Indications and High-grade Disease. *Eur. Urol. Focus.* **2023**. [CrossRef] [PubMed]

cancers

Review

Modern Kidney-Sparing Management of Upper Tract Urothelial Carcinoma

Alireza Ghoreifi [1], Reza Sari Motlagh [2] and Gerhard Fuchs [1,*]

1 Institute of Urology, University of Southern California, Los Angeles, CA 90089, USA; alireza.ghoreifi@med.usc.edu
2 Urology Department, University of Vienna, 1090 Vienna, Austria; reza.sarimotlagh@meduniwien.ac.at
* Correspondence: gerhard.fuchs@med.usc.edu; Tel.: +1-(323)-865-3700

Simple Summary: Upper tract urothelial carcinoma (UTUC) is a lethal cancer of the urinary tract. Radical nephroureterectomy with bladder cuff excision is the gold standard for the management of patients with UTUC. Nevertheless, less-invasive surgeries to preserve maximum kidney function, such as endoscopic ablation and segmental ureteral resection, have become the preferred options in select patients. In this paper, we reviewed the latest evidence on the kidney-sparing management of upper tract urothelial carcinoma. We showed that these approaches are acceptable for low- as well as select high-risk patients who are not eligible for radical treatments. The main advantages of such approaches include renal function preservation as well as decreased surgical morbidity associated with radical treatments.

Abstract: Purpose: To review the latest evidence on the modern techniques and outcomes of kidney-sparing surgeries (KSS) in patients with upper tract urothelial carcinoma (UTUC). Methods: A comprehensive literature search on the study topic was conducted before 30 April 2023 using electronic databases including PubMed, MEDLINE, and EMBASE. A narrative overview of the literature was then provided based on the extracted data and a qualitative synthesis of the findings. Results: KSS is recommended for low- as well as select high-risk UTUCs who are not eligible for radical treatments. Endoscopic ablation is a KSS option that is associated with similar oncological outcomes compared with radical treatments while preserving renal function in well-selected patients. The other option in this setting is distal ureterectomy, which has the advantage of providing a definitive pathological stage and grade. Data from retrospective studies support the superiority of this approach over radical treatment with similar oncological outcomes, albeit in select cases. Novel chemoablation agents have also been studied in the past few years, of which mitomycin gel has received FDA approval for use in low-risk UTUCs. Conclusion: KSSs are acceptable approaches for patients with low- and select high-risk UTUCs, which preserve renal function without compromising the oncological outcomes.

Keywords: kidney-sparing surgery; radical nephroureterectomy; upper tract urothelial cell carcinoma; ureteroscopy

1. Introduction

Upper tract urothelial carcinoma (UTUC) is an uncommon type of cancer with an estimated annual incidence of 1–2 cases per 100,000 [1,2]. The most common risk factors of UTUC in western countries are tobacco and aromatic amines exposure; however, 10–20% of cases are familial and can be linked to hereditary non-polyposis colorectal cancer spectrum disease (Lynch syndrome) [1]. Despite surgery with curative intent, the 5-year cancer-specific survival of UTUC is <50% for stage 2–3 and <10% for stage 4. Moreover, recurrence in the bladder and contralateral upper tract occurs in 22–47% and 2–6% of UTUC patients, respectively [1,3,4].

The incidence of UTUC has been increasing in the past few decades most likely due to improved diagnostic techniques, such as high-quality imaging and flexible ureteroscopy (URS) [2]. This also has led to an increased rate of diagnosis among older patients with an increasing need for less-invasive treatment approaches to preserve maximum renal function [1,2]. Radical nephroureterectomy (RNU) with bladder cuff excision is the gold standard for the management of UTUC regardless of tumor location [3,4]. Nevertheless, kidney-sparing techniques, including endoscopic ablation and segmental ureterectomy (SU), have become the preferred options in select patients, especially those with low-risk diseases [3,4]. Several studies have confirmed the efficacy of these approaches with comparable oncologic outcomes to radical treatments [5]. Nevertheless, recent development in surgical technologies, such as advanced robotic systems and modern ureteroscopes, as well as new ablative modalities, warrant re-reviewing this important topic.

The aim of this study is to review the latest evidence on the modern techniques and outcomes of kidney-sparing management in patients with UTUC.

2. Materials and Methods

The scientific paper offers a narrative review of the literature on modern kidney-sparing management strategies for UTUC. The authors conducted a comprehensive literature search on the studies published before 30 April 2023 using electronic databases including PubMed, MEDLINE, and EMBASE. We utilized specific keywords and Medical Subject Headings (MeSH) terms related to UTUC, kidney-sparing techniques, endoscopic treatments, and renal preservation to refine the search and retrieve relevant articles. Additionally, we included reference lists of identified articles for additional sources. Studies were selected based on the English language preference and their relevance to kidney-sparing management of UTUC, specifically focusing on various techniques such as ureteroscopic management, percutaneous approaches, segmental ureteral resection, and novel endoscopic technologies. The literature search identified 203 unique references. We excluded review articles, letters, editorials, and case reports as well as any study that was not relevant as described above. Consequently, 28 studies were included for qualitative synthesis according to the research topic, our inclusion criteria, and data availability. Data extraction involved retrieving important information from the selected studies. Based on the extracted data and a qualitative synthesis of the findings, we provide a narrative overview of the literature. We present the evidence coherently, highlighting the strengths and limitations of the reviewed studies.

3. Indications

Pretreatment staging in UTUC patients is challenging due to the limitations of currently available diagnostic tools [1]. The findings of URS/biopsy (tumor grade, focality, and shape), imaging (invasion, obstruction, and nodal status), as well as urine cytology will help in preoperative risk stratification to low vs. high risk for invasive disease (i.e., ≥pT2) [3,4]. Considering these factors, various nomograms and models have been proposed to predict low-risk disease and help with the optimal selection of patients for kidney-sparing surgery (KSS) [6–10]. Based on these data, the European Association of Urology (EAU) and American Urological Association (AUA) expert panels on UTUC proposed two models for pretreatment risk stratification of UTUC to support clinical decision-making (Figure 1). The new AUA guidelines also sub-stratify the patients into favorable and unfavorable to further facilitate risk-adapted management [3].

Current guidelines recommend KSS as a primary treatment option in patients with low-risk UTUC as well as select high-risk cases who have low-volume tumors or imperative indications precluding RNU (e.g., renal insufficiency, single kidney, or bilateral tumors) [3,4]. Taken together, patients who are considered for KSS should preferably have the following criteria: unifocal small-size papillary lesion, negative urine cytology, low-grade ureteroscopic biopsy, and absence of hydronephrosis or invasion in CT imaging [3,4].

In addition, technical feasibility of maximal tumor extirpation and patient compliance with a close follow-up schedule should be considered [11].

(A) EAU Risk Stratification	
Low-Risk*	**High-Risk****
Unifocal disease	Multi-focal disease
Tumor size < 2 cm	Tumor size ≥ 2 cm
Negative for high-grade cytology	High-grade cytology
Low-grade URS biopsy	High-grade URS biopsy
No invasive aspect on CT	Local invasion on CT
	Hydronephrosis
	Previous radical cystectomy for high-grade bladder cancer
	Histological subtype

* All these factors need to be present.
**Any of these factors need to be present.

(B) AUA Risk Stratification				
Feature	**Low-Risk**		**High-Risk**	
Biopsy grade	Low-Grade		High-Grade	
Sub-stratification	**Favorable**	**Unfavorable**	**Favorable**	**Unfavorable**
Cytology	Negative	No HGUC	Any cytology	HGUC
Radiology	No invasion	No invasion	No invasion	Invasion
	No obstruction	Obstruction	No obstruction	Obstruction
	Normal nodes	Normal nodes	Normal nodes	Suspicious nodes
Appearance	Unifocal	Multifocal	Unifocal	Multifocal
	Papillary	Papillary	Papillary	Sessile or Flat
Lower Tract Involvement*	No involvement	Involvement	No involvement	Involvement

* Concomitant or prior

Figure 1. (**A**) EAU and (**B**) AUA pretreatment risk stratification of non-metastatic UTUC. CT: computed tomography; URS: ureteroscopy; HGUC: high-grade urothelial carcinoma [3,4].

4. Endoscopic Ablation

Endoscopic ablation, as a KSS option in patients with UTUC, has gained popularity in the past two decades due to the evolution in technology with smaller deflecting endoscopes, advanced lasers, special instruments, and high-quality optics [12].

4.1. Techniques

Endoscopic ablation of a UTUC lesion can be performed via a retrograde or antegrade approach. Retrograde is the most common approach; however, the percutaneous method is preferred for larger tumors (>1.5 cm) and those that are difficult to access through a retrograde fashion (i.e., lower pole calyx lesion or prior urinary diversion) [3,4]. The retrograde approach is performed using a rigid or flexible ureteroscope. Using a ureteral access sheath can help with repeated scope passage and also decrease the rate of intravesical recurrence following ablation [13]. On the other hand, the antegrade approach requires establishment of a nephrostomy tract in the correct position [14]. Despite the promising oncologic results for this approach, there is still a lack of evidence regarding its safety profile [15].

The ablation techniques include bulk excision (using biopsy forceps or basket), resection of the tumor to its base (using ureteroscopic resectoscope), and ablation with electrocautery (e.g., Bugbee) or laser energy sources, including thulium (Tm)–yttrium aluminum garnet (YAG), holmium (Ho)–YAG, and neodymium (Nd)–YAG [16]. Ho–YAG is characterized by a longer wavelength and approximately 0.3–0.4 mm tissue penetration, which makes it suitable for use in superficial ureteral tumors. Nd–YAG has a deeper tissue penetration of up to 10 mm, which is a good option for bulkier tumors. However, its use in the ureter is limited due to the low safety margin that may increase its associated complications. Tm–YAG has gained more acceptance in this setting compared with other types of lasers due to the good coagulation and hemostasis features while having a short penetration depth of about 0.1–0.2 mm [17–20]. A recent systematic review on the use of Thulium lasers in UTUC reported no intraoperative complication and 10.5 to 38% rate of postoperative complications, most of which were mild and transient [21].

Novel endoscopic techniques, such as en bloc enucleation, have also been reported in the literature [22,23]. Although this approach was shown to be feasible in select cases with the advantage of improved histopathologic information, its indications and oncological safety have yet to be determined.

4.2. Adjuvant Instillation

Older studies on the use of adjuvant upper urinary tract instillation of BCG or mitomycin C following endoscopic ablation of UTUC have shown comparable results to unrented patients [24]. However, recent studies have demonstrated promising oncological outcomes in these patients. Gallioli et al. reported 52 UTUC patients treated by endoscopic ablation, of whom 26 received immediate adjuvant single-dose upper urinary tract instillation of mitomycin. On Cox regression, mitomycin instillation was associated with a 7.7-fold lower risk of urothelial recurrence [25]. In addition, Labbate et al. recently reported a 63% ipsilateral disease-free rate at 6.8 months following endoscopic ablation and adjuvant mitomycin gel instillation [26]. It is noteworthy that all available studies suffer from small sample size and lack of control groups. In addition, the rate of ureteral stenosis has been reported to be as high as 19% in recent series of adjuvant mitomycin gel instillation [24]. Therefore, the guidelines suggest adjuvant pelvicalyceal chemotherapy instillation following UTUC ablation, albeit as an optional part of routine practice, provided that there is no perforation in the urinary system [3,4].

4.3. Follow-Up

There is no high-level evidence regarding the optimal follow-up schedule in patients undergoing endoscopic ablation, and the recommendations are mostly based on experts' opinions. Current guidelines recommend repeat URS within three months following initial ablation to check for residual disease and/or recurrence [3,4]. In a study of 41 patients who underwent second-look URS, 6–8 weeks following endoscopic ablation for UTUC, cancer was detected in more than half of the patients, of whom 86% were in the same location as the first URS [27]. These findings underscore the importance of second-look URS following initial ablation. Surveillance URS should then be then continued every 3–6 months until no evidence of upper tract disease is identified (preferably up to 5 years). The surveillance intervals depend on tumor grade (low vs. high) and the indication of KSS (imperative vs. non-imperative); patients with high-grade UTUC and those with imperative indications will require closer follow-ups. In addition, CT urogram, cystoscopy, and urine cytology should be included in the follow-up workups [3,4].

4.4. Outcomes

The main goal of endoscopic ablation for UTUC is preserving renal function without compromising the oncological outcomes. There is no prospective study comparing endoscopic management with RNU for UTUC. However, the available data from retrospective studies have shown similar oncological outcomes between these two treatment modalities (Tables 1 and 2) [28–38]. In a recent systematic review and meta-analysis, including 13 studies, Kawada et al. reported that endoscopic management compared with RNU was associated with similar overall survival (OS) (Hazard Ratio: HR 1.27, 95% CI 0.75–2.16), cancer-specific survival (CSS) (HR 1.37, 95% CI 0.99–1.91), and bladder recurrence-free survival (BRFS) (HR 0.98, 95% CI 0.61–1.55). However, the results of this systematic review should be interpreted with caution given the retrospective nature of included studies as well as selection bias due to the heterogeneity of patient populations and inclusion criteria [39].

Table 1. Oncological outcomes of contemporary studies comparing endoscopic ablation vs. RNU for UTUC.

Study (yr) [Ref]	Patients (n)		Bladder Recurrence (%)		5 yr OS (%)			5 yr CSS (%)		
	EA	RNU	EA	RNU	EA	RNU	p Value	EA	RNU	p Value
Lucas et al. (2008) [28]	39	77	5	8	62	72	0.36	82	83	0.98
Cutress et al. (2012) [29]	59	70	42	33	64	75	0.02	85	92.1	0.21
Fajkovic et al. (2012) [30]	20	178	15	36	45	76	0.001	67	91	0.36
Seisen et al. (2016) [31]	42	128	NA	NA	74	73	0.06	83	87	0.18
Vemana et al. (2016) [32]	151	302	NA	NA	NA	NA	NA	88	92	NA
Chen et al. (2021) [33]	84	272	23	34	85	75	0.19	89	90	0.49
Shenhar et al. (2021) [34]	24	37	NA	NA	85	84	0.71	89	92	0.96
Shen et al. (2022) [35]	23	42	30	33	95	95	0.99	NA	NA	NA

EA: endoscopic ablation; RNU: radical nephroureterectomy; OS: overall survival; CSS: cancer-specific survival; NA: not available.

Table 2. Oncological outcomes of studies comparing endoscopic ablation vs. RNU for UTUC, stratified by tumor grade.

Study (yr) [Ref]	Patients (n)		Garde	5 yr OS (%)			5 yr CSS (%)			5 yr MFS (%)		
	EA	RNU		EA	RNU	p Value	EA	RNU	p Value	EA	RNU	p Value
Rouprêt et al. (2006) [36]	43	54	Low	NA	NA	NA	81	84	0.89	NA	NA	NA
Lucas et al. (2008) [28]	39	77	Low	75	66	0.28	86	87	0.91	NA	NA	NA
			High	45	72	0.08	69	75	0.53			
Gadzinski et al. (2010) [37]	34	62	Low	75	72	0.30	100	89	0.63	94	88	0.25
			High	25	48	0.62	86	72	0.94	86	64	0.79
Cutress et al. (2012) [29]	59	70	G1	75	86	0.62	100	100	0.65	NA	NA	NA
			G2	56	73	0.08	62	92	0.03			
			G3	33	75	0.001	83	89	0.26			
Grasso et al. (2012) [39]	80	80	Low	74	88	NA	87	93	NA	84	95	NA
			High	0	68	NA	0	78	NA	0	61	NA

EA: endoscopic ablation; RNU: radical nephroureterectomy; OS: overall survival; CSS: cancer-specific survival; MFS: metastasis-free survival; NA: not available.

Despite favorable oncological outcomes of endoscopic ablation, approximately 20–30% of patients may develop disease progression requiring salvage RNU [40]. In a study with a large sample size of 279 patients undergoing endoscopic management for UTUC, Chen et al. reported a 24% rate of salvage RNU. The authors showed that among patients with recurrence following endoscopic ablation, those undergoing salvage RNU compared with others had a better disease-free survival rate (92% vs. 77.5%) as well as a lower rate of UTUC-related death (7.8% vs. 22.5%) [41].

Endoscopic ablation is associated with a better or similar postoperative kidney function compared with RNU [30,33,34,42,43] (Table 3). In a study comparing 20 patients undergoing endoscopic ablation compared with 178 RNU cases, Fejkovic et al. reported better postoperative kidney function in the ablation group [30]. On the other hand, in a study comparing 84 cases of endoscopic ablation and 272 patients undergoing RNU, Chen et al. reported no significant difference in postoperative renal function, chronic kidney disease, or end-stage renal disease [33]. It is worth mentioning that all these studies are retrospective and their outcomes are affected by selection bias and short-term follow-ups.

Table 3. Renal function changes in contemporary studies comparing endoscopic ablation vs. RNU for UTUC.

Study (yr) [Ref]	Patients (n)		Renal Function			
	EA	RNU	Variable	EA	RNU	p Value
Fajkovic et al. (2013) [30]	20	178	Preoperative Cr (mg%) Postoperative Cr (mg%)	1.46 ± 0.52 1.3 ± 0.47	1.53 ± 1.2 1.64 ± 0.79	0.82 0.048
Hoffman et al. (2014) [42]	25	22	Preoperative eGFR Postoperative eGFR	66 62	68 58	>0.05 >0.05
Wen et al. (2018) [43]	32	107	Cr level POD1 (umol/L)	89 ± 7.5	123 ± 9.4	<0.01
Chen et al. (2021) [33]	84	272	Preoperative Cr (mg/dL) Postoperative Cr (1 mo) Postoperative Cr (final) ESRD	2.1 ± 1.9 3.57 ± 10.5 3.34 ± 3.01 29%	1.33 ± 2.82 1.61 ± 2.49 1.80 ± 2.73 27%	0.90 0.38 0.74 0.31
Shenhar et al. (2022) [34]	24	37	eGFR (mL/min/1.73 m^2) # CKD (GFR < 60) Severe CKD (GFR < 30)	58.7 ± 21.5 45% 9%	49.2 ± 22.1 70% 16%	0.12 0.59 0.44

All variables were measured at the end of follow-up (median 5 years). Cr: creatinine; GFR: glomerular filtration rate; CKD: chronic kidney disease; ESRD: end-stage renal disease; POD: postop day.

5. Segmental Ureterectomy

Although the feasibility of proximal and total ureterectomy has been shown in the literature [44,45], distal ureterectomy followed by ureteroneocystostomy ± psoas hitch/Boari flap forms the most common type of segmental resection in UTUC patients. It is indicated in low- as well as select high-risk UTUC tumors confined to the distal ureter [3,4]. The main advantage of this procedure over endoscopic ablation is that it provides a definitive pathological stage and grade while preserving ipsilateral renal function.

5.1. Technical Considerations

A distal ureterectomy can be performed through open, laparoscopic, and robotic approaches [46,47]. The robotic approach has gained more acceptance in recent years due to favorable perioperative outcomes while ensuring oncologic efficacy. In a study of 15 cases who underwent robotic SU, Campi et al. reported no intraoperative complications and no need for open conversion. Within a 30-day follow-up, 13% of patients experienced grade 3a, yet no ≥ grade 3b, Clavien complications [47].

Similar to RNU, a formal bladder cuff excision with watertight bladder closure is necessary during SU [48,49]. The absence of residual tumor should be confirmed by a negative frozen margin intraoperatively. Lymph node dissection is mandatory in high-risk yet optional in low-risk patients [3,4]. The appropriate template to yield maximal oncologic outcomes remains to be determined; however, dissection of the ipsilateral obturator and external iliac as well as (preferably) common and internal iliac lymph nodes is recommended in patients undergoing distal ureterectomy [50,51].

5.2. Outcomes

There is no randomized clinical trial comparing the outcomes of SU vs. RNU. Current data are based on retrospective studies with a high risk of selection, performance, and detection bias. There are two systematic reviews available comparing the outcomes of SU vs. RNU. The first includes 11 retrospective studies with 3963 patients (SU = 983 and RNU = 2980). The meta-analysis of adjusted data demonstrated similar CSS (HR = 0.90, $p = 0.47$), RFS (HR 1.06, $p = 0.72$), and BRFS (HR 1.35, $p = 0.39$) between the two groups [52]. A second systematic review and meta-analysis was recently performed by Veccia et al., which included 18 studies (all retrospective) comparing 1313 and 3484 patients undergoing SU vs. RNU, respectively. The authors showed no statistically significant difference between the two groups in terms of overall and bladder recurrences, metastases, and cancer-related death. On survival analyses, the SU group showed lower 5-year RFS but similar 5-year MFS and CSS compared with RNU [53]. Finally, a recent study of the national cancer database population, including 9016 RNU and 4045 SU cases, confirmed that long-term survival of SU is not inferior to RNU. In this study, female gender, advanced clinical T stage (cT4), and high-grade tumor were associated with a decreased likelihood of receiving SU, while age > 79 years was associated with an increased probability of undergoing SU [54].

In terms of renal function, available data support the superiority of SU over RNU. Feng et al., in a meta-analysis of the weighted mean changes in peri-operative estimated glomerular filtration rate (eGFR), reported a significant decrease of 9.32 mL/1.73 m^2 in patients undergoing RNU vs. SU [52]. Similarly, in their meta-analysis, Veccia et al. reported higher postoperative eGFR in patients receiving RNU compared with the SU group [53]. Although these findings are in favor of renal function preservation in patients undergoing SU, the results should be interpreted with caution due to the heterogeneity of cohorts and the effect of possible confounding factors, such as neoadjuvant and adjuvant systemic therapy.

6. Novel Chemoablation Therapies and Ongoing Trials

Bacillus Calmette–Guérin (BCG) and mitomycin C have been previously investigated for intracavitary management of UTUC, albeit mainly in the adjuvant setting following endoscopic ablation [55]. Nevertheless, the US Food and Drug Administration (FDA) recently approved mitomycin gel/UGN-101 (JELMYTO, UroGen Pharma) as a first-line treatment for patients with low-grade UTUC [56]. UGN-101 is a water-soluble mitomycin gel with reverse thermal properties that allow for local administration as a liquid with subsequent conversion to a semi-solid gel following instillation into the upper tract. The FDA approval was based on the results of the OLYMPUS trial, which was a phase III, open-label, multicenter study of patients with treatment-naïve or recurrent low-grade UTUC [57]. A total of 71 patients enrolled in this trial and received 6 weekly courses of mitomycin gel followed by URS evaluation. Complete response (primary endpoint, defined as negative endoscopic examination and cytology) was achieved in 58% of the patients, of whom 82% had a durable response in one year (secondary endpoint) [58]. While UGN-101 is approved for low-grade non-invasive UTUCs, a recent study showed promising results in patients with imperative indications, including those with high-grade disease. In this subgroup of high-grade UTUCs, 45% had no evidence of disease at the initial postinduction evaluation [59]. Long-term follow-up is needed to confirm the efficacy of UGN-101 in high-risk UTUC cases.

Ureteral stenosis was the most common treatment-associated adverse event in the OLYMPUS trial and was seen in 31/71 (44%) patients, of whom 6 (8%) required intervention (Clavien grade 3 complication). This was thought to be due to the retrograde approach for mitomycin gel instillation [57]. Using the antegrade approach, Rosen et al. reported a case series of patients receiving mitomycin gel. The authors reported similar oncological outcomes compared with the OLYMPUS trial, yet with a much lower rate of ureteral stricture (1/8 asymptomatic stricture) [60]. These findings were confirmed in a larger retrospective multicenter study of 132 patients who were treated with UGN-101 for low-grade UTUC via a retrograde vs. antegrade approach. In this study, complete response was achieved in 48% of retrograde and 60% of antegrade renal units (p = 0.1), while Clavien grade 3 ureteral strictures occurred in 32% of retrograde vs. 12% of antegrade cases ($p < 0.001$) [61].

The most novel modality for the ablation of UTUC lesions is photodynamic agents, which have been used in a phase I trial of WST-11/TOOKAD-Soluble for UTUC ablation. This was an open-label trial using padeliporfin to ablate UTUC lesions. This is a new investigational short-acting photodynamic agent, which produces a novel form of vascular-targeted photodynamic treatment. The results were promising with a 94% overall response within 30 days and a final complete pathologic response of 68%. The most common adverse events following padeliporfin administration were transient flank pain (79%) and hematuria (84%), with no ureteral strictures during follow-up [62].

Based on the results of phase I WSAT-11 trial, the multicenter Phase III ENdoluminal LIGHT ActivatED Treatment of UTUC (ENLIGHTED) trial (UCM301) has been initiated [63]. This is a single arm, non-randomized trial, including new or recurrent low-grade, non-invasive UTUCs. Patients receive 1–3 padeliporfin (vascular-targeted photodynamic) VTP treatments every 4 weeks as an induction therapy followed by repeated maintenance treatments for patients who show evidence of tumor recurrence that is deemed treatable. Primary outcome is the number of patients with complete response, defined as an absence of visual tumor on endoscopy, no evidence of tumor on biopsy (if feasible), and negative urinary cytology by instrumented collection. Secondary endpoints included the duration of response at the entire ipsilateral kidney as well as treatment area at 3, 6, 9, and 12 months postprimary response evaluation; overall renal function at 6 and 12 months; development of ureteral obstruction and/or ureteral stent placement; and duration of response/renal function on long-term follow-up. This trial is now in the recruiting phase, with an estimated enrollment of 100 participants.

7. Conclusions and Future Directions

KSSs, including endoscopic ablation and segmental ureterectomy, are acceptable approaches for patients with low-risk UTUC as well as select high-risk cases who are not eligible for radical treatments. The only level I evidence in this setting is the use of mitomycin gel in low-risk UTUCs. The feasibility and safety of other types of KSSs have been confirmed in several retrospective comparative studies. The main advantages of KSS include renal function preservation as well as decreased surgical morbidity associated with radical treatments. The key step in KSS is appropriate patient selection, which highly relies on preoperative risk stratification to find low-risk cases. Novel diagnostic and prognostic tools, such as urine-based methylation and blood-based liquid biopsy biomarkers, can help in optimizing preoperative risk stratification and proper patient selection for KSS [64,65]. In addition, these novel markers can be beneficial in the surveillance setting of patients with UTUC undergoing KSS to avoid unnecessary procedures (e.g., URS). On the other hand, the advent of new technologies, such as digital flexible ureteroscopes, as well as novel therapeutic agents, including mitomycin gel and photodynamic agents, may offer more-effective and less-invasive patient care. The efficacy of mitomycin gel was confirmed in a phase III trial that led to FDA approval as a first-line treatment for low-grade UTUC. In addition, the use of padeliporfin, a photodynamic agent, has shown promising results in a phase I trial; however, the phase III trial of this study is still ongoing. While the current data are mainly derived from retrospective studies, ongoing trials are eagerly awaited to shed light on this important topic.

Author Contributions: Conceptualization, A.G. and G.F.; methodology, A.G. and R.S.M.; investigation, A.G.; writing—original draft preparation, A.G. and R.S.M.; writing—review and editing, G.F.; supervision, G.F. All authors have read and agreed to the published version of the manuscript.

Funding: This research received no external funding.

Conflicts of Interest: The authors declare no conflict of interest.

References

1. Soria, F.; Shariat, S.F.; Lerner, S.P.; Fritsche, H.M.; Rink, M.; Kassouf, W.; Spiess, P.E.; Lotan, Y.; Ye, D.; Fernández, M.I.; et al. Epidemiology, diagnosis, preoperative evaluation and prognostic assessment of upper-tract urothelial carcinoma (UTUC). *World J. Urol.* **2017**, *35*, 379–387. [CrossRef]
2. Almås, B.; Halvorsen, O.J.; Johannesen, T.B.; Beisland, C. Higher than expected and significantly increasing incidence of upper tract urothelial carcinoma. A population based study. *World J. Urol.* **2021**, *39*, 3385–3391. [CrossRef] [PubMed]
3. Coleman, J.A.; Clark, P.E.; Bixler, B.R.; Buckley, D.I.; Chang, S.S.; Chou, R.; Hoffman-Censits, J.; Kulkarni, G.S.; Matin, S.F.; Pierorazio, P.M.; et al. Diagnosis and Management of Non-Metastatic Upper Tract Urothelial Carcinoma: AUA/SUO Guideline. *J. Urol.* **2023**, *209*, 1071–1081. [CrossRef] [PubMed]

4. Rouprêt, M.; Seisen, T.; Birtle, A.J.; Capoun, O.; Compérat, E.M.; Dominguez-Escrig, J.L.; Gürses Andersson, I.; Liedberg, F.; Mariappan, P.; Hugh Mostafid, A.; et al. European Association of Urology Guidelines on Upper Urinary Tract Urothelial Carcinoma: 2023 Update. *Eur. Urol.* **2023**, *84*, 49–64. [CrossRef] [PubMed]
5. Seisen, T.; Peyronnet, B.; Dominguez-Escrig, J.L.; Bruins, H.M.; Yuan, C.Y.; Babjuk, M.; Böhle, A.; Burger, M.; Compérat, E.M.; Cowan, N.C.; et al. Oncologic Outcomes of Kidney-sparing Surgery Versus Radical Nephroureterectomy for Upper Tract Urothelial Carcinoma: A Systematic Review by the EAU Non-muscle Invasive Bladder Cancer Guidelines Panel. *Eur. Urol.* **2016**, *70*, 1052–1068. [CrossRef]
6. Foerster, B.; Abufaraj, M.; Matin, S.F.; Azizi, M.; Gupta, M.; Li, W.M.; Seisen, T.; Clinton, T.; Xylinas, E.; Mir, M.C.; et al. Pretreatment Risk Stratification for Endoscopic Kidney-sparing Surgery in Upper Tract Urothelial Carcinoma: An International Collaborative Study. *Eur. Urol.* **2021**, *80*, 507–515. [CrossRef]
7. Marcq, G.; Foerster, B.; Abufaraj, M.; Matin, S.F.; Azizi, M.; Gupta, M.; Li, W.M.; Seisen, T.; Clinton, T.; Xylinas, E.; et al. Novel Classification for Upper Tract Urothelial Carcinoma to Better Risk-stratify Patients Eligible for Kidney-sparing Strategies: An International Collaborative Study. *Eur. Urol. Focus.* **2022**, *8*, 491–497. [CrossRef]
8. Favaretto, R.L.; Shariat, S.F.; Savage, C.; Godoy, G.; Chade, D.C.; Kaag, M.; Bochner, B.H.; Coleman, J.; Dalbagni, G. Combining imaging and ureteroscopy variables in a preoperative multivariable model for prediction of muscle-invasive and non-organ confined disease in patients with upper tract urothelial carcinoma. *BJU Int.* **2012**, *109*, 77–82. [CrossRef] [PubMed]
9. Brien, J.C.; Shariat, S.F.; Herman, M.P.; Ng, C.K.; Scherr, D.S.; Scoll, B.; Uzzo, R.G.; Wille, M.; Eggener, S.E.; Terrell, J.D.; et al. Preoperative hydronephrosis, ureteroscopic biopsy grade and urinary cytology can improve prediction of advanced upper tract urothelial carcinoma. *J. Urol.* **2010**, *184*, 69–73. [CrossRef]
10. Chromecki, T.F.; Cha, E.K.; Fajkovic, H.; Margulis, V.; Novara, G.; Scherr, D.S.; Lotan, Y.; Raman, J.D.; Kassouf, W.; Bensalah, K.; et al. The impact of tumor multifocality on outcomes in patients treated with radical nephroureterectomy. *Eur. Urol.* **2012**, *61*, 245–253. [CrossRef]
11. Lucca, I.; Klatte, T.; Rouprêt, M.; Shariat, S.F. Kidney-sparing surgery for upper tract urothelial cancer. *Curr. Opin. Urol.* **2015**, *25*, 100–104. [CrossRef]
12. Keller, E.X.; Doizi, S.; Villa, L.; Traxer, O. Which flexible ureteroscope is the best for upper tract urothelial carcinoma treatment? *World J. Urol.* **2019**, *37*, 2325–2333. [CrossRef]
13. Douglawi, A.; Ghoreifi, A.; Lee, R.; Yip, W.; Seyedian, S.S.L.; Ahmadi, H.; Cai, J.; Miranda, G.; Yu, W.; Bhanvadia, S.; et al. Bladder Recurrence Following Diagnostic Ureteroscopy in Patients Undergoing Nephroureterectomy for Upper Tract Urothelial Cancer: Is Ureteral Access Sheath Protective? *Urology.* **2022**, *160*, 142–146. [CrossRef] [PubMed]
14. Motamedinia, P.; Keheila, M.; Leavitt, D.A.; Rastinehad, A.R.; Okeke, Z.; Smith, A.D. The Expanded Use of Percutaneous Resection for Upper Tract Urothelial Carcinoma: A 30-Year Comprehensive Experience. *J. Endourol.* **2016**, *30*, 262–267. [CrossRef] [PubMed]
15. Laukhtina, E.; Kawada, T.; Quhal, F.; Yanagisawa, T.; Rajwa, P.; von Deimling, M.; Pallauf, M.; Bianchi, A.; Majdoub, M.; Enikeev, D.; et al. Oncologic and Safety Outcomes for Retrograde and Antegrade Endoscopic Surgeries for Upper Tract Urothelial Carcinoma: A Systematic Review and Meta-analysis. *Eur. Urol. Focus.* **2023**, *9*, 258–263. [CrossRef]
16. Shvero, A.; Zilberman, D.E.; Dotan, Z.A.; Laufer, M.; Fridman, E.; Winkler, H.; Kleinmann, N. Endoscopic management of upper tract urothelial carcinoma-tips and tricks. *Transl. Androl. Urol.* **2020**, *9*, 1815–1820. [CrossRef] [PubMed]
17. Proietti, S.; Rodríguez-Socarrás, M.E.; Eisner, B.H.; Lucianò, R.; Basulto Martinez, M.J.; Yeow, Y.; Rapallo, I.; Saitta, G.; Scarfò, F.; Gaboardi, F.; et al. Thulium:YAG Versus Holmium:YAG Laser Effect on Upper Urinary Tract Soft Tissue: Evidence from an Ex Vivo Experimental Study. *J. Endourol.* **2021**, *35*, 544–551. [CrossRef]
18. Doizi, S.; Germain, T.; Panthier, F.; Compérat, E.; Traxer, O.; Berthe, L. Comparison of Holmium:YAG and Thulium Fiber Lasers on Soft Tissue: An Ex Vivo Study. *J. Endourol.* **2022**, *36*, 251–258. [CrossRef]
19. Tada, Y.; Yokomizo, A.; Koga, H.; Seki, N.; Kuroiwa, K.; Tatsugami, K.; Yamaguchi, A.; Naito, S. Transurethral endoscopic treatment of patients with upper tract urothelial carcinomas using neodymium-YAG and/or holmium-YAG laser ablation. *BJU Int.* **2010**, *106*, 362–366. [CrossRef]
20. Korn, S.M.; Hübner, N.A.; Seitz, C.; Shariat, S.F.; Fajkovic, H. Role of lasers in urology. *Photochem. Photobiol. Sci.* **2019**, *18*, 295–303. [CrossRef]
21. Candela, L.; Ventimiglia, E.; Solano, C.; Chicaud, M.; Kutchukian, S.; Panthier, F.; Corrales, M.; Villa, L.; Briganti, A.; Montorsi, F.; et al. Endoscopic Conservative Treatment of Upper Urinary Tract Urothelial Carcinoma with a Thulium Laser: A Systematic Review. *J. Clin. Med.* **2023**, *12*, 4907. [CrossRef] [PubMed]
22. Shoen, E.; Zollinger, B.; Gresham, T.; Rezaei, K.M.; Whalen, M. Use of the T-1470 LiteTouch™ Laser in the En Bloc Resection of an Upper Tract Urothelial Cancer. *Case Rep. Urol.* **2021**, *2021*, 6623326. [CrossRef] [PubMed]
23. Jue, J.S.; Armenakas, N.A. Upper Tract Tumor En Bloc Enucleation: A Novel Approach to the Diagnosis and Management of Upper Tract Urothelial Carcinoma. *Urology.* **2023**, *174*, 196–200. [CrossRef]
24. Foerster, B.; D'Andrea, D.; Abufaraj, M.; Broenimann, S.; Karakiewicz, P.I.; Rouprêt, M.; Gontero, P.; Lerner, S.P.; Shariat, S.F.; Soria, F. Endocavitary treatment for upper tract urothelial carcinoma: A meta-analysis of the current literature. *Urol. Oncol.* **2019**, *37*, 430–436. [CrossRef] [PubMed]

25. Gallioli, A.; Boissier, R.; Territo, A.; Vila Reyes, H.; Sanguedolce, F.; Gaya, J.M.; Regis, F.; Subiela, J.D.; Palou, J.; Breda, A. Adjuvant Single-Dose Upper Urinary Tract Instillation of Mitomycin C After Therapeutic Ureteroscopy for Upper Tract Urothelial Carcinoma: A Single-Centre Prospective Non-Randomized Trial. *J. Endourol.* **2020**, *34*, 573–580. [CrossRef]
26. Labbate, C.; Woldu, S.; Murray, K.; Rose, K.; Sexton, W.; Tachibana, I.; Kaimakliotis, H.; Jacob, J.; Dickstein, R.; Linehan, J.; et al. Efficacy and Safety of Mitomycin Gel (UGN-101) as an Adjuvant Therapy After Complete Endoscopic Management of Upper Tract Urothelial Carcinoma. *J. Urol.* **2023**, *209*, 872–881. [CrossRef]
27. Villa, L.; Cloutier, J.; Letendre, J.; Ploumidis, A.; Salonia, A.; Cornu, J.N.; Montorsi, F.; Traxer, O. Early repeated ureteroscopy within 6–8 weeks after a primary endoscopic treatment in patients with upper tract urothelial cell carcinoma: Preliminary findings. *World J. Urol.* **2016**, *34*, 1201–1206. [CrossRef]
28. Lucas, S.M.; Svatek, R.S.; Olgin, G.; Arriaga, Y.; Kabbani, W.; Sagalowsky, A.I.; Lotan, Y. Conservative management in selected patients with upper tract urothelial carcinoma compares favourably with early radical surgery. *BJU Int.* **2008**, *102*, 172–176. [CrossRef]
29. Cutress, M.L.; Stewart, G.D.; Tudor, E.C.; Egong, E.A.; Wells-Cole, S.; Phipps, S.; Thomas, B.G.; Riddick, A.C.; McNeill, S.A.; Tolley, D.A. Endoscopic versus laparoscopic management of noninvasive upper tract urothelial carcinoma: 20-year single center experience. *J. Urol.* **2013**, *189*, 2054–2060. [CrossRef]
30. Fajkovic, H.; Klatte, T.; Nagele, U.; Dunzinger, M.; Zigeuner, R.; Hübner, W.; Remzi, M. Results and outcomes after endoscopic treatment of upper urinary tract carcinoma: The Austrian experience. *World J. Urol.* **2013**, *31*, 37–44. [CrossRef]
31. Seisen, T.; Nison, L.; Remzi, M.; Klatte, T.; Mathieu, R.; Lucca, I.; Bozzini, G.; Capitanio, U.; Novara, G.; Cussenot, O.; et al. Oncologic Outcomes of Kidney Sparing Surgery versus Radical Nephroureterectomy for the Elective Treatment of Clinically Organ Confined Upper Tract Urothelial Carcinoma of the Distal Ureter. *J. Urol.* **2016**, *195*, 1354–1361. [CrossRef]
32. Vemana, G.; Kim, E.H.; Bhayani, S.B.; Vetter, J.M.; Strope, S.A. Survival Comparison Between Endoscopic and Surgical Management for Patients With Upper Tract Urothelial Cancer: A Matched Propensity Score Analysis Using Surveillance, Epidemiology and End Results-Medicare Data. *Urology.* **2016**, *95*, 115–120. [CrossRef] [PubMed]
33. Chen, Y.T.; Yu, C.C.; Yeh, H.C.; Lee, H.Y.; Jiang, Y.H.; Lee, Y.K.; Kuei, C.H.; Wu, C.C.; Huang, C.Y.; Lin, W.Y.; et al. Endoscopic management versus radical nephroureterectomy for localized upper tract urothelial carcinoma in a high endemic region. *Sci. Rep.* **2021**, *11*, 4040. [CrossRef] [PubMed]
34. Shenhar, C.; Veredgorn, Y.; Bulis, S.; Aviv, T.; Darawsha, A.E.; Gilad, R.; Baniel, J.; Ehrlich, Y.; Lifshitz, D. Endoscopic Management of Low-Grade Upper Tract Urothelial Carcinoma: Characterizing the Long-term Burden of Care in Comparison to Radical Nephroureterectomy. *Urology.* **2022**, *159*, 152–159. [CrossRef]
35. Shen, C.Y.; Jou, Y.C.; Kan, W.C.; Tzai, T.S.; Tsai, Y.S. Outcome of Non-Muscle Invasive Upper Tract Urothelial Carcinoma Receiving Endoscopic Ablation: An Inverse Probability of Treatment Weighting Analysis. *J. Clin. Med.* **2022**, *11*, 1307. [CrossRef]
36. Rouprêt, M.; Hupertan, V.; Traxer, O.; Loison, G.; Chartier-Kastler, E.; Conort, P.; Bitker, M.O.; Gattegno, B.; Richard, F.; Cussenot, O. Comparison of open nephroureterectomy and ureteroscopic and percutaneous management of upper urinary tract transitional cell carcinoma. *Urology.* **2006**, *67*, 1181–1187. [CrossRef]
37. Gadzinski, A.J.; Roberts, W.W.; Faerber, G.J.; Wolf, J.S., Jr. Long-term outcomes of nephroureterectomy versus endoscopic management for upper tract urothelial carcinoma. *J. Urol.* **2010**, *183*, 2148–2153. [CrossRef] [PubMed]
38. Grasso, M.; Fishman, A.I.; Cohen, J.; Alexander, B. Ureteroscopic and extirpative treatment of upper urinary tract urothelial carcinoma: A 15-year comprehensive review of 160 consecutive patients. *BJU Int.* **2012**, *110*, 1618–1626. [CrossRef]
39. Kawada, T.; Laukhtina, E.; Quhal, F.; Yanagisawa, T.; Rajwa, P.; Pallauf, M.; von Deimling, M.; Bianchi, A.; Pradere, B.; Fajkovic, H.; et al. Oncologic and Safety Outcomes for Endoscopic Surgery Versus Radical Nephroureterectomy for Upper Tract Urothelial Carcinoma: An Updated Systematic Review and Meta-analysis. *Eur. Urol. Focus.* **2023**, *9*, 236–240. [CrossRef]
40. Knoedler, J.J. Outcomes of endoscopic management of upper tract urothelial carcinoma. *Transl. Androl. Urol.* **2020**, *9*, 1821–1830. [CrossRef]
41. Chen, Y.T.; Yeh, H.C.; Lee, H.Y.; Hsieh, P.F.; Chou, E.C.; Tsai, Y.C.; Hong, J.H.; Huang, C.Y.; Jiang, Y.H.; Lee, Y.K.; et al. Endoscopic management of upper tract urothelial cancer in a highly endemic area: A Taiwan nationwide collaborative study. *Asian J. Surg.* **2023**, *46*, 3058–3065. [CrossRef] [PubMed]
42. Hoffman, A.; Yossepowitch, O.; Erlich, Y.; Holland, R.; Lifshitz, D. Oncologic results of nephron sparing endoscopic approach for upper tract low grade transitional cell carcinoma in comparison to nephroureterectomy—A case control study. *BMC Urol.* **2014**, *14*, 97. [CrossRef] [PubMed]
43. Wen, J.; Ji, Z.G.; Li, H.Z. Treatment of upper tract urothelial carcinoma with ureteroscopy and thulium laser: A retrospective single center study. *BMC Cancer.* **2018**, *18*, 196. [CrossRef]
44. Ou, Y.C.; Hu, C.Y.; Cheng, H.L.; Yang, W.H. Long-term outcomes of total ureterectomy with ileal-ureteral substitution treatment for ureteral cancer: A single-center experience. *BMC Urol.* **2018**, *18*, 73. [CrossRef]
45. Wei, W.; Liu, J.; Wang, L.; Duan, X.; Ding, D. Segmental ureterectomy for high-risk ureteral carcinoma: A preliminary report. *BMC Urol.* **2023**, *23*, 103. [CrossRef]
46. Jia, Z.; Gong, Y.Q.; Zhang, C.J.; Bao, Z.Q.; Li, X.S.; Hao, H.; Xiong, G.Y.; Zhang, L.; Fang, D.; He, Z.S.; et al. Segmental ureterectomy can be performed safely in patients with urothelial carcinoma of distal ureter. *Can. Urol. Assoc. J.* **2019**, *13*, E202–E209. [CrossRef]

47. Campi, R.; Cotte, J.; Sessa, F.; Seisen, T.; Tellini, R.; Amparore, D.; Mormile, N.; Gobert, A.; Mari, A.; Porpiglia, F.; et al. Robotic radical nephroureterectomy and segmental ureterectomy for upper tract urothelial carcinoma: A multi-institutional experience. *World J. Urol.* **2019**, *37*, 2303–2311. [CrossRef]
48. Dalpiaz, O.; Ehrlich, G.; Quehenberger, F.; Pummer, K.; Zigeuner, R. Distal ureterectomy is a safe surgical option in patients with urothelial carcinoma of the distal ureter. *Urol. Oncol.* **2014**, *32*, e1–e8. [CrossRef] [PubMed]
49. Abrate, A.; Sessa, F.; Sebastianelli, A.; Preto, M.; Olivero, A.; Varca, V.; Benelli, A.; Campi, R.; Sessa, M.; Pavone, C.; et al. Segmental resection of distal ureter with termino-terminal ureteric anastomosis vs bladder cuff removal and ureteric re-implantation for upper tract urothelial carcinoma: Results of a multicentre study. *BJU Int.* **2019**, *124*, 116–123. [CrossRef]
50. Matin, S.F.; Sfakianos, J.P.; Espiritu, P.N.; Coleman, J.A.; Spiess, P.E. Patterns of Lymphatic Metastases in Upper Tract Urothelial Carcinoma and Proposed Dissection Templates. *J. Urol.* **2015**, *194*, 1567–1574. [CrossRef]
51. Campi, R.; Minervini, A.; Mari, A.; Hatzichristodoulou, G.; Sessa, F.; Lapini, A.; Sessa, M.; Gschwend, J.E.; Serni, S.; Roscigno, M.; et al. Anatomical templates of lymph node dissection for upper tract urothelial carcinoma: A systematic review of the literature. *Expert. Rev. Anticancer. Ther.* **2017**, *17*, 235–246. [CrossRef] [PubMed]
52. Fang, D.; Seisen, T.; Yang, K.; Liu, P.; Fan, X.; Singla, N.; Xiong, G.; Zhang, L.; Li, X.; Zhou, L. A systematic review and meta-analysis of oncological and renal function outcomes obtained after segmental ureterectomy versus radical nephroureterectomy for upper tract urothelial carcinoma. *Eur. J. Surg. Oncol.* **2016**, *42*, 1625–1635. [CrossRef] [PubMed]
53. Veccia, A.; Antonelli, A.; Checcucci, E.; Falagario, U.; Carrieri, G.; Guruli, G.; De Sio, M.; Simeone, C.; Porpiglia, F.; Autorino, R. Segmental Ureterectomy for Upper Tract Urothelial Carcinoma: A Systematic Review and Meta-analysis of Comparative Studies. *Clin Genitourin Cancer.* **2020**, *18*, e10–e20. [CrossRef]
54. Paciotti, M.; Alkhatib, K.Y.; Nguyen, D.D.; Yim, K.; Lipsitz, S.R.; Mossanen, M.; Casale, P.; Pierorazio, P.M.; Kibel, A.S.; Trinh, Q.D.; et al. Is Segmental Ureterectomy Associated with Inferior Survival for Localized Upper-Tract Urothelial Carcinoma of the Ureter Compared to Radical Nephroureterectomy? *Cancers.* **2023**, *15*, 1373. [CrossRef]
55. Kokorovic, A.; Matin, S.F. UGN-101 (mitomycin gel): A novel treatment for low-grade upper tract urothelial carcinoma. *Ther. Adv. Med. Oncol.* **2020**, *12*, 1758835920937950. [CrossRef] [PubMed]
56. Available online: https://www.fda.gov/drugs/resources-information-approved-drugs/fda-approves-mitomycin-low-grade-upper-tract-urothelial-cancer (accessed on 25 June 2023).
57. Kleinmann, N.; Matin, S.F.; Pierorazio, P.M.; Gore, J.L.; Shabsigh, A.; Hu, B.; Chamie, K.; Godoy, G.; Hubosky, S.; Rivera, M.; et al. Primary chemoablation of low-grade upper tract urothelial carcinoma using UGN-101, a mitomycin-containing reverse thermal gel (OLYMPUS): An open-label, single-arm, phase 3 trial. *Lancet Oncol.* **2020**, *21*, 776–785. [CrossRef]
58. Matin, S.F.; Pierorazio, P.M.; Kleinmann, N.; Gore, J.L.; Shabsigh, A.; Hu, B.; Chamie, K.; Godoy, G.; Hubosky, S.G.; Rivera, M.; et al. Durability of Response to Primary Chemoablation of Low-Grade Upper Tract Urothelial Carcinoma Using UGN-101, a Mitomycin-Containing Reverse Thermal Gel: OLYMPUS Trial Final Report. *J. Urol.* **2022**, *207*, 779–788. [CrossRef]
59. Rose, K.M.; Murray, K.S.; Labbate, C.; Woldu, S.; Linehan, J.; Jacob, J.; Kaimakliotis, H.; Dickstein, R.; Feldman, A.; Matin, S.F.; et al. Mitomycin Gel (UGN-101) as a Kidney-sparing Treatment for Upper Tract Urothelial Carcinoma in Patients with Imperative Indications and High-grade Disease. *Eur. Urol. Focus* **2023**, S2405-4569(23)00085-8, *Online ahead of print.* [CrossRef]
60. Rosen, G.H.; Nallani, A.; Muzzey, C.; Murray, K.S. Antegrade Instillation of UGN-101 (Mitomycin for Pyelocalyceal Solution) for Low-Grade Upper Tract Urothelial Carcinoma: Initial Clinical Experience. *J. Urol.* **2022**, *207*, 1302–1311. [CrossRef]
61. Linehan, J.; Gottlieb, J.; Woldu, S.L.; Labbate, C.; Rose, K.; Sexton, W.; Kaimakliotis, H.; Jacob, J.; Dickstein, R.; Nieder, A.; et al. Route of Administration for UGN-101 and Impact on Oncological and Safety Outcomes. *Eur. Urol. Focus* **2023**, S2405-4569(23)00123-2, *Online ahead of print.* [CrossRef] [PubMed]
62. Yip, W.; Sjoberg, D.D.; Nogueira, L.M.; Tracey, A.T.; Alvim, R.G.; Reisz, P.A.; Demac, Q.; Benfante, N.E.; Vanden Berg, R.W.; Kim, K.; et al. Final Results of a Phase I Trial of WST-11 (TOOKAD Soluble) Vascular-targeted Photodynamic Therapy for Upper Tract Urothelial Carcinoma. *J. Urol.* **2023**, *209*, 863–871. [CrossRef] [PubMed]
63. Available online: https://classic.clinicaltrials.gov/ct2/show/NCT04620239 (accessed on 25 June 2023).
64. Ghoreifi, A.; Ladi-Seyedian, S.S.; Piatti, P.; Chew, Y.C.; Jara, B.; Sanossian, L.; Bhasin, J.M.; Yamada, T.; Fuchs, G.; Bhanvadia, S.; et al. A Urine-based DNA Methylation Marker Test to Detect Upper Tract Urothelial Carcinoma: A Prospective Cohort Study. *J. Urol.* **2023**, *209*, 854–862. [CrossRef]
65. Shishido, S.N.; Ghoreifi, A.; Sayeed, S.; Courcoubetis, G.; Huang, A.; Ye, B.; Mrutyunjaya, S.; Gill, I.S.; Kuhn, P.; Mason, J.; et al. Liquid Biopsy Landscape in Patients with Primary Upper Tract Urothelial Carcinoma. *Cancers.* **2022**, *14*, 3007. [CrossRef]

cancers

MDPI

Review

Minimally Invasive Radical Nephroureterectomy: 5-Year Update of Techniques and Outcomes

Antonio Franco [1,2], Francesco Ditonno [1,3], Carol Feng [1], Celeste Manfredi [1,4], Morgan R. Sturgis [1], Mustafa Farooqi [1], Francesco Del Giudice [5], Christopher Coogan [1], Matteo Ferro [6], Chao Zhang [7], Zhenjie Wu [7], Bo Yang [7], Linhui Wang [7] and Riccardo Autorino [1,*]

1 Department of Urology, Rush University, Chicago, IL 60612, USA; antonio_franco@rush.edu (A.F.); francesco_ditonno@rush.edu (F.D.); carol_feng@rush.edu (C.F.); celeste_manfredi@rush.edu (C.M.); morgan_r_sturgis@rush.edu (M.R.S.); mustafafarooqi96@gmail.com (M.F.); christopher_coogan@rush.edu (C.C.)
2 Department of Urology, Sant'Andrea Hospital, Sapienza University, 00189 Rome, Italy
3 Department of Urology, Azienda Ospedaliera Universitaria Integrata Verona, University of Verona, 37126 Verona, Italy
4 Urology Unit, Department of Woman, Child and General and Specialized Surgery, University of Campania "Luigi Vanvitelli", 80138 Naples, Italy
5 Department of Maternal Infant and Urologic Sciences, Policlinico Umberto I Hospital, "Sapienza" University of Rome, 00161 Rome, Italy; francesco.delgiudice@uniroma1.it
6 Division of Urology, European Institute of Oncology (IEO), IRCCS, 20141 Milan, Italy; matteo.ferro@ieo.it
7 Department of Urology, Changhai Hospital, Naval Medical University, Shanghai 200433, China; tonyzhangchanghai@163.com (C.Z.); wuzhenjie17@163.com (Z.W.); boyangchanghai@163.com (B.Y.); wanglinhuicz@163.com (L.W.)
* Correspondence: riccardo_autorino@rush.edu

Simple Summary: Minimally invasive radical nephroureterectomy is gaining momentum among upper tract urothelial carcinoma management by offering oncological radicality and less surgical morbidity. Long-term oncological outcomes suggest that it is a safe and effective treatment option for upper tract urothelial cancer.

Abstract: The gold standard treatment for non-metastatic upper tract urothelial cancer (UTUC) is represented by radical nephroureterectomy (RNU). The choice of surgical technique in performing UTUC surgery continues to depend on several factors, including the location and extent of the tumor, the patient's overall health, and very importantly, the surgeon's skill, experience, and preference. Although open and laparoscopic approaches are well-established treatments, evidence regarding robot-assisted radical nephroureterectomy (RANU) is growing. Aim of our study was to perform a critical review on the evidence of the last 5 years regarding surgical techniques and outcomes of minimally invasive RNU, mostly focusing on RANU. Reported oncological and function outcomes suggest that minimally invasive RNU is safe and effective, showing similar survival rates compared to the open approach.

Keywords: kidney surgery; robotic urologic surgery; robot-assisted; upper tract urothelial carcinoma; ureterectomy

1. Introduction

Radical nephroureterectomy (RNU) continues to be the standard of care for upper tract urothelial carcinoma (UTUC) [1]. Historically, the procedure was performed using an open approach to access the kidney and ureter, however, there has been a major shift towards minimally invasive techniques over the past two decades [2]. First reported by Clayman in 1991 [3], laparoscopic nephroureterectomy was subsequently followed by robotic-assisted nephroureterectomy (RANU), with first case reported in 2006 [4].

Several potential benefits are associated with minimally invasive techniques, including reduced blood loss, shorter hospital stays, and faster recovery times [5]. With the introduction of the Xi platform (Intuitive Surgical, Sunnyvale, CA, USA), which is designed for "multi-quadrant" procedures, single stage RANU has been facilitated, which allowed to reduce operative time without the need to change patient's position and/or robot's docking. More recently, SP system hit the market [6,7] (da Vinci SP® surgical system, Intuitive, Sunnyvale, CA, USA) and it might allow further advances.

Regardless of the approach, distal ureter and bladder cuff management is a fundamental step of RNU, as it highly impacts oncological results. Poorer cancer specific and overall survival were observed in patients who did not undergo complete resection of a bladder cuff [8,9]. Furthermore, several factors might impact oncological outcomes of UTUC patients undergoing RNU [10].

The aim of the present critical review is to provide a comprehensive analysis of the latest techniques and innovative approaches of minimally invasive RNU in the last 5 years, as well as the related oncologic and functional outcomes.

2. Literature Search Methodology

A non-systematic literature review was conducted in June 2023. PubMed and Scopus databases were explored to retrieve publications related to minimally invasive RNU from 2018 to 2023. A different combination of the following keywords was used for a title/abstract search: "nephroureterectomy"; "robotic surgery"; "robotic kidney surgery"; "robot-assisted"; "minimally invasive"; "laparoscopic"; "segmental"; "distal"; "ureter"; "ureterectomy". Conference abstracts, review articles (except meta-analyses), editorials, commentaries, and letters to the editor were excluded from the search. Only English articles were included. Latest 5 years 'references from selected articles were also assessed for inclusion after careful evaluation by a senior author. An evidence-based critical analysis was conducted by focusing on the latest innovative techniques described in the literature, as well as oncological and renal functional outcomes.

3. Surgical Techniques

3.1. Single Stage Robotic Radical Nephroureterectomy

RANU is a multi-quadrant surgery, which in the early robotic era demanded patient repositioning and redocking to allow access to both upper and lower urinary tract [11]. Later, investigators implemented a linear port arrangement to perform a "single stage" RANU [12]. This was initially described for the Si system [13], but it has become more established with the introduction of the Xi system (Figure 1).

In 2022 Veccia et al. [6] described a series of Xi® single stage RANU in 148 patients through the ROBUUST multicenter collaborative group. Median operative time and estimated blood loss were 215.5 min and 100.0 mL, respectively; post-operative complications were 26 (17.7%) with 4 major ones (2.7%), while bladder cuff excision (BCE) and lymph node dissection were performed in 96% and 38.1% of the procedures, respectively [6]. An important aspect to be considered is the benefit and facilitation in performing one of the most challenging and fundamental RNU steps, the bladder cuff excision. In fact, a fully intracorporeal completion of this step was achieved in almost all the cases, proving that the utilization of the Xi® system effectively resolves the ongoing debate on how this aspect of the procedure should be approached, thereby excising en-bloc distal ureter, ureteral-vesical junction, and bladder cuff.

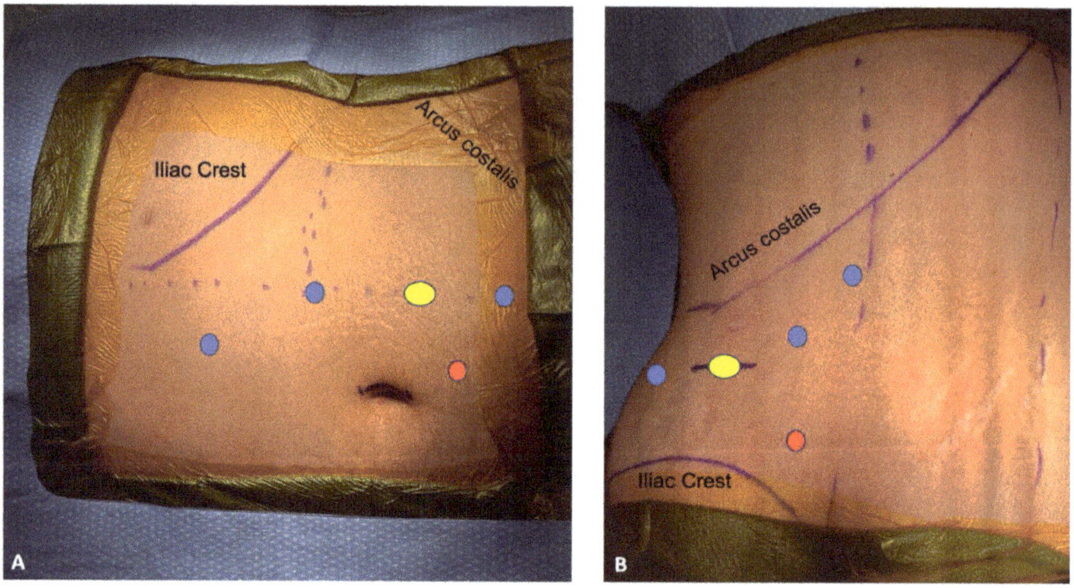

Figure 1. Robotic Nephroureterectomy (RANU) ports placement. (**A**) Single stage Transperitoneal RANU; (**B**) Retroperitoneal RANU, Blu circle: 8 mm Robotic Port; Yellow circle: 8 mm Camera Port; Red Circle: 12 mm Assistant Port.

3.2. Retroperitoneal Robotic Radical Nephroureterectomy

Despite some potential advantages of a retroperitoneal approach, this has been challenging in the case of RANU procedure, mainly because of limited working space [14,15].

Sparwasser et al. published the first series of completely retroperitoneal robot-assisted radical nephroureterectomy (RRNU) [16], and subsequently compared this technique to the standard transperitoneal approach [17]. In this scenario, ports placement starts from the Petit's triangle and then follows a line above the iliac crest (Figure 2). As the procedure advances towards the nephrectomy stage, the robot is docked parallel to the spine with the arms pointing towards the head; after releasing the middle ureter, re-docking is performed by 180°-twist of the main joint of the robot without the need for relocation, with the trajectory of the arms towards the leg. Interestingly, given the possibility to twist and rotate the whole robot system, the authors reported only a 7 min additional time for re-docking, while most series have cited an additional 30 to 60 min [15]. Regarding BCE, only in the case of RRNU, a V-Loc (Covidien, Dublin) suture is placed at the medial dissection margin of the bladder, to prevent the potential retraction of the bladder wall prior to BCE.

Perioperative outcomes demonstrated no significant differences in terms of complications nor survival. To note, RRNU showed significantly shorter surgery time and length of stay, compared to the transperitoneal approach [17]. On the other hand, trocar placement usually requires more time than the transperitoneal approach, due to the complexity of creating the retroperitoneal working space [18].

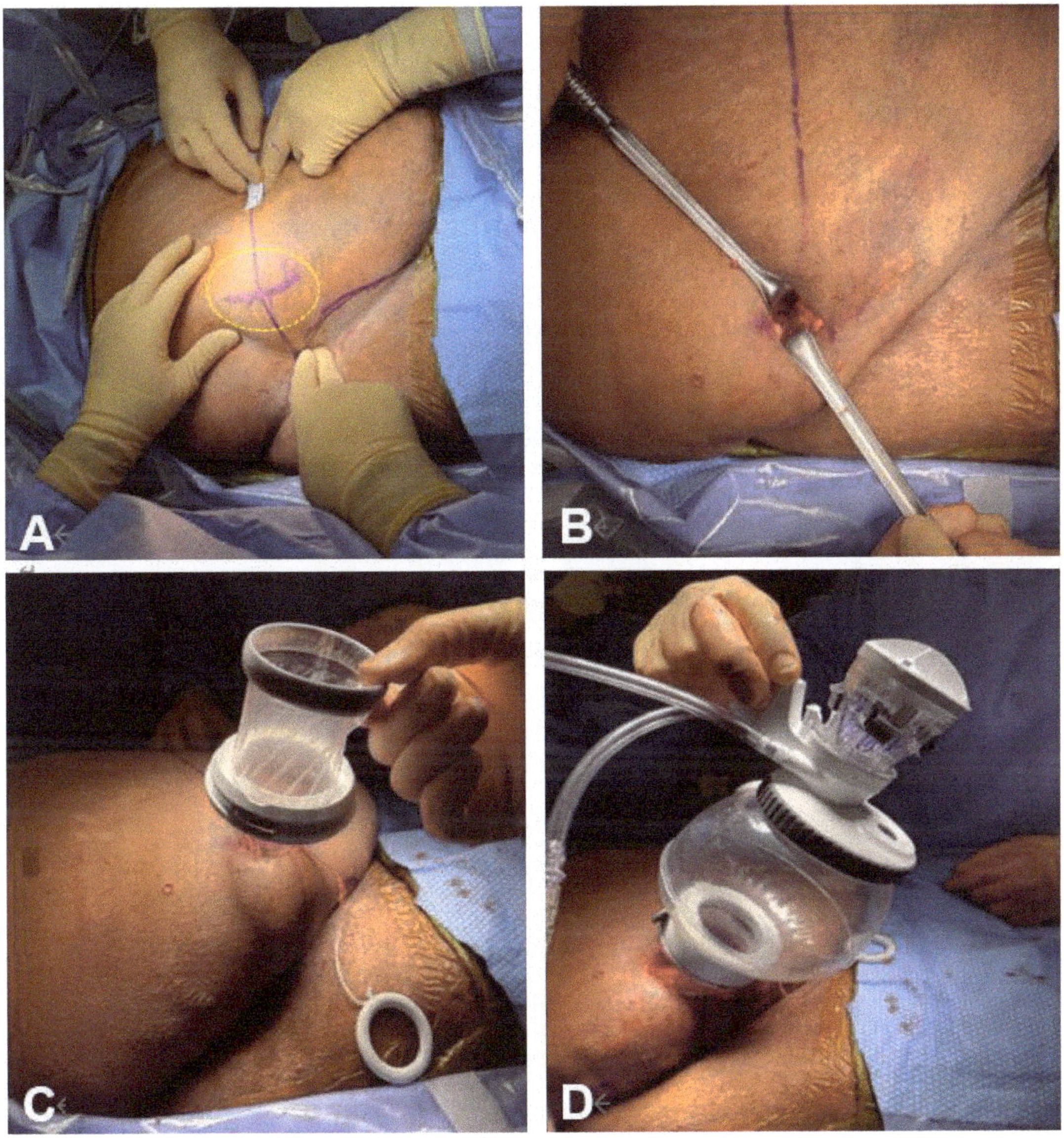

Figure 2. SARA access. (**A**) Incision site at McBurney point, 3 cm medial and 3 cm caudal to the anterior superior iliac spine; (**B**) 3 cm incision; (**C**) Wound retractor insertion; (**D**) SP access port placement. SARA: Supine Anterior Retroperitoneal Access; SP: Single Port.

3.3. Distal Ureterectomy and Bladder Cuff Excision

Various techniques have been outlined for BCE, such as open excision, transurethral resection of the ureteral orifice, ureteric intussusception, and pure laparoscopic or robotic approaches [19]. When attempting to compare outcomes between endoscopic, open or minimally invasive approaches for optimal BCE management, no clear consensus was gained [1]. However, some studies reported different findings in terms of intravesical recurrence, showing poorer outcomes for the endoscopic and laparoscopic [20–24].

Nevertheless, BCE by minimally invasive approaches have been implemented over the last decade. Recently, Wu et al. [25] proposed a modified retroperitoneoscopic technique that embraces the three goals for a safe and complete BCE: en-bloc excision, mucosa-to-mucosa reliable closure of the bladder opening, and no visible urine spillage. Compared to "blind" extravesical clamping techniques where essentially the distal ureter is clamped with Endo-GIA (Medtronic, Watford, UK) or Bulldogs without a proper individuation of the bladder plaque, this approach relies on maintaining tension on the ureter and meticulously incising through the bladder's muscular layer until a substantial funnel-shaped segment of the bladder mucosa is obtained in a circumferential manner. In doing so, the distal ureter along with the bladder cuff can be easily excised en-bloc, allowing a watertight suture of the bladder defect. BCE trifecta was observed in 95% of the patients, demonstrating oncological safety of the procedure. To note, even if only one patient experienced a bladder recurrence, follow-up of the study was too short (median: 7 months) to draw substantial conclusions [25].

Worth mentioning despite the small case series, is the keyhole technique proposed by the University of Southern California team [26]. Maintaining a single position and a single docking, the distal ureter is first clipped and then the ureteral-vesical junction (UVJ) is released. A keyhole incision is performed just above the UVJ, to better identify the ureteral orifice that is subsequently excised under direct vision. In doing so, resection margins are more precisely delineated, maintaining oncologic principles of en-bloc excision without necessitating secondary cystotomy incision or concomitant endoscopic procedure. Only three patients experienced bladder recurrence and one postoperative complication was reported [26]. Again, results should be interpreted with caution due to the relatively small sample size and the lack of a control group.

3.4. SP Robotic Radical Nephroureterectomy

Ongoing advancements led to the introduction of the Single-Port platform (da Vinci SP® surgical system, Intuitive, Sunnyvale, CA, USA). This novel platform accommodates all the robotic instruments and camera through a single multichannel 2.5 cm port inserted through a single skin incision.

To date, only a limited number of studies have documented Single-Port RNU, wherein dissection of the distal ureter and resection of the bladder cuff were conducted prior to the completion of nephrectomy, all without the need of altering the patient's position or re-docking of the robotic system [7,27]. In fact, the da Vinci SP platform can pivot 360° around the access port, facilitating easy access to both the renal and pelvic quadrants via the same single incision.

A novel approach named SARA (Supine Anterior Retroperitoneal access) for kidney surgery, including nephroureterectomy, was recently described by Pellegrino et al. in order to gain anterior access to the retroperitoneum [7]. A 3-cm incision at the McBurney point, 3 cm medial and 3 cm caudal to the anterior superior iliac spine is performed. Subsequently, dissection of the abdominal muscles facilitates the development of the retroperitoneal space for the insertion of the da Vinci SP access port. Delicate finger dissection is then employed to carefully separate the peritoneum's anterior reflection from the transversus abdominis muscle, creating sufficient room for the robotic access port placement (Figure 2). Advantages of the SARA technique primarily lies in the rapid access it provides to the renal hilum, as well as the easier dissection of the ureter. Regarding perioperative outcomes, the study reported a high rate of same-day discharges and a complete absence of narcotic administration, implying further potential benefits of this approach, that include reduced anesthesiologic complications thanks to the supine patient position [7].

4. Oncological Outcomes

Despite the above-mentioned progress in techniques, oncologic outcomes are still unsatisfactory, making UTUC a potentially deadly disease [28]. Risk of recurrence during follow-up, such as bladder, local, or distant recurrence can reach 47%, 18%, and 17% respectively [29,30], while 5-yr CSS rate are around <50% for pT2/pT3 and <10% for pT4 [31,32]. Several factors might impact the oncologic outcomes of UTUC patient, including type of treatment (open vs. minimally invasive, BCE vs. non-BCE), patient comorbidities (diabetes, acute/chronic kidney injury) and tumor features (grade, size, location, and histology) [33]. Latest oncological updates mainly involve the type of treatment used and histology variants (Table 1).

Table 1. Oncological outcomes of Radical Nephroureterectomy: literature overview.

Study Name	Year	Type of Study	*N* of Cases	Topic	Main Results
Inamoto [34]	2018	Retrospective two-arm comparative study	163	Variant Histology p-CIS vs. c-CIS	10 yrs CSS: p-CIS 111.8 months c-CIS 85.9 months
Upfill-Brown [35]	2019	Retrospective two-arm comparative study (NCDB Database)	16,783	Nephroureterectomy vs. Endoscopic Management	ET worse OS vs. RNU (HR 1.43; $p = 0.006$)
Nazzani [36]	2020	Retrospective two-arm comparative study (SEER Database)	4266	RNU + BCE vs. RNU	5 yrs CSM: BCE 19.7% vs. No BCE 23.5% ($p = 0.005$) ± BCE (HR 1.14; $p = 0.1$)
Peyronnet [22]	2019	Meta-analysis	7554	Laparoscopic vs. Open RNU	CSS, RFS, MFS: $p = 0.2$, $p = 0.86$, and $p = 0.12$ pT3/HG Open vs. Lap ($p < 0.05$)
Veccia [37]	2020	Meta-analysis	87,291	Robotic vs. Lap vs. Open RNU	RANU vs. Lap vs. Open RFS: 0.99; CSS: 0.83
Mori [38]	2020	Meta-analysis	12,865	Variant Histology	CSS: HR 2.00 OS: HR 1.76 RFS: HR 1.64
Kawada [39]	2023	Meta-analysis	N/A	Nephroureterectomy vs. Endoscopic Management	OS: HR 1.27 CSS: HR 1.37

4.1. *Bladder Cuff vs. Non-Bladder Cuff Excision*

Despite recommendations from both the National Comprehensive Cancer Network (NCCN) [40] and the European Association of Urology (EAU) [41] to perform RNU with BCE, studies showed controversial results, thus increasing research focusing on this topic [36,42].

Nazzani et al. [35] questioned the effect of BCE on survival and assessed rates of guidelines adherence and implementation by investigating the Surveillance, Epidemiology, and End Results (SEER) database. Interestingly, presence or absence of BCE at RNU did not influence cancer specific mortality (CSM) or other-cause mortality (OCM). Moreover, BCE rates did show an increasing trend over time, thereby proving enhanced guidelines' adherence in recent years.

However, as usually encountered when employing databases of this nature, information regarding type of surgical approach or BCE' techniques, as well as features on possible chemotherapy status or cancer recurrence are missing. Nevertheless, these findings showed an encouraging improvement in guidelines' adherence, but also revealed that more than 25% of RNUs are still performed without BCE [35].

4.2. Minimally Invasive vs. Open RNU

Despite the incremental diffusion of minimally invasive surgery during the last decade, controversy still exists on the differential perioperative and oncological outcomes of both robotic and laparoscopic versus open RNU [39,43,44].

According to the latest evidence, a recent systematic review of 7554 patients conducted by the EAU Guidelines panel suggests that laparoscopic bladder cuff excision appears to be associated with inferior oncologic outcomes, characterized by an increased rate of intravesical recurrence. Indeed, BCE in laparoscopic groups was performed via an open approach in most of the studies, and poorest outcomes were identified just in the former ones and in selected subgroups of patients with locally advanced (pT3/pT4) or high-grade disease, raising doubts on the importance of BCE rather than the proper type of surgical technique [45].

Regarding robotic approach, Veccia et al. [46] successfully evaluated over 87,000 RNU cases through a comprehensive and large metanalysis of 80 studies overall. Although most of each sample size was relatively small and randomized and prospective studies were lacking, results suggest that RANU appears to be a safe procedure, exhibiting the benefits of a minimally invasive approach without impairing the oncological outcomes. More specifically, when analyzing survival rates, no statistically significant differences were observed among hand-assisted laparoscopic nephroureterectomy (HALNU), laparoscopic and RANU in terms of 2- and 5-year recurrence free survival (RFS) and CSS. Noteworthy, no correlation between the surgical technique and RFS and CSS were found [46].

Notwithstanding these results, there is still an open debate regarding the best approach to adopt when dealing with locally advanced or invasive (T3/T4 and/or N+/M+) tumors. Some studies have reported atypical sites of recurrence such as port-sites metastases, peritoneal and abdominal wall implants after minimally invasive RNU [23,37]. On the other hand, cases of peritoneal cancer dissemination have been reported, but never reaching a statistical difference between the open and minimally invasive technique [47]. However, European guidelines still recommend an open approach to prevent tumor seeding in these advanced cases [38].

Despite the increasing popularity of minimally invasive RNU, persistent concerns regarding its use are pending, and the optimal surgical technique for RNU remains to be definitively established. Future clinical investigations are warranted to effectively address this issue.

4.3. Lymphadenectomy

The impact of Lymph Node Dissection (LND) on oncological outcomes in UTUC remains unclear [34,48]. Studies assessing the efficacy of LND during RNU, in terms of indication, extent and anatomical templates, are still controversial and debated in literature [34,41,49]. According to the latest update of the European guidelines, template based LND has a greater impact on patient survival, improving CSS and reducing the risk of local recurrence [38]. These data are further strengthened by one of the largest meta-analyses recently performed, which substantially confirmed the role of LND as a good staging procedure for UTUC disease, revealing an incidence of 13–40% of positive lymph nodes in cN0 $\geq$pT2 patients. Moreover, LND enhanced CSS in $\geq$pT2 renal pelvis tumors, thereby reducing the probability of regional lymph node metastases. However, this advantage was not evident in the case of ureteral tumors [50].

A multicenter retrospective analysis of the ROBUUST registry evaluated OS and RFS of three different cohorts who did not undergo LND (pNx), underwent LND with negative lymph nodes (pN0) and underwent LND with positive nodes (pN+), respectively. Results showed an important difference between pN+ cohort and the other two groups of patients in terms of 2 yrs OS (42% vs. 80%, 86%, $p < 0.001$) and RFS (35% vs. 53%, 61%, ($p < 0.001$). Therefore, LND during RNU in patients with positive lymph nodes provides prognostic data, but is not associated with improved OS; indeed, a poor prognosis is observed in this specific set of patients [51].

4.4. Impact of Histologic Variants

An additional significant factor that may influence oncological outcomes and survival rate after RNU is the presence of a histologic variant, for instance a micropapillary or sarcomatoid tumor. The incidence of such histologic variants has been documented between 7.9% to 11.8% [52].

Confirming this evidence through an extensive metanalysis, Mori et al. demonstrated a significant correlation with unfavorable outcomes for variant histology, in terms of CSS, OS and RFS. A subsequent subgroup analysis further revealed that specific variant histology, such as micropapillary and squamous and/or glandular variants, were particularly associated with poorer CSS [53].

A multi-institutional study conducted by the ROBUUST collaborative group evaluated the impact of histologic variants on oncological outcomes in patients who underwent RANU. According to the literature' incidence, the most common variant encountered was squamous followed by micropapillary and sarcomatoid, within a total of 70 patients out of 687 (10.2%). Oncologic outcomes revealed an increased risk of metastasis and death for patients with these variants. However, on multivariable analysis, OS rates and the risk of urothelial recurrence in the bladder or contralateral kidney were not affected by the presence of histologic variants [54].

Furthermore, RNU outcomes following a diagnosis of primary or concomitant carcinoma in situ (CIS) have been poorly explored. For this reason, the Nishinihon Uro-Oncology Collaborative Group [55] first attempted to compare prognostic features between primary and concomitant CIS in a multicenter study. Within a cohort of 163 patients diagnosed with either primary or concomitant CIS following RNU, intriguingly, they discovered that 10 yrs CSS was significantly longer in patients with pure/primary CIS rather than in concomitant CIS ones (111.8 vs. 85.89 months).

The current analysis represents the first description of the natural course of primary CIS in the upper tract managed by surgery [55]. According to the following outcomes, concomitant CIS in the upper tract might be a potential marker of aggressive alterations and therefore, patients presenting with such histology may benefit from multimodal therapeutic approaches, including the possibility of neoadjuvant or adjuvant chemotherapy.

5. Renal Functional Outcomes

Besides cancer control, preservation of renal function is one of the primary goals of UTUC management. Achieving renal function preservation in patient who underwent RNU can be notably challenging due to several factors, including prevalence of chronic kidney disease (CKD), renal associated comorbidities (hypertension, diabetes) and cisplatin-based chemotherapy, which is also an important consideration for patients with high-risk tumors [56,57].

Recent studies have investigated the role of renal function variation after RNU with the aim of predicting renal function recovery, to better counsel patient candidate to adjuvant treatment [58,59]. Dividing a cohort of patients undergoing RNU in relation to their eGFR, Lee et al. showed that cumulative incidence of eGFR recovery was significantly higher in patients with low baseline eGFR ($\leq$60 mL/min) compared to those with high baseline eGFR ($\geq$60), with recovery rates at 2 years of 56.6% and 27.7%, respectively. Interestingly, on multivariable analysis both preoperative hydronephrosis and eGFR $\leq$60 were significant predictors of renal function recovery [60].

These findings were partially confirmed later by a multicenter study conducted by the RaNeO research consortium [61], where the presence of hydronephrosis was associated with lower renal function reduction. A possible explanation of this phenomenon could rely on the fact that established contralateral compensatory kidney hypertrophy of the ipsilateral urinary tract facilitates the compensatory role of the remnant solitary kidney.

On the other hand, recent evidence suggests that preoperative eGFR $\leq$60 might have a negative impact on renal function recovery [62,63]. Moreover, a detrimental effect of postoperative acute kidney injury on eGFR can still be recognized at 6 and 12 months after surgery [61].

Notably, a nomogram predicting renal insufficiency for cisplatin-based adjuvant chemotherapy after minimally invasive RNU was developed. Including age, BMI, preoperative eGFR and hydronephrosis, this tool showed an accuracy of 77% after external validation, further implemented by dividing the cohort in low-risk and high-risk patients. In doing so, this prognostic tool might help in the discernment of treatment options in UTUC patients [64].

As a matter of fact, these results may prove important clinical implications: in the context of radical surgery as RNU, timely detection of patients who are at major risk of experiencing a reduction in eGFR and are no longer suitable candidates for adjuvant therapy, may take advantage from neoadjuvant treatment strategies, resulting in survival's increase. Conversely, patients who are ineligible for neoadjuvant therapy face an elevated risk of encountering a decline in renal function after RNU. For such individuals, kidney-sparing surgical interventions may be suggested, as they can mitigate the morbidity associated with radical surgery while preserving acceptable oncological outcomes.

6. Future Perspectives

As we continue to advance our understanding of UTUC management, several key areas of research and innovation emerge as critical for the future. These directions aim to further improve patient outcomes, refine surgical techniques, and enhance our understanding of the disease.

One of the most promising avenues for future research in UTUC is the development of precision medicine approaches. Identifying specific biomarkers that can predict treatment response and prognosis is crucial. Genomic and molecular profiling of UTUC tumors may help tailor treatments, such as targeted therapies or immunotherapies, to individual patients, especially the ones affected by Lynch syndrome [65,66].

Notably, variations in microsatellite instability (MSI) 678 frequency and hypermethylation status have been documented between UTUC and bladder urothelial carcinoma (BUC) [67,68]. Patients with Lynch syndrome face an elevated risk of developing UTUC more often than BUC when compared to the general population [66]. These distinctions could potentially offer additional prospects for clinical advantages from immune-checkpoint inhibitor therapy in a select group of individuals with MSI.

Furthermore, higher incidence of FGFR3 mutations in UTUC compared to BUC have been reported by earlier investigations [69,70]. This might be related to biological differences between the two types of urothelial cancer. In fact, UTUC more frequently exhibits gene expression patterns consistent with a luminal urothelial carcinoma molecular subtype, while BUC tends to express genes associated with urothelial basal cells and the basal-like subtype [65,69]. These biological distinctions may potentially impact the response to immune-checkpoint inhibition therapy and warrant the need of distinct clinical trials involving targeted therapies.

Another potential tool that is certainly crucial in UTUC treatment strategy, as suggested and confirmed by European Guidelines, is the use of prognostic models [41]. Among them, nomograms may serve as a user-friendly instrument for estimating an individual patient's risk of experiencing a particular event, such as tumor recurrence or mortality [71]. For instance, evaluating the risk before surgery aims to determine the most appropriate treatment approach for patients with localized disease: kidney sparing surgery for low-risk and radical nephroureterectomy for high-risk patients [72]. Furthermore, as previously reported, postoperative risk stratification may help deciding the administration of adjuvant chemotherapy and better defining the follow-up strategy [64]. Over the past decades, various nomograms have been developed for postoperative UTUC patient counseling [73]. However, there is still a lack of knowledge on the practicality and accuracy of these tools, with particular concern about their limited use in routine clinical practice.

Finally, collaboration between urologists, oncologists, pathologists, radiologists, and other experts is vital for advancing UTUC research. Multidisciplinary tumor boards should be established to discuss complex cases and develop personalized treatment plans. These collaborations can facilitate the translation of research findings into clinical practice.

7. Conclusions

Minimally invasive techniques have become well-established in the management of UTUC. RANU is rapidly becoming the new standard for minimally invasive RNU in many Centers. Both the transperitoneal and retroperitoneal approaches were shown to be effective and feasible, equally maintaining surgical radicality and safeness, although the choice of BCE technique remains key to maximize oncological results. Preserving renal function is mandatory since is the most common cause of cisplatin-based treatment ineligibility; therefore, the availability of predictive tools for assessing renal functions' decline should optimize perioperative management planning and helps in the identification of patients who most likely would benefit from neoadjuvant chemotherapy.

Author Contributions: Conceptualization, A.F. and C.F.; methodology, F.D. and C.M.; software, C.Z.; validation, Z.W., M.F. (Matteo Ferro) and C.C.; investigation, F.D.G.; resources, B.Y.; data curation, C.M.; writing—original draft preparation, A.F.; writing—review and editing, A.F. and M.F. (Mustafa Farooqi); visualization, M.R.S.; supervision, R.A.; project administration, L.W. and R.A. All authors have read and agreed to the published version of the manuscript.

Funding: This research received no external funding.

Conflicts of Interest: The authors declare no conflict of interest.

References

1. Alothman, K.I.; Mehmood, S.; Alzahrani, H.M.; Alotaibi, M.F.; Alkhudair, W.K.; Eldali, A.M. Surgical and oncological outcome after laparoscopic versus open nephroureterectomy for non-metastatic, upper-tract urothelial carcinoma: A single-centre experience. *Saudi Med. J.* **2020**, *41*, 25–33. [CrossRef] [PubMed]
2. Foerster, B.; Abufaraj, M.; Matin, S.F.; Azizi, M.; Gupta, M.; Li, W.-M.; Seisen, T.; Clinton, T.; Xylinas, E.; Mir, M.C.; et al. Pretreatment Risk Stratification for Endoscopic Kidney-sparing Surgery in Upper Tract Urothelial Carcinoma: An International Collaborative Study. *Eur. Urol.* **2021**, *80*, 507–515. [CrossRef]
3. Coleman, J.A.; Clark, P.E.; Bixler, B.R.; Buckley, D.I.; Chang, S.S.; Chou, R.; Hoffman-Censits, J.; Kulkarni, G.S.; Matin, S.F.; Pierorazio, P.M.; et al. Diagnosis and Management of Non-Metastatic Upper Tract Urothelial Carcinoma: AUA/SUO Guideline. *J. Urol.* **2023**, *209*, 1071–1081. [CrossRef]
4. Saini, S.; Pathak, R.A.; Hemal, A.K. Robotic nephroureterectomy in the management of upper tract urothelial cancer: Inching toward standard of care? *Int. Urol. Nephrol.* **2022**, *54*, 1777–1785. [CrossRef] [PubMed]
5. Clayman, R.V.; Kavoussi, L.R.; Figenshau, R.S.; Chandhoke, P.S.; Albala, D.M. Laparoscopic Nephroureterectomy: Initial Clinical Case Report. *J. Laparoendosc. Surg.* **1991**, *1*, 343–349. [CrossRef]
6. Nanigian, D.K.; Smith, W.; Ellison, L.M. Robot-Assisted Laparoscopic Nephroureterectomy. *J. Endourol.* **2006**, *20*, 463–466. [CrossRef]
7. Mullen, E.; Ahmed, K.; Challacombe, B. Systematic review of open versus laparoscopic versus robot-assisted nephroureterectomy. *Rev. Urol.* **2017**, *19*, 32–43. [PubMed]
8. Veccia, A.; Carbonara, U.; Derweesh, I.; Mehrazin, R.; Porter, J.; Abdollah, F.; Mazzone, E.; Sundaram, C.P.; Gonzalgo, M.; Mastroianni, R.; et al. Single-stage Xi® robotic radical nephroureterectomy for upper tract urothelial carcinoma: Surgical technique and outcomes. *Minerva Urol. Nephrol.* **2022**, *74*, 233–241. [CrossRef]
9. Pellegrino, A.A.; Chen, G.; Morgantini, L.; Calvo, R.S.; Crivellaro, S. Simplifying Retroperitoneal Robotic Single-port Surgery: Novel Supine Anterior Retroperitoneal Access. *Eur. Urol.* **2023**, *84*, 223–228. [CrossRef]
10. Kang, M.; Jeong, C.W.; Kwak, C.; Kim, H.H.; Ku, J.H. The Characteristics of Recurrent Upper Tract Urothelial Carcinoma after Radical Nephroureterectomy without Bladder Cuff Excision. *Yonsei Med. J.* **2015**, *56*, 375–381. [CrossRef]
11. Krabbe, L.-M.; Westerman, M.E.; Bagrodia, A.; Gayed, B.A.; Khalil, D.; Kapur, P.; Shariat, S.F.; Raj, G.V.; Sagalowsky, A.I.; Cadeddu, J.A.; et al. Surgical management of the distal ureter during radical nephroureterectomy is an independent predictor of oncological outcomes: Results of a current series and a review of the literature. *Urol. Oncol. Semin. Orig. Investig.* **2014**, *32*, 54.e19–54.e26. [CrossRef] [PubMed]
12. Kenigsberg, A.P.; Meng, X.; Ghandour, R.; Margulis, V. Oncologic outcomes of radical nephroureterectomy (RNU). *Transl. Androl. Urol.* **2020**, *9*, 1841–1852. [CrossRef] [PubMed]
13. Hemal, A.K.; Stansel, I.; Babbar, P.; Patel, M. Robotic-assisted Nephroureterectomy and Bladder Cuff Excision without Intraoperative Repositioning. *Urology* **2011**, *78*, 357–364. [CrossRef] [PubMed]

14. Zargar, H.; Krishnan, J.; Autorino, R.; Akca, O.; Brandao, L.F.; Laydner, H.; Samarasekera, D.; Ko, O.; Haber, G.-P.; Kaouk J.H.; et al. Robotic Nephroureterectomy: A Simplified Approach Requiring No Patient Repositioning or Robot Redocking. *Eur Urol.* **2014**, *66*, 769–777. [CrossRef] [PubMed]
15. Mittakanti, H.R.; Heulitt, G.; Li, H.-F.; Porter, J.R. Transperitoneal vs. retroperitoneal robotic partial nephrectomy: A matched-paired analysis. *World J. Urol.* **2020**, *38*, 1093–1099. [CrossRef]
16. Lim, S.; Teo, X.L. Robot-assisted nephroureterectomy: Current perspectives. *Robot. Surg. Res. Rev.* **2016**, *3*, 37–48. [CrossRef] [PubMed]
17. Sparwasser, P.; Epple, S.; Thomas, A.; Dotzauer, R.; Boehm, K.; Brandt, M.P.; Mager, R.; Borgmann, H.; Kamal, M.M.; Kurosch, M.; et al. First completely robot-assisted retroperitoneal nephroureterectomy with bladder cuff: A step-by-step technique. *World J. Urol.* **2022**, *40*, 1019–1026. [CrossRef] [PubMed]
18. Pathak, R.A.; Patel, M.; Hemal, A.K. Comprehensive Approach to Port Placement Templates for Robot-Assisted Laparoscopic Urologic Surgeries. *J. Endourol.* **2017**, *31*, 1269–1276. [CrossRef]
19. Sparwasser, P.; Frey, L.; Fischer, N.D.; Thomas, A.; Dotzauer, R.; Surcel, C.; Brandt, M.P.; Mager, R.; Höfner, T.; Haferkamp, A.; et al. First Comparison of Retroperitoneal Versus Transperitoneal Robot-Assisted Nephroureterectomy with Bladder Cuff: A Single Center Study. *Ann. Surg. Oncol.* **2023**, *30*, 4531–4539. [CrossRef]
20. Patel, M.N.; Aboumohamed, A.; Hemal, A. Does transition from the da Vinci Si® to Xi robotic platform impact single-docking technique for robot-assisted laparoscopic nephroureterectomy? *BJU Int.* **2015**, *116*, 990–994. [CrossRef]
21. Barton, G.J.; Tan, W.P.; Inman, B.A. The nephroureterectomy: A review of technique and current controversies. *Transl. Androl. Urol.* **2020**, *9*, 3168–3190. [CrossRef] [PubMed]
22. Li, W.-M.; Shen, J.-T.; Li, C.-C.; Ke, H.-L.; Wei, Y.-C.; Wu, W.-J.; Chou, Y.-H.; Huang, C.-H. Oncologic Outcomes Following Three Different Approaches to the Distal Ureter and Bladder Cuff in Nephroureterectomy for Primary Upper Urinary Tract Urothelial Carcinoma. *Eur. Urol.* **2010**, *57*, 963–969. [CrossRef] [PubMed]
23. Xylinas, E.; Rink, M.; Cha, E.K.; Clozel, T.; Lee, R.K.; Fajkovic, H.; Comploj, E.; Novara, G.; Margulis, V.; Raman, J.D.; et al Impact of Distal Ureter Management on Oncologic Outcomes Following Radical Nephroureterectomy for Upper Tract Urothelial Carcinoma. *Eur. Urol.* **2014**, *65*, 210–217. [CrossRef]
24. Luo, H.L.; Kang, C.H.; Chen, Y.T.; Chuang, Y.C.; Cheng, Y.T.; Lee, W.C.; Chiang, P.H. Oncological impact of endoscopic bladder cuff management during nephroureterectomy varies according to upper urinary tract tumor location. *Int. J. Urol.* **2014**, *21*, 366–369. [CrossRef] [PubMed]
25. Peyronnet, B.; Seisen, T.; Dominguez-Escrig, J.-L.; Bruins, H.M.; Yuan, C.Y.; Lam, T.; Maclennan, S.; N'dow, J.; Babjuk, M.; Comperat, E.; et al. Oncological Outcomes of Laparoscopic Nephroureterectomy Versus Open Radical Nephroureterectomy for Upper Tract Urothelial Carcinoma: An European Association of Urology Guidelines Systematic Review. *Eur. Urol. Focus* **2019**, *5*, 205–223. [CrossRef] [PubMed]
26. Katims, A.B.; Say, R.; Derweesh, I.; Uzzo, R.; Minervini, A.; Wu, Z.; Abdollah, F.; Sundaram, C.; Ferro, M.; Rha, K.; et al. Risk Factors for Intravesical Recurrence after Minimally Invasive Nephroureterectomy for Upper Tract Urothelial Cancer (ROBUUST Collaboration). *J. Urol.* **2021**, *206*, 568–576. [CrossRef]
27. Wu, Z.; Li, M.; Wang, J.; Veccia, A.; Xu, Y.; Zhang, C.; Ren, J.; Yin, L.; Chen, M.; Wang, J.; et al. Pure retroperitoneoscopic extravesical standardized seeable (PRESS) excision of distal ureter and bladder cuff in radical nephroureterectomy: Step-by-step technique. *Minerva Urol. Nephrol.* **2021**, *73*, 392–400. [CrossRef]
28. Medina, L.G.; Alsyouf, M.; Ghoreifi, A.; Sayegh, A.S.; Koh, K.; Yu, W.; Sobhani, S.; Douglawi, A.; Djaladat, H. Distal ureter and bladder cuff excision using the "Keyhole Technique" during Robotic Radical Nephroureterectomy. *Int. Braz. J. Urol.* **2022**, *48*, 876–877. [CrossRef]
29. Kim, K.H.; Ahn, H.K.; Kim, M.; Yoon, H. Technique and perioperative outcomes of single-port robotic surgery using the da Vinci SP platform in urology. *Asian J. Surg.* **2023**, *46*, 472–477. [CrossRef]
30. Martini, A.; Daza, J.; Poltiyelova, E.; Gul, Z.; Heard, J.R.; Ferket, B.S.; Waingankar, N.; Galsky, M.D.; Sfakianos, J.P. Pathological downstaging as a novel endpoint for the development of neoadjuvant chemotherapy for upper tract urothelial carcinoma. *BJU Int.* **2019**, *124*, 665–671. [CrossRef]
31. Xylinas, E.; Kluth, L.; Scherr, D.; Novara, G.; Comploj, E.; Pycha, A.; Fritsche, H.-M.; Trinh, Q.-D.; Karakiewicz, P.; Weizer, A.; et al. 573 Prediction of intravesical recurrence after radical nephroureterectomy: Development of a clinical decision-making tool. *Eur. Urol. Suppl.* **2013**, *12*, e573–e574. [CrossRef]
32. Tanaka, N.; Kikuchi, E.; Kanao, K.; Matsumoto, K.; Kobayashi, H.; Ide, H.; Miyazaki, Y.; Obata, J.; Hoshino, K.; Shirotake, S.; et al. Metastatic Behavior of Upper Tract Urothelial Carcinoma After Radical Nephroureterectomy: Association with Primary Tumor Location. *Ann. Surg. Oncol.* **2014**, *21*, 1038–1045. [CrossRef] [PubMed]
33. Jeldres, C.; Sun, M.; Isbarn, H.; Lughezzani, G.; Budäus, L.; Alasker, A.; Shariat, S.F.; Lattouf, J.-B.; Widmer, H.; Pharand, D.; et al. A Population-based Assessment of Perioperative Mortality After Nephroureterectomy for Upper-tract Urothelial Carcinoma. *Urology* **2010**, *75*, 315–320. [CrossRef]
34. Morselli, S.; Vitelli, F.D.; Verrini, G.; Sebastianelli, A.; Campi, R.; Liaci, A.; Spatafora, P.; Barzaghi, P.; Ferrari, G.; Gacci, M.; et al. Comparison of Tumor Seeding and Recurrence Rate After Laparoscopic vs. Open Nephroureterectomy for Upper Urinary Tract Transitional Cell Carcinoma. *Front. Surg.* **2021**, *8*, 769527. [CrossRef] [PubMed]

35. Capitanio, U.; Shariat, S.F.; Isbarn, H.; Weizer, A.; Remzi, M.; Roscigno, M.; Kikuchi, E.; Raman, J.D.; Bolenz, C.; Bensalah, K.; et al. Comparison of Oncologic Outcomes for Open and Laparoscopic Nephroureterectomy: A Multi-Institutional Analysis of 1249 Cases. *Eur. Urol.* **2009**, *56*, 1–9. [CrossRef]
36. Guo, R.; Zhu, Y.; Xiong, G.; Li, X.; Zhang, K.; Zhou, L. Role of lymph node dissection in the management of upper tract urothelial carcinomas: A meta-analysis. *BMC Urol.* **2018**, *18*, 24. [CrossRef] [PubMed]
37. Lughezzani, G.; Sun, M.; Perrotte, P.; Shariat, S.F.; Jeldres, C.; Buraus, L.; Alasker, A.; Duclos, A.; Widmer, H.; Latour, M.; et al. Should Bladder Cuff Excision Remain the Standard of Care at Nephroureterectomy in Patients with Urothelial Carcinoma of the Renal Pelvis? A Population-based Study. *Eur. Urol.* **2010**, *57*, 956–962. [CrossRef]
38. Veccia, A.; Antonelli, A.; Francavilla, S.; Simeone, C.; Guruli, G.; Zargar, H.; Perdoná, S.; Ferro, M.; Carrieri, G.; Hampton, L.J.; et al. Robotic versus other nephroureterectomy techniques: A systematic review and meta-analysis of over 87,000 cases. *World J. Urol.* **2020**, *38*, 845–852. [CrossRef]
39. Carrion, A.; Huguet, J.; García-Cruz, E.; Izquierdo, L.; Mateu, L.; Musquera, M.; Ribal, M.J.; Alcaraz, A. Intraoperative prognostic factors and atypical patterns of recurrence in patients with upper urinary tract urothelial carcinoma treated with laparoscopic radical nephroureterectomy. *Scand. J. Urol.* **2016**, *50*, 305–312. [CrossRef]
40. Rouprêt, M.; Hupertan, V.; Seisen, T.; Colin, P.; Xylinas, E.; Yates, D.R.; Fajkovic, H.; Lotan, Y.; Raman, J.D.; Zigeuner, R.; et al. Prediction of Cancer Specific Survival after Radical Nephroureterectomy for Upper Tract Urothelial Carcinoma: Development of an Optimized Postoperative Nomogram Using Decision Curve Analysis. *J. Urol.* **2013**, *189*, 1662–1669. [CrossRef]
41. Grob, G.; Rogers, D.; Pandolfo, S.D.; Vourganti, S.; Buscarini, M.; Mehrazin, R.; Grob, B.M.; Mir, M.C.; Perdonà, S.; Derweesh, I.H.; et al. Oncologic outcomes following radical nephroureterectomy for upper tract urothelial carcinoma: A literature review. *Transl. Androl. Urol.* **2023**, *12*, 1351–1362. [CrossRef] [PubMed]
42. Nazzani, S.; Preisser, F.; Mazzone, E.; Tian, Z.; Mistretta, F.A.; Soulières, D.; Montanari, E.; Acquati, P.; Briganti, A.; Shariat, S.F.; et al. Nephroureterectomy with or without Bladder Cuff Excision for Localized Urothelial Carcinoma of the Renal Pelvis. *Eur. Urol. Focus* **2020**, *6*, 298–304. [CrossRef] [PubMed]
43. Rouprêt, M.; Seisen, T.; Birtle, A.J.; Capoun, O.; Compérat, E.M.; Dominguez-Escrig, J.L.; Andersson, I.G.; Liedberg, F.; Mariappan, P.; Mostafid, A.H.; et al. European Association of Urology Guidelines on Upper Urinary Tract Urothelial Carcinoma: 2023 Update. *Eur. Urol.* **2023**, *84*, 49–64. [CrossRef] [PubMed]
44. Correia, J.; Mendes, G.; Texeira, B.; Madanelo, M.; Fraga, A.; Silva-Ramos, M. Perioperative and oncological outcomes of laparoscopic and open radical nephroureterectomy for locally advanced upper tract urothelial carcinoma: A single-center cohort study. *Cent. Eur. J. Urol.* **2022**, *75*, 257–264. [CrossRef]
45. Motzer, R.J.; Jonasch, E.; Bhayani, S.; Bro, W.P.; Chang, S.S.; Choueiri, T.K.; Costello, B.A.; Derweesh, I.H.; Ellis, R.; Fishman, M.; et al. *NCCN Guidelines Index Table of Contents Discussion. Kidney Cancer*; National Comprehensive Cancer Network: Plymouth Meeting, PA, USA, 2018.
46. Rouprêt, M.; Babjuk, M.; Burger, M.; Capoun, O.; Cohen, D.; Compérat, E.M.; Cowan, N.C.; Dominguez-Escrig, J.L.; Gontero, P.; Mostafid, A.H.; et al. European Association of Urology Guidelines on Upper Urinary Tract Urothelial Carcinoma: 2020 Update. *Eur. Urol.* **2021**, *79*, 62–79. [CrossRef]
47. Seisen, T.; Peyronnet, B.; Dominguez-Escrig, J.L.; Bruins, H.M.; Yuan, C.Y.; Babjuk, M.; Böhle, A.; Burger, M.; Compérat, E.M.; Cowan, N.C.; et al. Oncologic Outcomes of Kidney-sparing Surgery Versus Radical Nephroureterectomy for Upper Tract Urothelial Carcinoma: A Systematic Review by the EAU Non-muscle Invasive Bladder Cancer Guidelines Panel. *Eur. Urol.* **2016**, *70*, 1052–1068. [CrossRef]
48. Duquesne, I.; Ouzaid, I.; Loriot, Y.; Moschini, M.; Xylinas, E. Lymphadenectomy for Upper Tract Urothelial Carcinoma: A Systematic Review. *J. Clin. Med.* **2019**, *8*, 1190. [CrossRef] [PubMed]
49. Ouzzane, A.; Colin, P.; Ghoneim, T.P.; Zerbib, M.; De La Taille, A.; Audenet, F.; Saint, F.; Hoarau, N.; Adam, E.; Azemar, M.D.; et al. The impact of lymph node status and features on oncological outcomes in urothelial carcinoma of the upper urinary tract (UTUC) treated by nephroureterectomy. *World J. Urol.* **2013**, *31*, 189–197. [CrossRef]
50. Dominguez-Escrig, J.L.; Peyronnet, B.; Seisen, T.; Bruins, H.M.; Yuan, C.Y.; Babjuk, M.; Böhle, A.; Burger, M.; Compérat, E.M.; Gontero, P.; et al. Potential Benefit of Lymph Node Dissection During Radical Nephroureterectomy for Upper Tract Urothelial Carcinoma: A Systematic Review by the European Association of Urology Guidelines Panel on Non–muscle-invasive Bladder Cancer. *Eur. Urol. Focus* **2019**, *5*, 224–241. [CrossRef]
51. Hakimi, K.; Carbonara, U.; Djaladat, H.; Mehrazin, R.; Eun, D.; Reese, A.; Gonzalgo, M.L.; Margulis, V.; Uzzo, R.G.; Porter, J.; et al. Outcomes of Lymph Node Dissection in Nephroureterectomy in the Treatment of Upper Tract Urothelial Carcinoma: Analysis of the ROBUUST Registry. *J. Urol.* **2022**, *208*, 268–276. [CrossRef]
52. Chung, H.S.; Hwang, E.C.; Kim, M.S.; Yu, S.H.; Jung, S.I.; Kang, T.W.; Choi, C.; Choi, S.H.; Kwon, T.G.; Noh, J.H.; et al. Effects of Variant Histology on the Oncologic Outcomes of Patients with Upper Urinary Tract Carcinoma after Radical Nephroureterectomy: A Propensity Score-Matched Analysis. *Clin. Genitourin. Cancer* **2019**, *17*, e394–e407. [CrossRef] [PubMed]
53. Mori, K.; Janisch, F.; Parizi, M.K.; Mostafaei, H.; Lysenko, I.; Kimura, S.; Enikeev, D.V.; Egawa, S.; Shariat, S.F. Prognostic Value of Variant Histology in Upper Tract Urothelial Carcinoma Treated with Nephroureterectomy: A Systematic Review and Meta-Analysis. *J. Urol.* **2020**, *203*, 1075–1084. [CrossRef]

54. Douglawi, A.; Ghoreifi, A.; Carbonara, U.; Yip, W.; Uzzo, R.G.; Margulis, V.; Ferro, M.; De Cobelli, O.; Wu, Z.; Simone, G.; et al. Impact of Variant Histology on Oncological Outcomes in Upper Tract Urothelial Carcinoma: Results from the ROBUUST Collaborative Group. *Clin. Genitourin. Cancer* **2023**, *in press*. [CrossRef] [PubMed]
55. Inamoto, T.; Matsuyama, H.; Ibuki, N.; Komura, K.; Takahara, K.; Fujimoto, K.; Shiina, H.; Sakano, S.; Nagao, K.; Miyake, M.; et al. Biological Behavior and Long-Term Outcomes of Carcinoma In Situ in Upper Urinary Tract Managed by Radical Nephroureterectomy. *J. Urol.* **2018**, *199*, 933–939. [CrossRef] [PubMed]
56. Antonelli, A.; Minervini, A.; Sandri, M.; Bertini, R.; Bertolo, R.; Carini, M.; Furlan, M.; Larcher, A.; Mantica, G.; Mari, A.; et al. Below Safety Limits, Every Unit of Glomerular Filtration Rate Counts: Assessing the Relationship Between Renal Function and Cancer-specific Mortality in Renal Cell Carcinoma. *Eur. Urol.* **2018**, *74*, 661–667. [CrossRef]
57. Yamada, Y.; Nakagawa, T.; Miyakawa, J.; Kawai, T.; Tabata, M.; Kaneko, T.; Taguchi, S.; Naito, A.; Hikatsu, M.; Sato, Y.; et al. Smaller decline of renal function after nephroureterectomy predicts poorer prognosis of upper tract urothelial carcinoma: A multicentre retrospective study. *Jpn. J. Clin. Oncol.* **2021**, *51*, 1577–1586. [CrossRef]
58. Xylinas, E.; Rink, M.; Margulis, V.; Clozel, T.; Lee, R.K.; Comploj, E.; Novara, G.; Raman, J.D.; Lotan, Y.; Weizer, A.; et al. Impact of renal function on eligibility for chemotherapy and survival in patients who have undergone radical nephro-ureterectomy. *BJU Int.* **2013**, *112*, 453–461. [CrossRef]
59. Kaag, M.G.; O'Malley, R.L.; O'Malley, P.; Godoy, G.; Chen, M.; Smaldone, M.C.; Hrebinko, R.L.; Raman, J.D.; Bochner, B.; Dalbagni, G.; et al. Changes in Renal Function Following Nephroureterectomy May Affect the Use of Perioperative Chemotherapy. *Eur. Urol.* **2010**, *58*, 581–587. [CrossRef]
60. Lee, B.H.; Zabor, E.C.; Tennenbaum, D.; Furberg, H.; Benfante, N.; Coleman, J.A.; Jaimes, E.A.; Russo, P. Renal function recovery after radical nephroureterectomy for upper tract urothelial carcinoma. *World J. Urol.* **2018**, *36*, 257–263. [CrossRef]
61. Tafuri, A.; Marchioni, M.; Cerrato, C.; Mari, A.; Tellini, R.; Odorizzi, K.; Veccia, A.; Amparore, D.; Shakir, A.; Carbonara, U.; et al. Changes in renal function after nephroureterectomy for upper urinary tract carcinoma: Analysis of a large multicenter cohort (Radical Nephroureterectomy Outcomes (RaNeO) Research Consortium). *World J. Urol.* **2022**, *40*, 2771–2779. [CrossRef]
62. Hashimoto, T.; Ohno, Y.; Nakashima, J.; Gondo, T.; Nakagami, Y.; Namiki, K.; Horiguchi, Y.; Yoshioka, K.; Ohori, M.; Tachibana, M. Prediction of renal function after nephroureterectomy in patients with upper tract urothelial carcinoma. *Jpn. J. Clin. Oncol.* **2015**, *45*, 1064–1068. [CrossRef]
63. Rodríguez Faba, O.; Palou, J.; Breda, A.; Maroto, P.; Gómez, J.F.; Wong, A.; Villavicencio, H. Predictive Factors for Impaired Renal Function following Nephroureterectomy in Upper Urinary Tract Urothelial Cell Carcinoma. *Urol. Int.* **2014**, *92*, 169–173. [CrossRef] [PubMed]
64. Wu, Z.; Chen, Q.; Djaladat, H.; Minervini, A.; Uzzo, R.G.; Sundaram, C.P.; Rha, K.H.; Gonzalgo, M.L.; Mehrazin, R.; Mazzone, E.; et al. A Preoperative Nomogram to Predict Renal Function Insufficiency for Cisplatin-based Adjuvant Chemotherapy Following Minimally Invasive Radical Nephroureterectomy (ROBUUST Collaborative Group). *Eur. Urol. Focus* **2022**, *8*, 173–181. [CrossRef]
65. Necchi, A.; Madison, R.; Pal, S.K.; Ross, J.S.; Agarwal, N.; Sonpavde, G.; Joshi, M.; Yin, M.; Miller, V.A.; Grivas, P.; et al. Comprehensive Genomic Profiling of Upper-tract and Bladder Urothelial Carcinoma. *Eur. Urol. Focus* **2021**, *7*, 1339–1346. [CrossRef] [PubMed]
66. Lim, A.; Rao, P.; Matin, S.F. Lynch syndrome and urologic malignancies: A contemporary review. *Curr. Opin. Urol.* **2019**, *29*, 357–363. [CrossRef]
67. Catto, J.W.; Azzouzi, A.-R.; Rehman, I.; Feeley, K.M.; Cross, S.S.; Amira, N.; Fromont, G.; Sibony, M.; Cussenot, O.; Meuth, M.; et al. Promoter Hypermethylation Is Associated with Tumor Location, Stage, and Subsequent Progression in Transitional Cell Carcinoma. *J. Clin. Oncol.* **2005**, *23*, 2903–2910. [CrossRef] [PubMed]
68. Amira, N.; Rivet, J.; Soliman, H.; Cancel-Tassin, G.; LE Duc, A.; Janin, A.; Cussenot, O. Microsatellite Instability in Urothelial Carcinoma of the Upper Urinary Tract. *J. Urol.* **2003**, *170*, 1151–1154. [CrossRef]
69. Sfakianos, J.P.; Cha, E.K.; Iyer, G.; Scott, S.N.; Zabor, E.C.; Shah, R.H.; Ren, Q.; Bagrodia, A.; Kim, P.H.; Hakimi, A.A.; et al. Genomic Characterization of Upper Tract Urothelial Carcinoma. *Eur. Urol.* **2015**, *68*, 970–977. [CrossRef]
70. Le, D.T.; Uram, J.N.; Wang, H.; Bartlett, B.R.; Kemberling, H.; Eyring, A.D.; Skora, A.D.; Luber, B.S.; Azad, N.S.; Laheru, D.; et al. PD-1 Blockade in Tumors with Mismatch-Repair Deficiency. *N. Engl. J. Med.* **2015**, *372*, 2509–2520. [CrossRef]
71. Iasonos, A.; Schrag, D.; Raj, G.V.; Panageas, K.S. How To Build and Interpret a Nomogram for Cancer Prognosis. *J. Clin. Oncol.* **2008**, *26*, 1364–1370. [CrossRef]
72. Favaretto, R.L.; Shariat, S.F.; Chade, D.C.; Godoy, G.; Adamy, A.; Kaag, M.; Bochner, B.H.; Coleman, J.; Dalbagni, G. The Effect of Tumor Location on Prognosis in Patients Treated with Radical Nephroureterectomy at Memorial Sloan-Kettering Cancer Center. *Eur. Urol.* **2010**, *58*, 574–580. [CrossRef] [PubMed]
73. Pallauf, M.; König, F.; D'andrea, D.; Laukhtina, E.; Mostafaei, H.; Motlagh, R.S.; Quhal, F.; Aydh, A.; Yanagisawa, T.; Kawada, T.; et al. A Systematic Review and Meta-Analysis of Prognostic Nomograms After UTUC Surgery. *Front. Oncol.* **2022**, *12*, 907975. [CrossRef] [PubMed]

cancers MDPI

Review

Upper Tract Urothelial Carcinoma: A Narrative Review of Current Surveillance Strategies for Non-Metastatic Disease

Jakob Klemm [1,2,*,†], Kensuke Bekku [2,3,†], Mohammad Abufaraj [2,4], Ekaterina Laukhtina [2,5], Akihiro Matsukawa [2,6], Mehdi Kardoust Parizi [2], Pierre I. Karakiewicz [7] and Shahrokh F. Shariat [2,5,8,9,10,11,12]

1 Department of Urology, University Medical Center Hamburg-Eppendorf, 20251 Hamburg, Germany
2 Department of Urology, Comprehensive Cancer Center, Medical University of Vienna, 1090 Vienna, Austria; gmd421030@s.okayama-u.ac.jp (K.B.); dr.abufaraj@gmail.com (M.A.); katyalaukhtina@gmail.com (E.L.); akihiro.matsukawa@meduniwien.ac.at (A.M.); mehdi.kardoustparizi@meduniwien.ac.at (M.K.P.); shahrokh.shariat@meduniwien.ac.at (S.F.S.)
3 Department of Urology, Okayama University Graduate School of Medicine, Dentistry and Pharmaceutical Sciences, Okayama 700-8525, Japan
4 Division of Urology, Department of Special Surgery, Jordan University Hospital, The University of Jordan, Amman 11733, Jordan
5 Institute for Urology and Reproductive Health, Sechenov University, 119991 Moscow, Russia
6 Department of Urology, Jikei University School of Medicine, Tokyo 105-8461, Japan
7 Cancer Prognostics and Health Outcomes Unit, University of Montreal Health Centre, Montreal, QC H2X 3E4, Canada; pierre.karakiewicz@umontreal.ca
8 Hourani Center for Applied Scientific Research, Al-Ahliyya Amman University, Amman 11942, Jordan
9 Karl Landsteiner Institute of Urology and Andrology, 1090 Vienna, Austria
10 Department of Urology, Weill Cornell Medical College, New York, NY 10065, USA
11 Department of Urology, University of Texas Southwestern, Dallas, TX 75390, USA
12 Department of Urology, Second Faculty of Medicine, Charles University, 252 50 Prague, Czech Republic
* Correspondence: jakob.klemm@gmx.net
† These authors contributed equally to this work.

Simple Summary: Upper tract urinary carcinoma (UTUC) is a rare type of cancer affecting the urinary system. Patients with UTUC often undergo surgeries like kidney-sparing surgery or radical nephroureterectomy. However, even after treatment, there remains a risk of the cancer recurring in different parts of the body. This narrative review aims to better understand the frequency and locations of such recurrences, which is crucial for effectively monitoring patients after their initial treatment. Currently, there is limited information on the optimal methods for tracking patients post-surgery, and on how early detection of cancer, before the appearance of symptoms, might improve health outcomes. This article presents the most important current guideline recommendations and elucidates the evidence behind them. Exploring new imaging technologies and improving methods for assessing patient risk, can potentially lead to more personalized and effective monitoring plans in the near future.

Abstract: Non-metastatic upper urinary tract carcinoma (UTUC) is a comparatively rare condition, typically managed with either kidney-sparing surgery (KSS) or radical nephroureterectomy (RNU). Irrespective of the chosen therapeutic modality, patients with UTUC remain at risk of recurrence in the bladder; in patients treated with KSS, the risk of recurrence is high in the remnant ipsilateral upper tract system but there is a low but existent risk in the contralateral system as well as in the chest and in the abdomen/pelvis. For patients treated with RNU for high-risk UTUC, the risk of recurrence in the chest, abdomen, and pelvis, as well as the contralateral UT, depends on the tumor stage, grade, and nodal status. Hence, implementing a risk-stratified, location-specific follow-up is indicated to ensure timely detection of cancer recurrence. However, there are no data on the type and frequency/schedule of follow-up or on the impact of the recurrence type and site on outcomes; indeed, it is not well known whether imaging-detected asymptomatic recurrences confer a better outcome than recurrences detected due to symptoms/signs. Novel imaging techniques and more precise risk stratification methods based on time-dependent probabilistic events hold significant promise for making a cost-efficient individualized, patient-centered, outcomes-oriented follow-up strategy possible. We show and discuss the follow-up protocols of the major urologic societies.

Keywords: upper tract urothelial carcinoma; urothelial carcinoma; surveillance; follow-up

1. Introduction

Upper urinary tract carcinoma (UTUC) is a relatively rare malady, constituting approximately 5–10% of urothelial carcinomas [1]. The treatment of non-metastatic UTUC is based on risk stratification into low- vs. high-risk tumors, with preferred therapeutic options being kidney-sparing surgery (KSS) or radical nephroureterectomy (RNU) with perioperative platinum-based chemotherapy when possible and indicated [2]. Indeed, the current guidelines from the European Association of Urology (EAU), the American Urological Association (AUA), and the National Comprehensive Cancer Network (NCCN) recommend offering neoadjuvant or adjuvant chemotherapy to high-risk UTUC patients, as they have been shown to improve disease-free survival (DFS), at least in non-metastatic UTUC patients [2–5]. Recognizing the potential for metachronous bladder tumors, local recurrences, or distant metastases after RNU or KSS, the EAU, AUA, and NCCN guidelines advocate robust surveillance protocols for UTUC patients [2–4]. However, evidence on follow-up strategies after definitive treatment for non-metastatic UTUC is low. For this reason, this article aims to summarize the available evidence on surveillance after surgery for non-metastatic UTUC with curative intent.

2. Evidence Acquisition

We searched the PubMed database up to 1 October 2023 using pre-defined search criteria as follows: (Upper Tract Urothelial Carcinoma) OR (Renal Pelvic Urothelial Cancer) OR (Ureteral Urothelial Cancer) AND (Surveillance) OR (Follow-up). In addition, we assessed the references in the EAU, AUA, and NCCN guidelines.

3. Prognostic Factors for UTUC

Assessment of established prognostic factors can help better understand which patients are at risk for disease recurrence and/or progression after definitive surgical therapy with curative intent for non-metastatic UTUC. However, it is essential to recognize that UTUC and bladder urothelial carcinoma are distinct entities, characterized by unique clinical, pathological, practical, and molecular factors [6].

3.1. Patient Related Factors

Advanced age and worse performance status have been significantly associated with decreased CSS in several studies including a systematic review including all published articles until December 2014 (Hazard ratio (HR) 1.02) [7]. Studies including a SEER database UTUC cohort analysis revealed that stage, grade, age, and sex were significantly associated with Cancer-Specific Survival (CSS) in 9208 non-metastatic UTUC patients treated with RNU [8–11]. However, as opposed to bladder cancer, sex was not associated with CSS in UTUC patients according to individual studies and a meta-analysis of 39,759 UTUC patients (pooled HR 0.94, 95% confidence interval (CI) = 0.89–1.00) [11,12]. Moreover, being a smoker at diagnosis has been shown to increase the risk of recurrence and mortality. In a retrospective study involving 864 clinically non-metastatic UTUC patients treated with RNU, of whom 202 were identified as heavy long-term smokers, the study found that heavy long-term smoking was significantly associated with advanced disease, disease recurrence, and worse CSS [13].

Although Lynch syndrome patients are at higher risk of developing UTUC [14], high microsatellite instability (MSI), which is a screening tool for Lynch syndrome in UTUC patients, seems to be associated with better overall survival [15].

Furthermore, residing in Balkan endemic nephropathy (BEN) areas has been independently linked to an increased risk of bladder recurrence following RNU for UTUC, with patients from these regions experiencing higher rates compared to those outside BEN areas (HR 1.81; $p = 0.01$) [16]. Additionally, a propensity-matched survival analysis revealed that patients in Taiwan and China who have undergone kidney transplantation are at a higher risk of developing UTUC than those without such a transplant history [17].

3.2. Tumor Stage and Grade

Despite the insights gained from these patient-related prognostic factors, the TNM stage and tumor grade continue to be the most influential prognostic indicators for UTUC [8,9,18–20]. A large retrospective study, including 13,314 patients with primary UTUC in the Netherlands between 1993 and 2017, reported five-year CSSs of 86% (95% CI = 84–87), 70% (95% CI = 68–72), and 44% for Ta/Tis, T1-T2, and non-organ confined tumors, respectively [21]. Simultaneously, a survival analysis of 6826 patients who underwent RNU for non-metastatic UTUC from the SEER database revealed a decreasing five-year CSS with increasing T stage: 86% for T1 high-grade N0 disease, 78% for T2 N0 disease, 63% for T3 N0, and 39% for T4 N0 or any N1–3 disease [22].

Moreover, M0 UTUC patients with lymph node involvement experience very poor five-year OS rates of approximately 15–30% [23–25]. In addition, extracapsular extension and lymph node density have been reported to be strong predictors of survival outcomes in N+ UTUC patients [26].

3.3. Tumor Characteristics

Tumor location has been shown to be associated with worse outcomes in univariable analyses [27]. According to a systematic review of 14,895 RNU patients, ureteral tumor location has a negative impact on CSS compared to pelvicalyceal tumors after adjusting for covariates (pooled HR of 1.52, $p < 0.001$) [28]. Multifocality is another factor that has been associated with disease recurrence and CSS in 2492 RNU patients, of whom 590 had multifocal tumors (HR 1.43, $p = 0.019$ and HR 1.46, $p = 0.027$, respectively) [29]. Furthermore, clinical tumor size has been linked to T stage, as shown by a large multi-institutional retrospective study of 932 RNUs for non-metastatic UTUC. The study demonstrated that a tumor size of 2 cm was the optimal cutoff to identify patients at risk for >T2 disease (decision curve analysis: clinical net benefit of 0.09 and a net reduction of 8 per 100 patients) [30]. An analysis of 4657 patients from the SEER database confirmed these findings: each 1 cm increase in tumor size translated into an adjusted odds ratio of 1.25 ($p > 0.001$) [31].

3.4. Other Pathological Features

Similarly to bladder UC, histological subtypes including micropapillary, squamous, and/or sarcomatoid were associated with worse CSS in a systematic review including 12,865 UTUC patients (pooled HR 2.00, 95% CI = 1.57–2.56) [32]. Additionally, lymphovascular invasion (LVI) was demonstrated to be an independent predictor of CSS in a large multicenter series including 763 UTUC patients who underwent RNU without neoadjuvant chemotherapy (HR 3.3, $p = 0.005$) [33]. Finally, as with other malignancies, positive surgical margins are associated with an increased risk of disease recurrence after RNU (HR 2.7, $p = 0.001$) [34].

In summary, risk factors serve as key indicators in forecasting the likelihood for a patient to experience recurrence of a disease, and, as such, they are integral to risk stratification [35], which in turn can help in patient counseling and shared decision-making based on evidence regarding intensification or deintensification of adjuvant therapy and surveillance. Indeed, prognostic tools integrating the above risk factors are the data-driven backbone to the development of effective and cost-serving surveillance protocols.

4. Current Surveillance Protocols after RNU

Leading urological and oncological associations such as the NCCN, AUA, and EAU propose surveillance protocols for both KSS- and RNU-treated patients. These protocols typically encompass a combination of regular cystoscopy, cytology, and imaging (Tables 1–3) [2–4]. The specific follow-up protocol for UTUC is generally determined based on the risk stratification group and the type of definitive therapy performed (i.e., KSS or RNU). Tables 1–3 provide an overview of the exact surveillance protocols of the EAU, AUA, and NCCN guidelines. Although little evidence exists on the value of these follow-up protocols, there is a rationale behind each of the surveillance modalities and regimens. In general, evidence shows that patients with asymptomatically detected recurrence have better overall survival, CSS, and recurrence-free survival than symptomatic UTUC patients [36].

Table 1. Displaying the current EAU guideline surveillance protocol.

EAU	Months	3	6	9	12	15	18	21	24	30	36	42	48	54	60	
low risk after RNU	cytology								not mandatory							
	cystoscopy	○			○				○		○		○		○	
	CT/MR urography								not mandatory							
high risk after RNU	cytology	○	○	○	○	○	○	○	○	○	○	○	○	○	○	annually thereafter
	cystoscopy	○	○	○	○	○	○	○	○	○	○	○	○	○	○	annually thereafter
	CT/MR urography		○		○		○		○		○		○		○	annually thereafter
	Chest CT		○		○		○		○							
low risk after KSS	cytology															
	cystoscopy	○	○		○				○		○		○		○	
	CT/MR urography	○	○		○				○		○		○		○	
	URS	○														
high risk after KSS	cytology	○	○													
	cystoscopy															
	CT/MR urography															
	URS	○	○													
low risk	unifocal, tumor size < 2 cm, low-grade cytology, low-grade URS biopsy, no invasive aspect on CT urography (all of these)															
high risk	hydronephrosis, tumor size $\geq$ 2 cm, high-grade cytology, high-grade URS biopsy, multifocal, previous RC for MIBC, variant histology (any of these)															

CT = computed tomography; MR = magnet resonance; URS = ureterorenoscopy. ○ = recommended.

Table 2. Displaying the current AUA guideline surveillance protocol.

AUA	Months	3	6	9	12	15	18	21	24	30	36	42	48	54	60
<pT2 N0/M0 after RNU	cystoscopy, cytology	○	○		○		○		○		○		○		○
	cross-sectional imaging *		○		○		○		○		○		x		x
	chest imaging				○										
	BMP **	○			○		○		○		○		○		○
>pT2 Nx/0 after RNU	cystoscopy, cytology	○	○		○		○		○	○	○		○		○
	cross-sectional imaging *	○	○		○		○		○		○		○		○
	chest imaging	○	○		○		○		○		○		○		○
	BMP **	○			○		○		○		○		○		○
low risk after KSS	cystoscopy, cytology	○	○		○		○		○		○		○		○
	URS	○	○		○										
	cross-sectional imaging *	○			○		○		○		○		○		○
	chest imaging				○										
	BMP **				○				○		○		○		○

Table 2. *Cont.*

AUA	Months	3	6	9	12	15	18	21	24	30	36	42	48	54	60
high risk after KSS	cystoscopy, cytology	○	○		○		○		○	○	○		○		○
	URS	○	○		○										
	cross-sectional imaging *	○	○		○		○		○	○	○		○		○
	chest imaging		○		○		○		○		○				
	BMP **				○				○		○		○		○
low risk		Bx: low-grade; cytology: no HGUC, <cT2 N0M0, no sessile or flat tumors													
high risk		BX: high-grade; cytology: HGUC, ≥cT2 N+													

* Cross-sectional imaging of the abdomen and pelvis should be performed with contrast when possible; ** basic metabolic panel. ○ = recommended; x = optional.

Table 3. Displaying the current NCCN guideline surveillance protocol.

NCCN		3	6	9	12	15	18	21	24	30	36	42	48	54	60	months
pT0–1 after RNU	cytology	○	○	○	○	longer intervals not specified										
	cystoscopy	○	○	○	○											
	cross-sectional imaging *	not specifically recommended														
pT2–4, pN+ after RNU	cytology	○	○	○	○	longer intervals not specified										
	cystoscopy	○	○	○	○											
	cross-sectional imaging *	not specifically recommended														
	chest imaging															
pT0–1 after KSS	cytology	○	○	○	○	longer intervals not specified										
	cystoscopy	○	○	○	○											
	cross-sectional imaging *	3–12-month intervals														
	URS															
pT2–4, pN+ after KSS	cytology	○	○	○	○	longer intervals not specified										
	cystoscopy	○	○	○	○											
	cross-sectional imaging *	3–12-month intervals														
	chest imaging															
	URS															

* Abdominal/pelvic CT or MRI with and without contrast. ○ = recommended.

4.1. Bladder Recurrence

Since bladder recurrence is common after definitive treatment for UTUC, cystoscopy is an integral part of the follow-up. The risk of bladder recurrence was assessed by two studies that created a nomogram to predict bladder recurrence at different time points. The UTUC collaboration group analyzed 1839 UTUC patients treated with open or laparoscopic RNU and found an intravesical recurrence in 31% of the patients with a median follow-up of 45 months [19]. Similarly, a retrospective study from Japan showed an intravesical recurrence rate of 29% after 5 years in 754 UTUC patients treated with RNU [37]. Nonetheless, no specific thresholds were found regarding intravesical recurrence risk and endoscopic surveillance.

Conditional survival analyses take into account that a patient's likelihood of bladder recurrence decreases with increasing recurrence-free survival. For example, Shigeta et al. analyzed 364 UTUC patients treated with open or laparoscopic RNU and found a 5-year intravesical recurrence-free survival (IVRFS) rate of 41.5%. However, the 5-year conditional IVRFS rate after 4 years of survivorship was 96.7% [38]. Similarly, the 5-year IVRFS rate of 3544 UTUC patients who underwent RNU was 55% but the conditional 5-year IVRFS rate increased to 90% after 4 years of survivorship [39]. These data support that the guideline recommendations cover a timeframe of 5 years. However, the retrospective study design and the relatively small patient cohort of the Shigeta study represent major limitations, meaning that no clear conclusions can be drawn regarding endoscopic surveillance protocols.

Martini et al. recommended continuing cystoscopy follow-up for more than 10 years, especially for patients with a prior history of bladder cancer. This recommendation is supported by Weibull regression models for the hazard rate of recurrence and other-cause mortality, which indicate a higher risk of recurrence than other-cause mortality for patients under 70 years of age [40]. The impact of a single dose of intravesical post-operative chemotherapy lowers the risk of intravesical recurrence [41] and could lead to a de-escalation of cystoscopies, but it is unclear to what extent. After KSS, the rate of IVR is likely to be higher due to many interventions with ureteroscopies, which have been shown to lead to higher rate of IVR due to presumed seeding [42].

4.2. Local and Distant Recurrence

Unlike intravesical recurrences, which can be effectively monitored through frequent cystoscopies, the emergence of loco-regional and distant recurrences necessitates regular abdominopelvic and chest imaging. Generally, local recurrence rates after RNU are reported to range from 5 to 32% in retrospective studies [43–48]. In a study conducted by Martini et al., the risk of non-bladder recurrence was assessed in 1378 prospectively collected UTUC patients treated with RNU across various European academic centers. Patients were classified into two groups based on their prior history of bladder cancer. After 2 years, the risk of non-bladder recurrence was 42% for patients without and 47% for those with a history of prior bladder cancer. Considering that European guidelines advocate a deintensification of imaging after 2 years, the authors suggest maintaining a semiannual imaging schedule until after the fourth year when the risk curve for non-bladder recurrence post RNU significantly plateaus [40].

A study from Japan that followed 733 UTUC patients post RNU found a non-bladder recurrence rate of 34% within 5 years, with most recurrences occurring within the first 3 years following treatment [49]. The study also indicated a correlation between the location of the primary tumor and patterns of recurrence or metastasis. Lower and middle ureter tumors were more prone to local recurrence in the pelvic cavity, while tumors in the renal pelvis or upper ureter were more likely to metastasize to the lungs or liver [49].

In terms of metastatic patterns in UTUC patients, primary metastatic UTUC patients are most likely to experience lung (36.1%) bone (27%), or liver (19.1%) metastasis, with brain metastasis only in 1.6% of cases (SEER: 9436 primary UTUC patients) [50]. These patterns were corroborated by Tanaka et al., who found that 30% of 733 low- and high-risk UTUC patients experienced recurrence within 3 years post RNU, with distant recurrences accounting for 56% of these cases. The predominant sites of metastasis were the lungs, liver, and bones [49]. Other studies have reported similar metastasis rates post RNU, ranging from 8.3% to 46% [44–48,51]. Consequently, abdominal and chest imaging are part of the surveillance protocols of the NCCN, AUA, and EAU guidelines, allowing for the detection of these metastasis patterns.

4.3. Risk Stratification and Surveillance

Risk stratification plays a crucial role in striking the right equilibrium between the intensity and frequency of surveillance modalities tailored for each patient. A retrospective analysis of 1029 UTUC patients who underwent RNU in Canada revealed that 73% of patients experienced recurrence at any site (urothelial, local, and distant recurrences) within the first two years [52]. Based on these findings, the authors suggested a surveillance protocol based on three risk groups: low risk (pTa-T1, pN0, low grade, no LVI, unifocality), intermediate risk (pTa-T1, pN0, +/− high grade, +/− LVI, +/− multifocality), and high risk (≥pT2 and/or pN+), with the first two years post RNU demanding heightened surveillance, particularly for high-risk patients [52].

In a retrospective analysis of 426 UTUC patients who underwent RNU, Momota et al. sought to assess the cost-effectiveness of surveillance protocols. Initially, a pathology-based surveillance protocol (normal risk: ≤pT2N0; high risk: N0 with pT3 or LVI+; very high risk: pT4, positive surgical margin, or lymph node involvement (cN+ or pN+)) was utilized;

however, it fell short in its ability to effectively distinguish between patients with a high risk of recurrence and those without. The authors subsequently improved cost-effectiveness by implementing a risk-score-based surveillance protocol which weighted different risk factors, resulting in a 55% reduction in the cost of 5-year surveillance [53]. However, it should be noted that the authors did not include grading in their risk stratification, resulting in risk groups with mixed grading.

In a retrospective analysis of 714 UTUC patients who underwent RNU, Shigeta et al. found that smokers had a higher risk of UTUC-related death compared to non-smokers according to Weibull model estimates. The authors suggest that extending surveillance may be necessary for this population to detect and manage potential recurrences or metastases [54]. Yet, similar to the Momota study, this study also had a major limitation in risk stratification, as it was not based on the standard pathological features or risk groups recommended by guidelines.

The key questions are the optimal protocol and the duration of surveillance. Lindner et al. studied time-to-tumor recurrence in 54 UTUC patients post RNU and 14 UTUC patients post KSS. They discovered that 38.9% of patients post RNU developed distant metastasis, with the vast majority (85.7%) occurring within the first year post surgery. Only 9.5% and 4.8% occurred in the second and third years, respectively [55]. These findings underscore the rationale of the EAU guidelines' recommendation to de-intensify imaging after the first two years post RNU.

Finally, the delivery of adjuvant systemic therapy with platinum-based combination has shown to lower recurrence rates and may impact the intensity of surveillance imaging [56].

In conclusion, considering their elevated risk of recurrence, patients with UTUC post RNU necessitate a meticulous follow-up regimen. This should encompass routine chest and abdominopelvic imaging, supplemented with periodic cystoscopy. It is particularly crucial to maintain an intensified monitoring schedule during the initial two years of surveillance.

5. Current Surveillance Protocols after Endoscopic Treatment

A kidney-sparing approach is generally recommended to reduce morbidity associated with radical surgery [2] for UTUC tumors with low-risk features including all of the following: unifocal disease, tumor size < 2 cm, negative cytology, low-grade ureterorenoscopy (URS) biopsy, and no invasive aspect on computed tomography (CT). Current surveillance strategies for UTUC patients after KSS (either for low-risk tumors or for imperative indications such as solitary kidney, bilateral UTUC, chronic kidney disease, or any other comorbidity compromising the use of RNU) include imaging and periodic cystoscopy but also URS as a standard (Tables 1–3) [2].

5.1. Recurrence Rates

The design of surveillance strategies is fundamentally shaped by recurrence rates and patterns. This principle is illustrated in a recent systematic review that scrutinized the oncologic outcome of endoscopic surgeries for UTUC including 1091 patients from twenty studies with mostly low-grade tumors. The authors found a pooled bladder recurrence rate of 35% (95% CI 28–42.3: I^2 = 48%) after retrograde URS and 17.7% (95% CI 6.5–32.1: I^2 = 29%) after antegrade URS. Additionally, the pooled rate of upper urinary tract recurrence was 56.4% (95% CI 41.2–70.9: I^2 = 93%) after retrograde treatment and 36.2% (95% CI 25.5–47.6: I^2 = 57%) after antegrade treatment [57].

Interestingly, Mohapatra et al. retrospectively analyzed patients who initially received endoscopic treatment at two large tertiary referral centers in the U.S. for low- and high-risk UTUC and found that 80% of their cohort experienced disease progression to high-risk UTUC, triggering an RNU within 5 years [58].

Given these results, it is crucial to implement a rigorous follow-up schedule involving repeated cystoscopy and ureteroscopy, particularly after endoscopic treatment. This strategy ensures timely detection of any disease recurrence or progression, and keeps the option for RNU open, preserving the critical window of opportunity for intervention if required.

5.2. Cytology

Urinary cytology serves as a crucial tool for diagnosing UTUC and its subsequent surveillance, particularly in high-risk tumors, regardless of the definitive therapy approach. This tool is widely recommended across various guidelines due to its high specificity and non-invasive nature [2–4]. The adoption of the Paris System for Reporting Urinary Cytology (TPS) has led to varying results with respect to sensitivity and specificity. Studies have reported sensitivity ranging from 19% to 82%, while specificity ranges from 86% to 100% for primary diagnosis [59]. Interestingly, these results align with a meta-analysis from the pre-TPS era, which demonstrated a pooled sensitivity of 53% (95% CI = 42–64; I^2 = 86%) and a pooled specificity of 90% (95% CI = 85–93; I^2 = 0%) for UTUC detection in upper urinary tract cytology during primary diagnosis [60].

Given these findings, cytology is also recommended for UTUC follow-up. However, it is important to note that the impact of the Paris System on sensitivity and specificity during surveillance is yet to be determined.

5.3. Second-Look URS and Endoscopic Follow-Up

EAU and AUA guidelines agree on an early repeated URS which should be performed one to three and six months after KSS [2,3]. Villa et al. demonstrated a high cancer detection rate of 51.2% during the second URS 6–8 weeks after initial URS treatment in 41 UTUC patients with high- or low-risk UTUC. Patients who had a positive result during the second URS had an 81.3% likelihood of also having a positive result during the third URS, in contrast to a cancer detection rate of 41.2% for the third URS following a negative second URS result [61]. The authors therefore strongly recommend a second-look URS within 6–8 weeks after initial endoscopic management.

Several studies provide further evidence for the importance of close endoscopic follow-up in UTUC patients who undergo KSS. Kawada et al. conducted a systematic review and found that endoscopically managed tumors had similar oncologic outcomes to those managed with RNU, but recurrence in the upper urothelial tract was observed in 28–85% of patients across the studies [62]. Lindner et al. reported a stable recurrence rate after KSS (endoscopic treatment and ureterectomy) at 12.5% to 20.5% per year during the first 5 years after surgery, with six upper urinary tract recurrences, two bladder recurrences, and two lymph node and/or distant metastases in 14 KSS patients (57.1% high-grade tumors). As most of the recurrences after KSS concerned the bladder or upper urinary tract (six upper urinary tract recurrences, two bladder recurrences), the authors suggest, contrary to the current EAU, AUA, and NCCN guidelines, that cystoscopies and URS should not be deintensified after 2 years of follow-up [55].

This is further emphasized by Seisen et al., who analyzed 42 primary endoscopically treated patients with mostly low-grade tumors. The local recurrence-free survival defined as recurrence in the operation site was 35.7% after endoscopic treatment. Additionally, Kaplan–Meier curves showed a consistent incidence of local recurrence over the 5-year follow-up period [63]. Moreover, Hendriks et al. found a higher IVR rate for high-risk UTUC patients treated with KSS (endoscopic treatment and ureterectomy) compared to RNU in a propensity-score-matched cohort based on EAU risk stratification (52% for KSS vs. 32% for RNU; $p = 0.029$) [64].

In conclusion, while the existing evidence may be of a low level, it, nonetheless, underscores the necessity for rigorous surveillance, including URS, following the endoscopic management of UTUC.

Specifically, because KSS is an alternative to RNU, it has promise to be safe while retaining the renal unit.

6. Current Surveillance Protocols after Segmental or Distal Ureterectomy

Segmental and distal ureterectomy represent non-endoscopic kidney-sparing approaches that are recommended for low-risk UTUC tumors [2]. Seisen et al. assessed oncologic outcomes of ureterectomies compared with RNU in a systematic review including 586 segmental ureterectomy patients from comparative studies and reported no differences in CSS, OS, and RFS between the two groups [65]. Seisen also showed that the 5-year local RFS, defined as recurrence in the operation site, ranged from 37% to 91% across studies [66–69]. Similarly, Fang et al. included 983 ureterectomy patients from comparative studies and reported no differences in oncologic outcomes between ureterectomy and RNU (CSS: HR 0.90, $p = 0.33$, OS: HR 0.98, $p = 0.93$, and RFS: HR 1.06, $p = 0.72$). However, patients undergoing ureterectomy were more likely to harbor favorable pathological features. The cumulative recurrence rate 5 years after surgery ranged from 16% to 72% across three studies comprising 165 patients [66,68,70,71].

Due to ureteroureterostomy or ureteroneocystostomy, which complicate endoscopic follow-up, surveillance after ureterectomy was frequently based on the follow-up regimen of RNUs across retrospective studies [66,68]. Yet, Kim et al. retrospectively analyzed 394 RNU patients and 44 segmental ureterectomy patients and found no significant differences regarding 3-year PFS and IVRFS (68% vs. 73%: $p = 0.9$ and 42% vs. 37%: $p = 0.8$, respectively). Interestingly, the authors stated the use of semiannual ureteroscopy in their follow-up regimen for patients treated with segmental ureterectomy [72]. While ureterectomies are considered kidney-sparing approaches for UTUC, the surveillance protocols recommended by guidelines do not distinguish between endoscopic management and ureterectomy, leading to non-compliance with guideline protocols, especially after ureterectomy. As of now, this issue has not been addressed in the guidelines.

7. Discussion

The existing guideline recommendations for surveillance following definitive therapy for UTUC largely rely on expert opinions and low-level evidence due to the relative rarity of this disease, which has led to a dearth of large prospective randomized clinical trials that could bolster the evidence. The available data frequently hail from retrospective studies involving small cohorts. Most existing data on surveillance, recurrence, and progression center around RNU. Given that UTUC patients, particularly those in the high-risk category, are generally at substantial risk of recurrence or progression, frequent follow-up examinations seem necessary.

The challenge for healthcare providers lies in delivering an appropriate surveillance protocol with the correct frequency to suit each individual patient and tumor type. As highlighted by Momota et al., risk stratification plays a pivotal role in selecting the appropriate patient and surveillance protocol, and it significantly impacts healthcare system costs, resource utilization, and patient convenience/quality of life [53]. Currently, risk stratification largely depends on tumor T and N stage as well as grade. However, the advent of next-generation sequencing (NGS) in recent years has led to the discovery of molecular subtypes of various tumor entities, which are gradually being incorporated into clinical practice. Additionally, liquid biopsies, which utilize blood or other body fluids like urine, are being explored and show promise in the detection of UTUC [73]. The utilization of biomarkers, in general, has the potential to enhance surveillance protocols. The integration of biomarkers and liquid biopsies could lead to less-invasive disease monitoring, improved detection accuracy, and the identification of novel therapeutic targets, thereby potentially reducing the risk of recurrence. Incorporating such biomarkers into routine surveillance could transform patient management, allowing for more personalized and effective monitoring strategies.

A systematic review assessing UTUC alterations revealed significant differences between UTUC and urothelial bladder cancer, particularly in areas such as activated FGFR3 signaling, the extent of altered somatic expression of DNA mismatch repair genes, and individual UTUC molecular subtypes [74]. The impact of these discoveries on future treatments and, consequently, future surveillance protocols in UTUC is in its burgeoning phase and much is expected.

Furthermore, emerging urinary biomarkers might offer the potential to reduce patient discomfort by providing equivalent diagnostic value without necessitating invasive ureterorenoscopy during follow-up. Territo et al. evaluated the diagnostic worth of EpiCheck, a urine test based on the analysis of 15 DNA methylation biomarkers, and the results were promising with a sensitivity/negative predictive value (NPV) for high-grade tumors of 96%/97%, compared to 71%/86% for cytology [75]. However, additional evidence is required to integrate these novel urinary biomarkers into surveillance protocols.

Additionally, by enhancing precise imaging techniques, patients can not only be directed towards the treatment approach that best suits their individual needs, but also the accuracy of risk stratification can be improved. This enhancement may help circumvent unnecessary and invasive surveillance methods such as URS. Moreover, advancements in imaging such as PET/CT and PET/MRI, which seem to be promising imaging tools for the detection of lymph nodes and distant metastases in urothelial bladder cancer, hold the potential to change surveillance protocols and risk stratification by offering a more accurate nodal and distant assessment of the disease [76].

8. Conclusions

The evidence supporting surveillance protocols following definitive therapy for UTUC is currently sparse, and predominantly reliant on low-level evidence and expert opinion. Given the rarity of UTUC, conducting large prospective randomized clinical trials may prove challenging, underscoring the need for refined risk stratification methods. Surveillance protocols may be optimized in the future to meet the individual needs of each patient by enhancing risk stratification accuracy through more precise imaging and/or the implementation of novel urine and blood-based biomarkers.

Author Contributions: Conceptualization J.K., K.B., S.F.S. and P.I.K.; methodology J.K., K.B., E.L., A.M., M.A. and M.K.P.; literature research J.K., K.B. and E.L.; writing—original draft preparation J.K., K.B. and M.A.; writing—review and editing S.F.S., P.I.K., E.L., A.M. and M.K.P.; supervision S.F.S., M.A. and P.I.K. All authors have read and agreed to the published version of the manuscript.

Funding: This research received no external funding.

Conflicts of Interest: The authors declare no conflict of interest.

References

1. Siegel, R.L.; Miller, K.D.; Fuchs, H.E.; Jemal, A. Cancer Statistics, 2021. *CA Cancer J. Clin.* **2021**, *71*, 7–33. [CrossRef]
2. Rouprêt, M.; Seisen, T.; Birtle, A.J.; Capoun, O.; Compérat, E.M.; Dominguez-Escrig, J.L.; Gürses Andersson, I.; Liedberg, F.; Mariappan, P.; Hugh Mostafid, A.; et al. European Association of Urology Guidelines on Upper Urinary Tract Urothelial Carcinoma: 2023 Update. *Eur. Urol.* **2023**, *84*, 49–64. [CrossRef]
3. Coleman, J.A.; Clark, P.E.; Bixler, B.R.; Buckley, D.I.; Chang, S.S.; Chou, R.; Hoffman-Censits, J.; Kulkarni, G.S.; Matin, S.F.; Pierorazio, P.M.; et al. Diagnosis and Management of Non-Metastatic Upper Tract Urothelial Carcinoma: AUA/SUO Guideline. *J. Urol.* **2023**, *209*, 1071–1081. [CrossRef]
4. Flaig, T.W.; Spiess, P.E.; Agarwal, N.; Bangs, R.; Boorjian, S.A.; Buyyounouski, M.K.; Chang, S.; Downs, T.M.; Efstathiou, J.A.; Friedlander, T.; et al. Bladder Cancer, Version 3.2020, NCCN Clinical Practice Guidelines in Oncology. *J. Natl. Compr. Cancer Netw.* **2020**, *18*, 329–354. [CrossRef]
5. Leow, J.J.; Chong, Y.L.; Chang, S.L.; Valderrama, B.P.; Powles, T.; Bellmunt, J. Neoadjuvant and Adjuvant Chemotherapy for Upper Tract Urothelial Carcinoma: A 2020 Systematic Review and Meta-analysis, and Future Perspectives on Systemic Therapy. *Eur. Urol.* **2021**, *79*, 635–654. [CrossRef]
6. Robinson, B.D.; Vlachostergios, P.J.; Bhinder, B.; Liu, W.; Li, K.; Moss, T.J.; Bareja, R.; Park, K.; Tavassoli, P.; Cyrta, J.; et al. Upper tract urothelial carcinoma has a luminal-papillary T-cell depleted contexture and activated FGFR3 signaling. *Nat. Commun.* **2019**, *10*, 2977. [CrossRef]
7. Kim, H.S.; Jeong, C.W.; Kwak, C.; Kim, H.H.; Ku, J.H. Association between demographic factors and prognosis in urothelial carcinoma of the upper urinary tract: A systematic review and meta-analysis. *Oncotarget* **2017**, *8*, 7464–7476. [CrossRef]
8. Collà Ruvolo, C.; Nocera, L.; Stolzenbach, L.F.; Wenzel, M.; Cucchiara, V.; Tian, Z.; Shariat, S.F.; Saad, F.; Longo, N.; Montorsi, F.; et al. Incidence and Survival Rates of Contemporary Patients with Invasive Upper Tract Urothelial Carcinoma. *Eur. Urol. Oncol.* **2021**, *4*, 792–801. [CrossRef]

9. Lughezzani, G.; Jeldres, C.; Isbarn, H.; Sun, M.; Shariat, S.F.; Alasker, A.; Pharand, D.; Widmer, H.; Arjane, P.; Graefen, M.; et al. Nephroureterectomy and segmental ureterectomy in the treatment of invasive upper tract urothelial carcinoma: A population-based study of 2299 patients. *Eur. J. Cancer* **2009**, *45*, 3291–3297. [CrossRef]
10. Lughezzani, G.; Sun, M.; Perrotte, P.; Shariat, S.F.; Jeldres, C.; Budäus, L.; Latour, M.; Widmer, H.; Duclos, A.; Bénard, F.; et al. Gender-related differences in patients with stage I to III upper tract urothelial carcinoma: Results from the Surveillance, Epidemiology, and End Results database. *Urology* **2010**, *75*, 321–327. [CrossRef]
11. Shariat, S.F.; Favaretto, R.L.; Gupta, A.; Fritsche, H.M.; Matsumoto, K.; Kassouf, W.; Walton, T.J.; Tritschler, S.; Baba, S.; Matsushita, K.; et al. Gender differences in radical nephroureterectomy for upper tract urothelial carcinoma. *World J. Urol.* **2011**, *29*, 481–486. [CrossRef] [PubMed]
12. Mori, K.; Mostafaei, H.; Enikeev, D.V.; Lysenko, I.; Quhal, F.; Kimura, S.; Karakiewicz, P.I.; Egawa, S.; Shariat, S.F. Differential Effect of Sex on Outcomes after Radical Surgery for Upper Tract and Bladder Urothelial Carcinoma: A Systematic Review and Meta-Analysis. *J. Urol.* **2020**, *204*, 58–62. [CrossRef] [PubMed]
13. Rink, M.; Xylinas, E.; Margulis, V.; Cha, E.K.; Ehdaie, B.; Raman, J.D.; Chun, F.K.; Matsumoto, K.; Lotan, Y.; Furberg, H.; et al. Impact of smoking on oncologic outcomes of upper tract urothelial carcinoma after radical nephroureterectomy. *Eur. Urol.* **2013**, *63*, 1082–1090. [CrossRef] [PubMed]
14. Lonati, C.; Necchi, A.; Gómez Rivas, J.; Afferi, L.; Laukhtina, E.; Martini, A.; Ventimiglia, E.; Colombo, R.; Gandaglia, G.; Salonia, A.; et al. Upper Tract Urothelial Carcinoma in the Lynch Syndrome Tumour Spectrum: A Comprehensive Overview from the European Association of Urology—Young Academic Urologists and the Global Society of Rare Genitourinary Tumors. *Eur. Urol. Oncol.* **2022**, *5*, 30–41. [CrossRef] [PubMed]
15. Rouprêt, M.; Fromont, G.; Azzouzi, A.-R.; Catto, J.W.; Vallancien, G.; Hamdy, F.C.; Cussenot, O. Microsatellite instability as predictor of survival in patients with invasive upper urinary tract transitional cell carcinoma. *Urology* **2005**, *65*, 1233–1237. [CrossRef] [PubMed]
16. Milojevic, B.; Dzamic, Z.; Grozdic Milojevic, I.; Bumbasirevic, U.; Santric, V.; Kajmakovic, B.; Janicic, A.; Durutovic, O.; Dragicevic, D.; Bojanic, N.; et al. Prognostic value of Balkan endemic nephropathy and gender on upper tract urothelial carcinoma outcomes after radical nephroureterectomy: A cohort study. *Urol. Oncol.* **2021**, *39*, 786.e9–786.e16. [CrossRef] [PubMed]
17. Luo, H.L.; Chiang, P.H.; Cheng, Y.T.; Chen, Y.T. Propensity-Matched Survival Analysis of Upper Urinary Tract Urothelial Carcinomas between End-Stage Renal Disease with and without Kidney Transplantation. *BioMed Res. Int.* **2019**, *2019*, 2979142. [CrossRef]
18. Mbeutcha, A.; Rouprêt, M.; Kamat, A.M.; Karakiewicz, P.I.; Lawrentschuk, N.; Novara, G.; Raman, J.D.; Seitz, C.; Xylinas, E.; Shariat, S.F. Prognostic factors and predictive tools for upper tract urothelial carcinoma: A systematic review. *World J. Urol.* **2017**, *35*, 337–353. [CrossRef]
19. Xylinas, E.; Kluth, L.; Passoni, N.; Trinh, Q.-D.; Rieken, M.; Lee, R.K.; Fajkovic, H.; Novara, G.; Margulis, V.; Raman, J.D.; et al. Prediction of Intravesical Recurrence After Radical Nephroureterectomy: Development of a Clinical Decision-making Tool. *Eur. Urol.* **2014**, *65*, 650–658. [CrossRef]
20. Compérat, E.M.; Burger, M.; Gontero, P.; Mostafid, A.H.; Palou, J.; Rouprêt, M.; van Rhijn, B.W.G.; Shariat, S.F.; Sylvester, R.J.; Zigeuner, R.; et al. Grading of Urothelial Carcinoma and The New "World Health Organisation Classification of Tumours of the Urinary System and Male Genital Organs 2016". *Eur. Urol. Focus* **2019**, *5*, 457–466. [CrossRef]
21. van Doeveren, T.; van der Mark, M.; van Leeuwen, P.J.; Boormans, J.L.; Aben, K.K.H. Rising incidence rates and unaltered survival rates for primary upper urinary tract urothelial carcinoma: A Dutch population-based study from 1993 to 2017. *BJU Int.* **2021**, *128*, 343–351. [CrossRef] [PubMed]
22. Rosiello, G.; Palumbo, C.; Knipper, S.; Pecoraro, A.; Luzzago, S.; Deuker, M.; Mistretta, F.A.; Tian, Z.; Fossati, N.; Gallina, A.; et al. Contemporary conditional cancer-specific survival after radical nephroureterectomy in patients with nonmetastatic urothelial carcinoma of upper urinary tract. *J. Surg. Oncol.* **2020**, *121*, 1154–1161. [CrossRef] [PubMed]
23. Pelcovits, A.; Mueller-Leonhard, C.; Mega, A.; Amin, A.; Kim, S.P.; Golijanin, D.; Gershman, B. Outcomes of upper tract urothelial carcinoma with isolated lymph node involvement following surgical resection: Implications for multi-modal management. *World J. Urol.* **2020**, *38*, 1243–1252. [CrossRef] [PubMed]
24. Roscigno, M.; Brausi, M.; Heidenreich, A.; Lotan, Y.; Margulis, V.; Shariat, S.F.; Van Poppel, H.; Zigeuner, R. Lymphadenectomy at the time of nephroureterectomy for upper tract urothelial cancer. *Eur. Urol.* **2011**, *60*, 776–783. [CrossRef] [PubMed]
25. Lughezzani, G.; Jeldres, C.; Isbarn, H.; Shariat, S.F.; Sun, M.; Pharand, D.; Widmer, H.; Arjane, P.; Graefen, M.; Montorsi, F.; et al. A critical appraisal of the value of lymph node dissection at nephroureterectomy for upper tract urothelial carcinoma. *Urology* **2010**, *75*, 118–124. [CrossRef] [PubMed]
26. Fajkovic, H.; Cha, E.K.; Jeldres, C.; Donner, G.; Chromecki, T.F.; Margulis, V.; Novara, G.; Lotan, Y.; Raman, J.D.; Kassouf, W.; et al. Prognostic value of extranodal extension and other lymph node parameters in patients with upper tract urothelial carcinoma. *J. Urol.* **2012**, *187*, 845–851. [CrossRef]
27. Isbarn, H.; Jeldres, C.; Shariat, S.F.; Liberman, D.; Sun, M.; Lughezzani, G.; Widmer, H.; Arjane, P.; Pharand, D.; Fisch, M.; et al. Location of the primary tumor is not an independent predictor of cancer specific mortality in patients with upper urinary tract urothelial carcinoma. *J. Urol.* **2009**, *182*, 2177–2181. [CrossRef] [PubMed]
28. Kaczmarek, K.; Lemiński, A.; Gołąb, A.; Słojewski, M. Survival differences of patients with ureteral versus pelvicalyceal tumours: A systematic review and meta-analysis. *Arch. Med. Sci.* **2021**, *17*, 603–612. [CrossRef]

29. Chromecki, T.F.; Cha, E.K.; Fajkovic, H.; Margulis, V.; Novara, G.; Scherr, D.S.; Lotan, Y.; Raman, J.D.; Kassouf, W.; Bensalah, K.; et al. The impact of tumor multifocality on outcomes in patients treated with radical nephroureterectomy. *Eur. Urol.* **2012**, *61*, 245–253. [CrossRef]
30. Foerster, B.; Abufaraj, M.; Mari, A.; Seisen, T.; Bandini, M.; Schweitzer, D.; Czech, A.K.; Moschini, M.; D'Andrea, D.; Bianchi, M.; et al. The Performance of Tumor Size as Risk Stratification Parameter in Upper Tract Urothelial Carcinoma (UTUC). *Clin. Genitourin. Cancer* **2021**, *19*, 272.e1–272.e7. [CrossRef]
31. Collà Ruvolo, C.; Nocera, L.; Stolzenbach, L.F.; Wenzel, M.; Califano, G.; Tian, Z.; Verze, P.; Shariat, S.F.; Saad, F.; Briganti, A.; et al. Tumor Size Predicts Muscle-invasive and Non–organ-confined Disease in Upper Tract Urothelial Carcinoma at Radical Nephroureterectomy. *Eur. Urol. Focus* **2022**, *8*, 498–505. [CrossRef] [PubMed]
32. Mori, K.; Janisch, F.; Parizi, M.K.; Mostafaei, H.; Lysenko, I.; Kimura, S.; Enikeev, D.V.; Egawa, S.; Shariat, S.F. Prognostic Value of Variant Histology in Upper Tract Urothelial Carcinoma Treated with Nephroureterectomy: A Systematic Review and Meta-Analysis. *J. Urol.* **2020**, *203*, 1075–1084. [CrossRef] [PubMed]
33. Novara, G.; Matsumoto, K.; Kassouf, W.; Walton, T.J.; Fritsche, H.M.; Bastian, P.J.; Martínez-Salamanca, J.I.; Seitz, C.; Lemberger, R.J.; Burger, M.; et al. Prognostic role of lymphovascular invasion in patients with urothelial carcinoma of the upper urinary tract: An international validation study. *Eur. Urol.* **2010**, *57*, 1064–1071. [CrossRef] [PubMed]
34. Colin, P.; Ouzzane, A.; Yates, D.R.; Audenet, F.; Pignot, G.; Arvin-Berod, A.; Merigot de Treigny, O.; Laurent, G.; Valeri, A.; Irani, J.; et al. Influence of positive surgical margin status after radical nephroureterectomy on upper urinary tract urothelial carcinoma survival. *Ann. Surg. Oncol.* **2012**, *19*, 3613–3620. [CrossRef] [PubMed]
35. Shariat, S.F.; Capitanio, U.; Jeldres, C.; Karakiewicz, P.I. Can nomograms be superior to other prediction tools? *BJU Int.* **2009**, *103*, 492–495; discussion 495–497. [CrossRef] [PubMed]
36. Horiguchi, H.; Hatakeyama, S.; Anan, G.; Kubota, Y.; Kodama, H.; Momota, M.; Kido, K.; Yamamoto, H.; Tobisawa, Y.; Yoneyama, T.; et al. Detecting asymptomatic recurrence after radical nephroureterectomy contributes to better prognosis in patients with upper urinary tract urothelial carcinoma. *Oncotarget* **2018**, *9*, 8746–8755. [CrossRef] [PubMed]
37. Ishioka, J.; Saito, K.; Kijima, T.; Nakanishi, Y.; Yoshida, S.; Yokoyama, M.; Matsuoka, Y.; Numao, N.; Koga, F.; Masuda, H.; et al. Risk stratification for bladder recurrence of upper urinary tract urothelial carcinoma after radical nephroureterectomy. *BJU Int.* **2015**, *115*, 705–712. [CrossRef] [PubMed]
38. Shigeta, K.; Kikuchi, E.; Hagiwara, M.; Ando, T.; Mizuno, R.; Abe, T.; Mikami, S.; Miyajima, A.; Nakagawa, K.; Oya, M. The Conditional Survival with Time of Intravesical Recurrence of Upper Tract Urothelial Carcinoma. *J. Urol.* **2017**, *198*, 1278–1285. [CrossRef]
39. Ploussard, G.; Xylinas, E.; Lotan, Y.; Novara, G.; Margulis, V.; Rouprêt, M.; Matsumoto, K.; Karakiewicz, P.I.; Montorsi, F.; Remzi, M.; et al. Conditional Survival After Radical Nephroureterectomy for Upper Tract Carcinoma. *Eur. Urol.* **2015**, *67*, 803–812. [CrossRef]
40. Martini, A.; Lonati, C.; Nocera, L.; Fallara, G.; Raggi, D.; Herout, R.; Zamboni, S.; Ploussard, G.; Predere, B.; Mattei, A.; et al. Oncologic Surveillance After Radical Nephroureterectomy for High-risk Upper Tract Urothelial Carcinoma. *Eur. Urol. Oncol.* **2022**, *5*, 451–459. [CrossRef]
41. Hwang, E.C.; Sathianathen, N.J.; Jung, J.H.; Kim, M.H.; Dahm, P.; Risk, M.C. Single-dose intravesical chemotherapy after nephroureterectomy for upper tract urothelial carcinoma. *Cochrane Database Syst. Rev.* **2019**, *5*, Cd013160. [CrossRef]
42. Yonese, I.; Ito, M.; Waseda, Y.; Kobayashi, S.; Toide, M.; Takazawa, R.; Koga, F. Impact of diagnostic ureteral catheterization on intravesical tumour recurrence following radical nephroureterectomy for upper tract urothelial carcinoma. *World J. Urol.* **2023**, *41*, 1869–1875. [CrossRef]
43. Cha, E.K.; Shariat, S.F.; Kormaksson, M.; Novara, G.; Chromecki, T.F.; Scherr, D.S.; Lotan, Y.; Raman, J.D.; Kassouf, W.; Zigeuner, R.; et al. Predicting clinical outcomes after radical nephroureterectomy for upper tract urothelial carcinoma. *Eur. Urol.* **2012**, *61*, 818–825. [CrossRef]
44. Gao, J.; Liu, J.; Liu, J.; Lin, S.; Ding, D. Survival and risk factors among upper tract urothelial carcinoma patients after radical nephroureterectomy in Northeast China. *Front. Oncol.* **2022**, *12*, 1012292. [CrossRef]
45. Taweemonkongsap, T.; Nualyong, C.; Amornvesukit, T.; Leewansangtong, S.; Srinualnad, S.; Chaiyaprasithi, B.; Sujijantararat, P.; Tantiwong, A.; Soontrapa, S. Outcomes of surgical treatment for upper urinary tract transitional cell carcinoma: Comparison of retroperitoneoscopic and open nephroureterectomy. *World J. Surg. Oncol.* **2008**, *6*, 3. [CrossRef]
46. Yoo, S.; You, D.; Jeong, I.G.; Hong, B.; Hong, J.H.; Ahn, H.; Kim, C.-S. Impact of Tumor Location on Local Recurrence After Nephroureterectomy for Upper Tract Urothelial Carcinoma: Implications for Adjuvant Radiotherapy. *Clin. Genitourin. Cancer* **2017**, *15*, e199–e204. [CrossRef]
47. Li, X.; Cui, M.; Gu, X.; Fang, D.; Li, H.; Qin, S.; Yang, K.; Zhu, T.; Li, X.; Zhou, L.; et al. Pattern and risk factors of local recurrence after nephroureterectomy for upper tract urothelial carcinoma. *World J. Surg. Oncol.* **2020**, *18*, 114. [CrossRef]
48. Chen, T.S.; Chen, Y.T.; Wang, H.J.; Chiang, P.H.; Yang, W.C.; Lee, W.C.; Chuang, Y.C.; Cheng, Y.T.; Kang, C.H.; Lee, W.C.; et al. The Prognostic Impact of Tumor Location in pT3N0M0 Upper Urinary Tract Urothelial Carcinoma: A Retrospective Cohort Study. *Front. Oncol.* **2022**, *12*, 850874. [CrossRef]
49. Tanaka, N.; Kikuchi, E.; Kanao, K.; Matsumoto, K.; Kobayashi, H.; Ide, H.; Miyazaki, Y.; Obata, J.; Hoshino, K.; Shirotake, S.; et al. Metastatic Behavior of Upper Tract Urothelial Carcinoma After Radical Nephroureterectomy: Association with Primary Tumor Location. *Ann. Surg. Oncol.* **2014**, *21*, 1038–1045. [CrossRef]

50. Hu, X.H.; Miao, J.; Qian, L.; Zhang, D.H.; Wei, H.B. The predictors and surgical outcomes of different distant metastases patterns in upper tract urothelial carcinoma: A SEER-based study. *Front. Surg.* **2022**, *9*, 1045831. [CrossRef]
51. Colin, P.; Ghoneim, T.P.; Nison, L.; Seisen, T.; Lechevallier, E.; Cathelineau, X.; Ouzzane, A.; Zerbib, M.; Long, J.A.; Ruffion, A.; et al. Risk stratification of metastatic recurrence in invasive upper urinary tract carcinoma after radical nephroureterectomy without lymphadenectomy. *World J. Urol.* **2014**, *32*, 507–512. [CrossRef]
52. Locke, J.A.; Hamidizadeh, R.; Kassouf, W.; Rendon, R.A.; Bell, D.; Izawa, J.; Chin, J.; Kapoor, A.; Shayegen, B.; Lattouf, J.B.; et al. Surveillance guidelines based on recurrence patterns for upper tract urothelial carcinoma. *Can. Urol. Assoc. J.* **2018**, *12*, 243–251. [CrossRef]
53. Momota, M.; Hatakeyama, S.; Yamamoto, H.; Iwamura, H.; Tobisawa, Y.; Yoneyama, T.; Yoneyama, T.; Hashimoto, Y.; Koie, T.; Iwabuchi, I.; et al. Risk-stratified surveillance protocol improves cost-effectiveness after radical nephroureterectomy in patients with upper tract urothelial carcinoma. *Oncotarget* **2018**, *9*, 23047–23057. [CrossRef]
54. Shigeta, K.; Kikuchi, E.; Abe, T.; Hagiwara, M.; Ogihara, K.; Anno, T.; Umeda, K.; Baba, Y.; Sanjo, T.; Shojo, K.; et al. A Novel Risk-based Approach Simulating Oncological Surveillance After Radical Nephroureterectomy in Patients with Upper Tract Urothelial Carcinoma. *Eur. Urol. Oncol.* **2020**, *3*, 756–763. [CrossRef]
55. Lindner, A.K.; Pichler, M.; Maier, S.; Ulmer, H.; Gorreri, T.; Luger, A.K.; Barth, D.A.; Seeber, A.; Kocher, F.; Pichler, R. Optimization of postoperative surveillance protocols in upper tract urothelial cancer: A retrospective cohort study. *Front. Oncol.* **2023**, *13*, 1143030. [CrossRef]
56. Birtle, A.; Johnson, M.; Chester, J.; Jones, R.; Dolling, D.; Bryan, R.T.; Harris, C.; Winterbottom, A.; Blacker, A.; Catto, J.W.F.; et al. Adjuvant chemotherapy in upper tract urothelial carcinoma (the POUT trial): A phase 3, open-label, randomised controlled trial. *Lancet* **2020**, *395*, 1268–1277. [CrossRef]
57. Laukhtina, E.; Kawada, T.; Quhal, F.; Yanagisawa, T.; Rajwa, P.; von Deimling, M.; Pallauf, M.; Bianchi, A.; Majdoub, M.; Enikeev, D.; et al. Oncologic and Safety Outcomes for Retrograde and Antegrade Endoscopic Surgeries for Upper Tract Urothelial Carcinoma: A Systematic Review and Meta-analysis. *Eur. Urol. Focus* **2023**, *9*, 258–263. [CrossRef]
58. Mohapatra, A.; Strope, S.A.; Liu, N.; Winer, A.; Benfante, N.E.; Coleman, J.A.; Vetter, J.; Murray, K.S. Importance of long-term follow-up after endoscopic management for upper tract urothelial carcinoma and factors leading to surgical management. *Int. Urol. Nephrol.* **2020**, *52*, 1465–1469. [CrossRef]
59. Zhang, M.L.; Miki, Y.; Hang, J.-F.; Vohra, M.; Peyton, S.; McIntire, P.J.; VandenBussche, C.J.; Vohra, P. A review of upper urinary tract cytology performance before and after the implementation of The Paris System. *Cancer Cytopathol.* **2021**, *129*, 264–274. [CrossRef]
60. Potretzke, A.M.; Knight, B.A.; Vetter, J.M.; Anderson, B.G.; Hardi, A.C.; Bhayani, S.B.; Figenshau, R.S. Diagnostic Utility of Selective Upper Tract Urinary Cytology: A Systematic Review and Meta-analysis of the Literature. *Urology* **2016**, *96*, 35–43. [CrossRef]
61. Villa, L.; Cloutier, J.; Letendre, J.; Ploumidis, A.; Salonia, A.; Cornu, J.N.; Montorsi, F.; Traxer, O. Early repeated ureteroscopy within 6-8 weeks after a primary endoscopic treatment in patients with upper tract urothelial cell carcinoma: Preliminary findings. *World J. Urol.* **2016**, *34*, 1201–1206. [CrossRef]
62. Kawada, T.; Laukhtina, E.; Quhal, F.; Yanagisawa, T.; Rajwa, P.; Pallauf, M.; von Deimling, M.; Bianchi, A.; Pradere, B.; Fajkovic, H.; et al. Oncologic and Safety Outcomes for Endoscopic Surgery Versus Radical Nephroureterectomy for Upper Tract Urothelial Carcinoma: An Updated Systematic Review and Meta-analysis. *Eur. Urol. Focus* **2023**, *9*, 236–240. [CrossRef]
63. Seisen, T.; Nison, L.; Remzi, M.; Klatte, T.; Mathieu, R.; Lucca, I.; Bozzini, G.; Capitanio, U.; Novara, G.; Cussenot, O.; et al. Oncologic Outcomes of Kidney Sparing Surgery versus Radical Nephroureterectomy for the Elective Treatment of Clinically Organ Confined Upper Tract Urothelial Carcinoma of the Distal Ureter. *J. Urol.* **2016**, *195*, 1354–1361. [CrossRef]
64. Hendriks, N.; Baard, J.; Beerlage, H.P.; Schout, B.M.A.; Doherty, K.S.G.; Pelger, R.C.M.; Kamphuis, G.M. Survival and Long-term Effects of Kidney-sparing Surgery Versus Radical Nephroureterectomy on Kidney Function in Patients with Upper Urinary Tract Urothelial Carcinoma. *Eur. Urol. Open Sci.* **2022**, *40*, 104–111. [CrossRef]
65. Seisen, T.; Peyronnet, B.; Dominguez-Escrig, J.L.; Bruins, H.M.; Yuan, C.Y.; Babjuk, M.; Böhle, A.; Burger, M.; Compérat, E.M.; Cowan, N.C.; et al. Oncologic Outcomes of Kidney-sparing Surgery Versus Radical Nephroureterectomy for Upper Tract Urothelial Carcinoma: A Systematic Review by the EAU Non-muscle Invasive Bladder Cancer Guidelines Panel. *Eur. Urol.* **2016**, *70*, 1052–1068. [CrossRef]
66. Dalpiaz, O.; Ehrlich, G.; Quehenberger, F.; Pummer, K.; Zigeuner, R. Distal ureterectomy is a safe surgical option in patients with urothelial carcinoma of the distal ureter. *Urol. Oncol.* **2014**, *32*, 34.e3–34.e8. [CrossRef]
67. Fukushima, H.; Saito, K.; Ishioka, J.; Matsuoka, Y.; Numao, N.; Koga, F.; Masuda, H.; Fujii, Y.; Sakai, Y.; Arisawa, C.; et al. Equivalent survival and improved preservation of renal function after distal ureterectomy compared with nephroureterectomy in patients with urothelial carcinoma of the distal ureter: A propensity score-matched multicenter study. *Int. J. Urol.* **2014**, *21*, 1098–1104. [CrossRef]
68. Bagrodia, A.; Kuehhas, F.E.; Gayed, B.A.; Wood, C.G.; Raman, J.D.; Kapur, P.; Derweesh, I.H.; Bensalah, K.; Sagalowsky, A.I.; Shariat, S.F.; et al. Comparative analysis of oncologic outcomes of partial ureterectomy vs radical nephroureterectomy in upper tract urothelial carcinoma. *Urology* **2013**, *81*, 972–977. [CrossRef]

69. Colin, P.; Ouzzane, A.; Pignot, G.; Ravier, E.; Crouzet, S.; Ariane, M.M.; Audouin, M.; Neuzillet, Y.; Albouy, B.; Hurel, S.; et al. Comparison of oncological outcomes after segmental ureterectomy or radical nephroureterectomy in urothelial carcinomas of the upper urinary tract: Results from a large French multicentre study. *BJU Int.* **2012**, *110*, 1134–1141. [CrossRef]
70. Fang, D.; Seisen, T.; Yang, K.; Liu, P.; Fan, X.; Singla, N.; Xiong, G.; Zhang, L.; Li, X.; Zhou, L. A systematic review and meta-analysis of oncological and renal function outcomes obtained after segmental ureterectomy versus radical nephroureterectomy for upper tract urothelial carcinoma. *Eur. J. Surg. Oncol.* **2016**, *42*, 1625–1635. [CrossRef]
71. Hung, S.Y.; Yang, W.C.; Luo, H.L.; Hsu, C.C.; Chen, Y.T.; Chuang, Y.C. Segmental ureterectomy does not compromise the oncologic outcome compared with nephroureterectomy for pure ureter cancer. *Int. Urol. Nephrol.* **2014**, *46*, 921–926. [CrossRef] [PubMed]
72. Kim, T.H.; Lee, C.U.; Kang, M.; Jeon, H.G.; Jeong, B.C.; Seo, S.I.; Jeon, S.S.; Lee, H.M.; Sung, H.H. Comparison of oncologic and functional outcomes between radical nephroureterectomy and segmental ureterectomy for upper urinary tract urothelial carcinoma. *Sci. Rep.* **2021**, *11*, 7828. [CrossRef] [PubMed]
73. Duquesne, I.; Abou Chakra, M.; Hage, L.; Pinar, U.; Loriot, Y. Liquid biopsies for detection, surveillance, and prognosis of urothelial cancer: A future standard? *Expert. Rev. Anticancer Ther.* **2023**, *23*, 995–1007. [CrossRef] [PubMed]
74. Hassler, M.R.; Bray, F.; Catto, J.W.F.; Grollman, A.P.; Hartmann, A.; Margulis, V.; Matin, S.F.; Roupret, M.; Sfakianos, J.P.; Shariat, S.F.; et al. Molecular Characterization of Upper Tract Urothelial Carcinoma in the Era of Next-generation Sequencing: A Systematic Review of the Current Literature. *Eur. Urol.* **2020**, *78*, 209–220. [CrossRef]
75. Territo, A.; Gallioli, A.; Diana, P.; Boissier, R.; Fontana, M.; Gaya, J.M.; Sanguedolce, F.; Calderón, J.; Piana, A.; Fontanet, S.; et al. DNA Methylation Urine Biomarkers Test in the Diagnosis of Upper Tract Urothelial Carcinoma: Results from a Single-Center Prospective Clinical Trial. *J. Urol.* **2022**, *208*, 570–579. [CrossRef]
76. Muin, D.; Laukhtina, E.; Hacker, M.; Shariat, S.F. PET in bladder cancer imaging. *Curr. Opin. Urol.* **2023**, *33*, 206–210. [CrossRef]

cancers

MDPI

Article

Clinical Determinants of Extraurinary Tract Recurrence and Survival after Radical Surgery for pT2 Upper Tract Urothelial Carcinoma

Yun-Ching Huang [1,2], Jui-Ming Liu [3,4], Hui-Ying Liu [5], Yin-Lun Chang [5], Chih-Shou Chen [1], Dong-Ru Ho [1], Chun-Te Wu [6], Miao-Fen Chen [7], Hung-Jen Wang [5,*] and Hao-Lun Luo [5,8,*]

1 Department of Urology, Chang Gung Memorial Hospital, Chiayi 613, Taiwan; dr5326@cgmh.org.tw (Y.-C.H.); cv7589@cgmh.org.tw (C.-S.C.); redox@cgmh.org.tw (D.-R.H.)
2 Department of Medicine, College of Medicine, Chang Gung University, Taoyuan 333, Taiwan
3 Department of Urology, Taoyuan General Hospital, Ministry of Health and Welfare, Taoyuan 330, Taiwan; m5134@mail.tygh.gov.tw
4 Department of Obstetrics and Gynecology, Tri-Service General Hospital, National Defense Medical Center, Taipei 114, Taiwan
5 Department of Urology, Kaohsiung Chang Gung Memorial Hospital, Chang Gung University College of Medicine, Kaohsiung 833, Taiwan; ying1011@cgmh.org.tw (H.-Y.L.); tailanylyl@cgmh.org.tw (Y.-L.C.)
6 Department of Urology, Chang Gung Memorial Hospital, Linkou, Taoyuan 333, Taiwan; chuntewu@cgmh.org.tw
7 Department of Radiation Oncology, Chang Gung Memorial Hospital, Linkou, Taoyuan 333, Taiwan; miaofen@cgmh.org.tw
8 Center for Shockwave Medicine and Tissue Engineering, Kaohsiung Chang Gung Memorial Hospital, Chang Gung University College of Medicine, Kaohsiung 833, Taiwan
* Correspondence: wang6107@cgmh.org.tw (H.-J.W.); alesy@cgmh.org.tw (H.-L.L.); Tel.: +886-7-7317123 (ext. 8094) (H.-J.W. & H.-L.L.); Fax: +886-7-7354309 (H.-J.W. & H.-L.L.)

Simple Summary: Although upper tract urothelial carcinoma (UTUC) is a relatively rare malignancy in Western countries, recurrence and distant metastasis are common even after definitive surgery. Many prognostic factors have been identified from previous studies, allowing clinicians to better stratify risk to select patients for perioperative systemic therapy; however, the applicability of adjuvant chemotherapy for patients with stage II UTUC after radical surgery remains unclear. In this study, we found that patients with primary tumor location at ureter or renal pelvis plus synchronous ureter had more frequent disease relapse and worse long-term oncological outcomes than other patients. Male sex, older age, history of previous bladder cancer, and positive surgical margins remain important unfavorable prognostic factors for recurrence and survival. Additional treatment and closer surveillance in patients with these negative prognostic factors are warranted despite complete pathological removal of the tumor.

Abstract: Background: Oncologic outcomes for pT2N0M0 upper tract urothelial carcinoma (UTUC) after nephroureterectomy are not well defined, with most previous studies focused on a heterogeneous population. Therefore, we aimed to investigate the clinical determinants of extraurinary tract recurrence and survival after radical surgery in patients with localized UTUC. Methods: We retrospectively identified 476 patients with pT2N0M0 UTUC who underwent radical nephroureterectomy or ureterectomy between October 2002 and March 2022. To evaluate the prognostic impact, patients were divided into renal pelvic, ureteral, and both-region (renal pelvis plus synchronous ureter) groups based on tumor location. The outcomes included recurrence-free survival (RFS), cancer-specific survival (CSS), and overall survival (OS). Associations were evaluated using multivariable Cox regression analyses for prognostic factors and Kaplan–Meier analyses for survival curves. Results: The renal pelvic, ureteral, and both-region groups consisted of 151 (31.7%), 314 (66.0%), and 11 (2.3%) patients, respectively. Kaplan–Meier analyses comparing the three tumor types showed significant differences in 5-year RFS (83.6% vs. 73.6% vs. 52.5%, $p = 0.013$), CSS (88.6% vs. 80.7% vs. 51.0%, $p = 0.011$), and OS (83.4% vs. 70.1% vs. 45.6%, $p = 0.002$). Multivariable analyses showed that age > 60 years, previous bladder cancer history, ureteral involvement (ureteral and both-regional groups), and positive surgical margins were significant negative prognostic factors for the studied outcomes. Conclusions: Patients with pT2 UTUC and presence of ureteral involvement had more frequent disease relapse. Subsequent adjuvant therapy regimens and close follow-up in patients with negative prognostic factors are warranted despite complete pathological removal of the tumor.

Keywords: upper tract urothelial carcinoma; nephroureterectomy; ureterectomy; recurrence; survival

1. Introduction

Urothelial carcinoma is characterized by neoplastic growth of the entire urothelium, including the upper (renal pelvis and ureter) and the lower (bladder and urethra) urinary tract. Although upper tract urothelial carcinoma (UTUC) is a relatively uncommon malignancy in Western countries, making up only 5–10% of all urothelial carcinomas [1,2], it has a more advanced stage and worse differentiation than bladder cancer, as 62% of UTUCs are muscle-invasive at diagnosis compared to 35% of bladder cancers [3].

Locoregional control of non-muscle-invasive UTUC is satisfactory in definitive surgical series, with extraurinary tract recurrence and distant metastasis being rare [4]. However, in muscle-invasive UTUC, recurrence and distant metastasis are common even after radical nephroureterectomy [4]. A series from the UTUC collaboration showed 5-year recurrence-free survival (RFS) of 92%, 88%, 71%, 48%, and 5% for pTa/Tis, pT1, pT2, pT3, and pT4, respectively [5]. Therefore, adjuvant therapy should be considered for patients with muscle-invasive UTUC after definitive surgical therapy.

Many significant prognostic factors have been proposed based on previously published data [4], allowing clinicians to better stratify risk to select patients for subsequent adjuvant management; however, the use of adjuvant chemotherapy for patients with pT2 UTUC after radical surgery remains controversial. The 2022 National Comprehensive Cancer Network guidelines state that "adjuvant chemotherapy should be considered for patients with no platinum-based neoadjuvant treatment administered and pT3–4 or pN+ disease after surgery" [6]. Contrastingly, a phase 3, open-label, randomized controlled trial that enrolled 260 patients with pT2–4 or pN+ UTUC, of whom 74 (28%) had stage pT2 disease, concluded that adjuvant platinum-based chemotherapy after nephroureterectomy significantly improved disease-free survival [7].

Due to the lack of data on the utility of adjuvant therapy and population heterogeneity in previously published studies, prognostic predictors to identify patients with pT2 UTUC who are more likely to have extraurinary tract recurrence and should receive adjuvant chemotherapy and/or radiotherapy remain insufficient [4,8]. Therefore, this retrospective study aimed to evaluate the association between clinical characteristics and RFS, cancer-specific survival (CSS), and overall survival (OS) of the pT2 UTUC population and provide information to guide the postoperative management and prognostication of patients with pT2 UTUC after radical surgery. We hypothesized that the known risk factors for disease recurrence and survival after radical surgery would apply to the localized UTUC population.

2. Materials and Methods

2.1. Patient Selection

This study was performed with the approval and oversight of the Institutional Review Board (IRB No. 202100779B0). We retrospectively reviewed the medical charts of 476 consecutive patients with pT2 UTUC who were treated with radical nephroureterectomy or ureterectomy between October 2002 and March 2022 at three main branches of Chang Gung Memorial Hospital (Figure 1), which span northern to southern regions of Taiwan with high overall disease coverage [9]. Radical nephroureterectomy with bladder cuff excision is our institution's standard treatment for patients with pT2 UTUC, with segmental ureteral resection performed in patients with distal ureteral tumors, serious renal insufficiency, or a solitary kidney. Patients with neoadjuvant chemotherapy, radiographic metastases, or retroperitoneal lymph node size > 1 cm were excluded. All patients underwent cystoscopy, chest radiography, and computed tomography (CT) urography or magnetic resonance urography (e.g., if any contraindications to CT urography were present) for preoperative risk stratification. In selected patients, diagnostic ureteroscopy, chest CT, and bone scan were used.

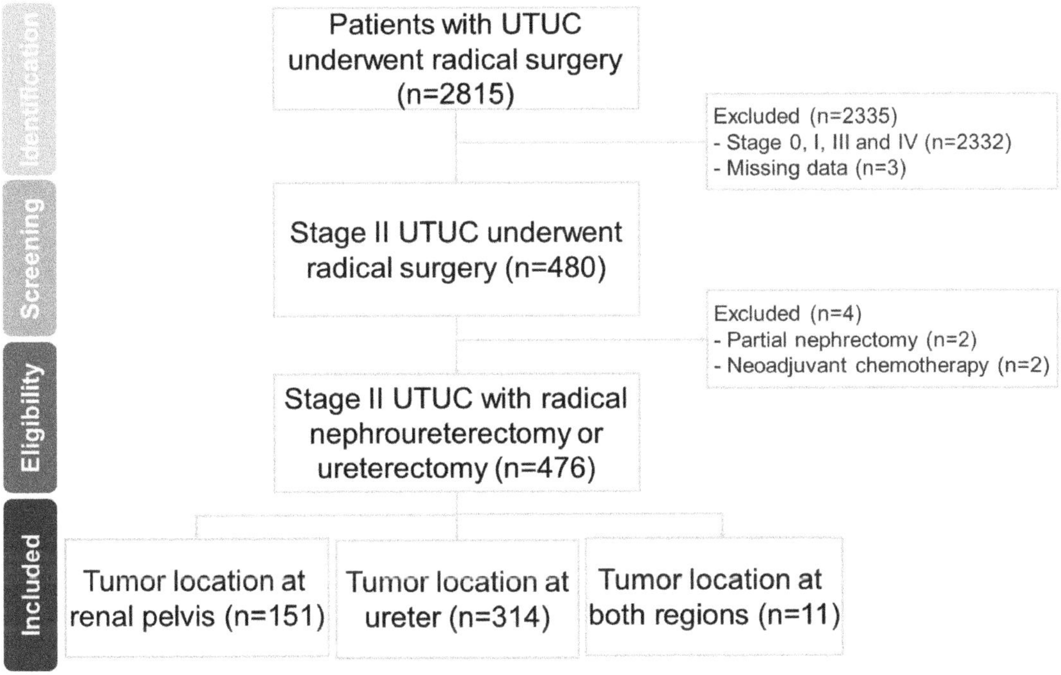

Figure 1. Flow chart for creation of the patient cohort dataset.

2.2. Pathological Evaluation

All the surgical specimens were examined by urologic pathologists at our institution. Tumors were staged according to the 2017 TNM classification by the American Joint Committee on Cancer for UTUC. Tumor grading was assessed according to the 2016 World Health Organization/International Society of Urological Pathology consensus classification. The pathological characteristics collected for predicting prognosis included tumor location, tumor grade, multifocal disease, carcinoma in situ (CIS), lymphovascular invasion (LVI), and surgical margin.

2.3. Outcome Measures

After surgery, patients were generally seen every three months for the first two years, every six months from the third through fifth year, and annually thereafter. Follow-up generally consisted of medical history, physical examination, blood laboratory tests, urinary cytology, renal ultrasound, and cystoscopic evaluation. Diagnostic imaging of both chest radiography and CT urography were used at least annually to detect locoregional recurrence and distant metastasis. Chest CT and bone scans were performed when clinically indicated.

The following clinical characteristics that may be associated with the outcomes were collected: sex, age at surgery, contralateral UTUC history (previous/synchronous/metachronous), bladder cancer history (previous/synchronous/metachronous), hydronephrosis grade,

American Society of Anesthesiologists (ASA) score, diagnostic ureteroscopy (with/without biopsy), surgical approach (open/laparoscopic/robotic), surgical procedure (nephroureterectomy/ureterectomy), and estimated glomerular filtration rate (eGFR). Hydronephrosis grade was assessed by preoperative imaging, including CT, excretory urography, and renal ultrasonography. Hydronephrosis was reported as grade 0, no caliceal or pelvic dilatation; 1, pelvic dilatation only; 2, mild caliceal dilatation; 3, severe caliceal dilatation; and 4, caliceal dilatation accompanied by renal parenchymal atrophy [10]. eGFR was calculated using the 2021 Chronic Kidney Disease Epidemiology creatinine-based equation [11], which was the most widely used equation and recommended by the National Kidney Foundation and the American Society of Nephrology [12].

To evaluate the impact of clinical features on recurrence and survival, patients were divided into renal pelvic, ureteral, and both-region (renal pelvis plus synchronous ureter) groups based on the location of the muscle-invasive tumor at radical surgery (pT2).

Disease recurrence was defined as locoregional failure or distant metastases. Metachronous UC in the remnant genitourinary tract was not considered in the analysis of recurrence [13,14]. RFS interval was defined as the time between radical surgery and the first extraurinary tract recurrence, CSS interval was defined as the time between radical surgery and death from UTUC, and OS interval was defined as the time between radical surgery and death from any cause. Additionally, patients who died within 30 days of radical surgery or during hospital admission were censored at the time of death for the CSS and OS analysis [15].

2.4. Statistical Analysis

Continuous and categorical variables are presented as median values with interquartile ranges (IQR) and proportions, respectively. One-way ANOVA followed by the Tukey–Kramer test for post hoc comparisons [16] and chi-square test were used to compare continuous and categorical variables in the three groups, respectively. Survival curves were analyzed using the Kaplan–Meier method, and differences were determined using the log-rank test. The prognostic factors for RFS, CSS, and OS were estimated using the Cox proportional hazards regression model in the univariate and multivariate analyses. Only those factors with $p < 0.05$ in univariable analysis were further evaluated in multivariable analysis. All reported p values were two-sided, and statistical significance was set at $p < 0.05$. All statistical analyses were performed using SPSS version 20 (IBM Corp, Armonk, NY, USA) or Prism version 9 (GraphPad Software, San Diego, CA, USA).

3. Results

3.1. Baseline Characteristics

Patients' clinical and pathological features stratified by tumor location are presented in Table 1. In the studied cohort, the renal pelvic, ureteral, and both-region groups comprised 151 (31.7%), 314 (66.0%), and 11 (2.3%) patients, respectively. The median age was 70.7 years (IQR, 62.4–77.0 years), and the proportion of female patients was 52.9% in the study population.

The proportion of patients with synchronous bladder cancer, metachronous bladder cancer, and extraurinary tract recurrence was significantly higher in the ureteral and both-region groups than in the renal pelvic group ($p = 0.003$, 0.004, and 0.025, respectively). Hydronephrosis, ureteroscopic biopsy, and ureterectomy were more commonly performed in the ureteral group than in the renal pelvic and both-region groups ($p < 0.001$, 0.001, and <0.001, respectively). Patients in the both-region group had a significantly higher proportion of multifocal disease than those in the renal pelvic and ureteral groups ($p < 0.001$). LVI was more common in the renal pelvic and both-region groups than in the ureteral group ($p = 0.013$). No statistically significant differences were observed in sex, age, contralateral UTUC history, previous bladder cancer history, ASA score, surgical approach, tumor grade, CIS, positive surgical margin, and eGFR between the groups (all, $p > 0.05$).

Table 1. Clinical and pathological characteristics.

	Total (n = 476)	Main Tumor Location			p Value
		Renal Pelvis (n = 151)	Ureter (n = 314)	Both Regions (n = 11)	
Gender					0.236
Female	252 (52.9)	87 (57.6)	161 (51.3)	4 (36.4)	
Male	224 (47.1)	64 (42.4)	153 (48.7)	7 (63.6)	
Age, years, median (IQR)	70.7 (62.4–77.0)	69.2 (61.2–76.1)	70.8 (62.7–77.5)	68.9 (58.5–74.0)	0.224
<60	94 (19.7)	34 (22.5)	56 (17.8)	4 (36.4)	0.439
60–70	133 (27.9)	44 (29.1)	87 (27.7)	2 (18.2)	
70–80	180 (37.8)	51 (33.8)	124 (39.5)	5 (45.5)	
>80	69 (14.5)	22 (14.6)	47 (15.0)	0 (0)	
Contralateral UTUC history					0.370
Previous	23 (4.8)	10 (6.6)	13 (4.1)	0 (0)	
Synchronous	7 (1.5)	2 (1.3)	4 (1.3)	1 (9.1)	
Metachronous	32 (6.7)	10 (6.6)	21 (6.7)	1 (9.1)	
Bladder cancer history					
Previous	58 (12.2)	16 (10.6)	39 (12.4)	3 (27.3)	0.258
Synchronous	93 (19.5)	18 (11.9)	70 (22.3)	5 (45.5)	0.003
Metachronous	158 (33.2)	37 (24.5)	114 (36.3)	7 (63.6)	0.004
Hydronephrosis grade					<0.001
0	41 (8.6)	25 (16.6)	15 (4.8)	1 (9.1)	
1	59 (12.4)	38 (25.2)	19 (6.1)	2 (18.2)	
2	114 (23.9)	39 (25.8)	71 (22.6)	4 (36.4)	
3	121 (25.4)	25 (16.6)	96 (30.6)	0 (0)	
4	130 (27.3)	21 (13.9)	105 (33.4)	4 (36.4)	
Unknown	11 (2.3)	3 (2.0)	8 (2.5)	0 (0)	
ASA score, median (IQR)	3 (2–3)	3 (2–3)	3 (2–3)	3 (2–3)	0.542
≤2	189 (39.7)	64 (42.4)	122 (38.9)	3 (27.3)	0.533
≥3	287 (60.3)	87 (57.6)	192 (61.1)	8 (72.7)	
Diagnostic ureteroscopy					0.001
Ureteroscopic biopsy	125 (26.3)	22 (14.6)	100 (31.8)	3 (27.3)	
Ureteroscopy without biopsy	100 (21.0)	31 (20.5)	68 (21.7)	1 (9.1)	
Surgical approach					0.608
Open	247 (51.9)	76 (50.3)	164 (52.2)	7 (63.6)	
Laparoscopic	213 (44.7)	72 (47.7)	137 (43.6)	4 (36.4)	
Robotic	16 (3.4)	3 (2.0)	13 (4.1)	0 (0)	
Surgical procedure					<0.001
Nephroureterectomy	440 (92.4)	151 (100.0)	278 (88.5)	11 (100.0)	
Ureterectomy	36 (7.6)	0 (0)	36 (11.5)	0 (0)	
Tumor grade					0.307
Low	25 (5.3)	11 (7.3)	13 (4.1)	1 (9.1)	
High	451 (94.7)	140 (92.7)	301 (95.9)	10 (90.9)	
Multifocal disease	141 (29.6)	38 (25.2)	92 (29.3)	11 (100.0)	<0.001
Carcinoma in situ	125 (26.3)	35 (23.2)	85 (27.1)	5 (45.5)	0.230
Lymphovascular invasion	54 (11.3)	26 (17.2)	26 (8.3)	2 (18.2)	0.013
Positive surgical margin	18 (3.8)	2 (1.3)	16 (5.1)	0 (0)	0.109
eGFR, mL/min/1.73 m^2, median (IQR)	44.9 (24.3–57.0)	43.3 (20.8–56.8)	46.2 (27.2–57.1)	35.3 (0–53.9)	0.156
<60	362 (76.1)	117 (77.5)	235 (74.8)	10 (90.9)	0.315
≥60	97 (20.4)	26 (17.2)	70 (22.3)	1 (9.1)	
Unknown	17 (3.6)	8 (5.3)	9 (2.9)	0 (0)	
Recurrence	107 (22.5)	23 (15.2)	80 (25.5)	4 (36.4)	0.025
Locoregional failure	42 (8.8)	7 (4.6)	33 (10.5)	2 (18.2)	0.111
Distant metastasis	51 (10.7)	14 (9.3)	36 (11.5)	1 (9.1%)	
Locoregional + distant metastasis	14 (2.9)	2 (1.3)	11 (3.5)	1 (9.1)	

Data are n (%), unless otherwise stated. IQR: interquartile range, UTUC: upper urinary tract urothelial carcinoma, ASA: American Society of Anesthesiologists, eGFR: estimated glomerular filtration rate. Hydronephrosis grading scale, including grade 0—no caliceal or pelvic dilation, grade 1—pelvic dilatation only, grade 2—mild caliceal dilatation, grade 3—severe caliceal dilatation, and grade 4—renal parenchymal atrophy.

3.2. Recurrence and Survival

Median follow-up for the entire study cohort after surgery was 57.3 months (IQR, 24.1–100.2 months). At the end of the follow-up, 107 (21.0%) patients experienced extraurinary tract recurrence, 79 (18.9%) died of cancer-related causes, and 63 (12.6%) died of other causes. Of the 107 (21.0%) patients who had extraurinary tract recurrence, 42 (8.8%) had locoregional failure, 51 (10.7%) had distant metastasis, and 14 (2.9%) had locoregional failure plus synchronous distant metastasis, suggesting that the relatively common relapse pattern was distant metastasis (Table 1).

3.2.1. Extraurinary Tract Recurrence

Extraurinary tract recurrence occurred in 23 (15.2%), 80 (25.5%), and 4 (36.4%) patients in the renal pelvic, ureteral, and both-region groups, respectively ($p = 0.025$). The median time interval of recurrence after radical surgery was 15.5 months (IQR, 7.4–32.9 months), and 73 (68.2%) patients with disease recurrence were identified within two years. The 5-year RFS was significantly higher in the renal pelvic group than in the ureteral and both-region groups (83.6% vs. 73.6% vs. 52.5%, $p = 0.013$; Figure 2).

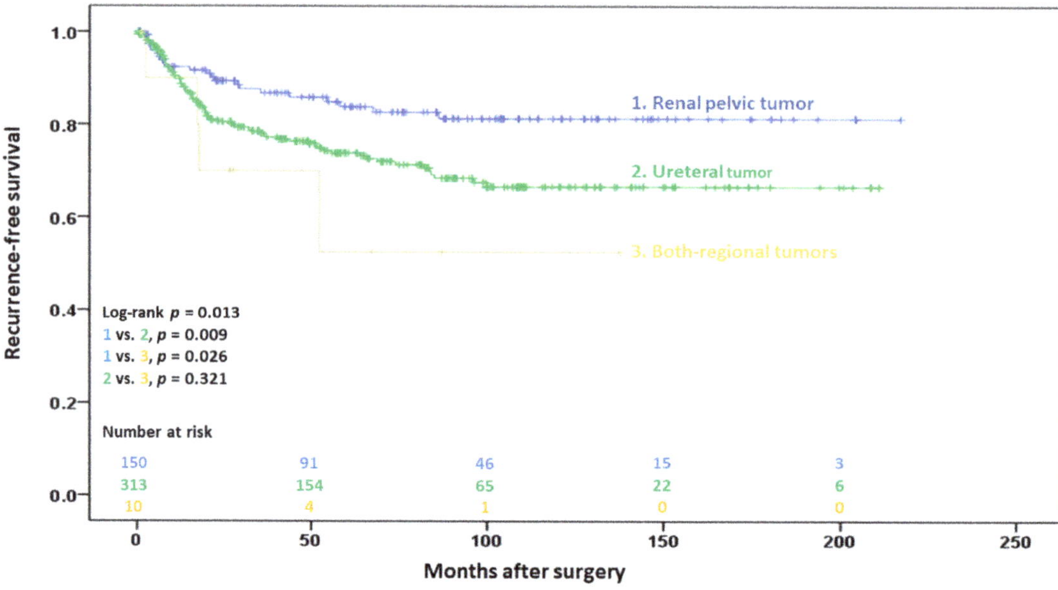

Figure 2. Kaplan–Meier estimates of extraurinary tract recurrence-free survival in 476 patients following radical surgery for pT2 upper urinary tract urothelial carcinoma, with stratification by tumor location.

In the multivariable analysis, previous bladder cancer history ($p = 0.002$), ureteral involvement, including ureteral and both-region groups ($p = 0.022$), and positive surgical margin ($p < 0.001$) were independent unfavorable prognostic factors for extraurinary tract recurrence (Table 2).

Table 2. Univariate and multivariate analysis predicting prognostic factors for recurrence-free survival in the patients with pT2 UTUC after radical surgery.

	Recurrence-Free Survival			
	Univariate		Multivariate	
	HR (95% CI)	p Value	HR (95% CI)	p Value
Male gender (referent: female)	1.54 (1.05–2.26)	0.026	1.41 (0.96–2.08)	0.080
Age (referent: <60 years)		0.085		0.056
60–70 years	1.84 (1.02–3.34)	0.044	2.12 (1.16–3.88)	0.015
70–80 years	1.70 (0.95–3.04)	0.073	1.86 (1.03–3.37)	0.040
>80	2.38 (1.20–4.74)	0.013	2.42 (1.21–4.87)	0.013
Contralateral UTUC (referent: absent)		0.766		
Previous	1.37 (0.64–2.96)	0.418		
Synchronous	0.69 (0.10–4.96)	0.713		
Metachronous	0.81 (0.38–1.75)	0.592		
Bladder cancer (referent: absent)				
Previous	2.20 (1.39–3.50)	0.001	2.12 (1.31–3.42)	0.002
Synchronous	1.28 (0.81–2.01)	0.289		
Metachronous	1.44 (0.98–2.11)	0.062		
Hydronephrosis grade (referent: grade 0)		0.209		
1	0.42 (0.16–1.11)	0.081		
2	0.98 (0.47–2.01)	0.945		
3	1.14 (0.56–2.32)	0.715		
4	0.88 (0.43–1.81)	0.725		
ASA score $\geq$ 3 (referent: ASA $\leq$ 2)	0.97 (0.67–1.43)	0.892		
Diagnostic ureteroscopy (referent: no)		0.453		
Ureteroscopic biopsy	1.27 (0.82–1.97)	0.282		
Ureteroscopy without biopsy	0.94 (0.57–1.54)	0.793		
Surgical approach (referent: open)		0.173		
Laparoscopic	1.11 (0.75–1.64)	0.610		
Robotic	2.24 (0.96–5.22)	0.062		
Ureterectomy procedure (referent: NU)	1.70 (0.93–3.10)	0.083		
Tumor location (referent: renal pelvis)		0.015		0.022
Ureter	1.85 (1.16–2.94)	0.010	1.77 (1.11–2.83)	0.016
Synchronous renal pelvis and ureter	3.09 (1.07–8.94)	0.038	3.18 (1.07–9.41)	0.037
Tumor grade (referent: low grade)	1.45 (0.53–3.94)	0.466		
Multifocal disease (referent: absent)	1.12 (0.75–1.69)	0.579		
Carcinoma in situ (referent: absent)	0.82 (0.52–1.28)	0.374		
Lymphovascular invasion (referent: absent)	1.50 (0.88–2.55)	0.135		
Positive surgical margin (referent: absent)	4.48 (2.33–8.61)	<0.001	3.79 (1.95–7.35)	<0.001
Chronic kidney disease [a] (referent: absent)	0.86 (0.54–1.35)	0.499		

Hydronephrosis grading scale, including grade 0—no caliceal or pelvic dilation, grade 1—pelvic dilatation only, grade 2—mild caliceal dilatation, grade 3—severe caliceal dilatation, and grade 4—renal parenchymal atrophy. [a] Chronic kidney disease was defined as estimated glomerular filtration rate less than 60 mL/min/1.73 m^2. UTUC: upper urinary tract urothelial carcinoma; HR: hazard ratio; CI: confidence interval; ASA: American Society of Anesthesiologists; NU: nephroureterectomy.

3.2.2. Cancer-Specific Survival

Cancer-specific death occurred in 17 (11.3%), 58 (18.5%), and 4 (36.4%) patients in the renal pelvic, ureteral, and both-region groups, respectively ($p = 0.030$). The 5-year CSS was significantly higher in the renal pelvic group than in the ureteral and both-region groups (88.6% vs. 80.7% vs. 51.0%, $p = 0.011$; Figure 3). Multivariate analysis showed that male sex ($p = 0.034$), age > 60 years ($p < 0.001$), previous bladder cancer history ($p = 0.001$), ureteral involvement ($p = 0.008$), and positive surgical margins ($p = 0.026$) were significant negative prognostic factors for cancer-specific death (Table 3).

Table 3. Univariate and multivariate analysis predicting prognostic factors for cancer-specific survival in the patients with pT2 UTUC after radical surgery.

	Cancer-Specific Survival			
	Univariate		Multivariate	
	HR (95% CI)	*p* Value	HR (95% CI)	*p* Value
Male gender (referent: female)	1.72 (1.10–2.69)	0.017	1.64 (1.04–2.59)	0.034
Age (referent: <60 years)		0.001		<0.001
60–70 years	3.87 (1.69–8.85)	0.001	4.89 (2.10–11.4)	<0.001
70–80 years	2.96 (1.29–6.78)	0.010	3.66 (1.57–8.52)	0.003
>80	5.86 (2.37–14.5)	<0.001	6.78 (2.69–17.1)	<0.001
Contralateral UTUC (referent: absent)		0.929		
Previous	1.35 (0.54–3.34)	0.523		
Synchronous	0.93 (0.13–6.67)	0.938		
Metachronous	1.10 (0.50–2.39)	0.817		
Bladder cancer (referent: absent)				
Previous	2.54 (1.50–4.32)	0.001	2.49 (1.44–4.32)	0.001
Synchronous	1.64 (1.0–2.71)	0.051		
Metachronous	1.30 (0.83–2.03)	0.249		
Hydronephrosis grade (referent: grade 0)		0.350		
1		0.555		
2	0.72 (0.24–2.14)	0.776		
3	0.87 (0.33–2.27)	0.474		
4	1.39 (0.57–3.39)	0.472		
ASA score $\geq$ 3 (referent: ASA $\leq$ 2)	1.41 (0.89–2.22)	0.146		
Diagnostic ureteroscopy (referent: no)		0.511		
Ureteroscopic biopsy	1.19 (0.71–1.98)	0.510		
Ureteroscopy without biopsy	0.81 (0.45–1.46)	0.483		
Surgical approach (referent: open)		0.365		
Laparoscopic	0.95 (0.60–1.49)	0.809		
Robotic	2.01 (0.72–5.60)	0.185		
Ureterectomy procedure (referent: NU)	1.10 (0.48–2.53)	0.823		
Tumor location (referent: renal pelvis)		0.015		0.008
Ureter	1.79 (1.04–3.08)	0.035	1.75 (1.01–3.02)	0.045
Synchronous renal pelvis and ureter	4.35 (1.46–13.0)	0.008	5.39 (1.76–16.5)	0.003
Tumor grade (referent: low grade)	1.36 (0.43–4.33)	0.598		
Multifocal disease (referent: absent)	1.34 (0.84–2.13)	0.221		
Carcinoma in situ (referent: absent)	0.97 (0.59–1.60)	0.971		
Lymphovascular invasion (referent: absent)	1.57 (0.85–2.90)	0.151		
Positive surgical margin (referent: absent)	3.48 (1.51–8.03)	0.004	2.64 (1.13–6.17)	0.026
Chronic kidney disease [a] (referent: absent)	0.81 (0.49–1.35)	0.424		

Hydronephrosis grading scale, including grade 0—no caliceal or pelvic dilation, grade 1—pelvic dilatation only, grade 2—mild caliceal dilatation, grade 3—severe caliceal dilatation, and grade 4—renal parenchymal atrophy. [a] Chronic kidney disease was defined as estimated glomerular filtration rate less than 60 mL/min/1.73 m^2. UTUC: upper urinary tract urothelial carcinoma; HR: hazard ratio; CI: confidence interval; ASA: American Society of Anesthesiologists; NU: nephroureterectomy.

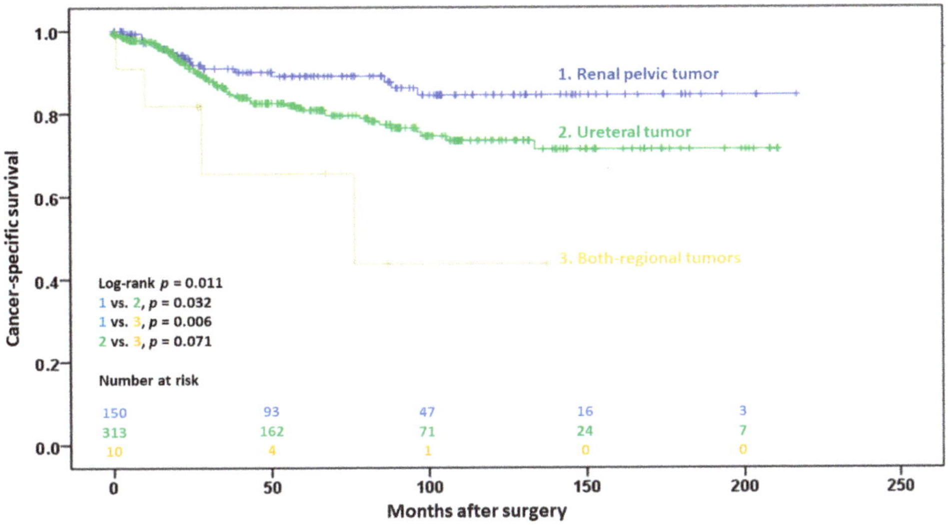

Figure 3. Kaplan–Meier estimates of cancer-specific survival in 476 patients following radical surgery for pT2 upper urinary tract urothelial carcinoma, with stratification by tumor location.

3.2.3. Overall Survival

Death from any cause occurred in 33 (21.9%), 103 (32.8%), and 6 (54.5%) patients in the renal pelvic, ureteral, and both-region groups, respectively ($p = 0.010$). The 5-year OS was significantly higher in the renal pelvic group than in the ureteral and both-region groups (83.4% vs. 70.1% vs. 45.6%, $p = 0.002$; Figure 4). Age > 60 years ($p < 0.001$), previous bladder cancer history ($p = 0.001$), ureteral involvement ($p = 0.005$), and positive surgical margins ($p = 0.009$) were independently associated with OS in the multivariate Cox regression models (Table 4).

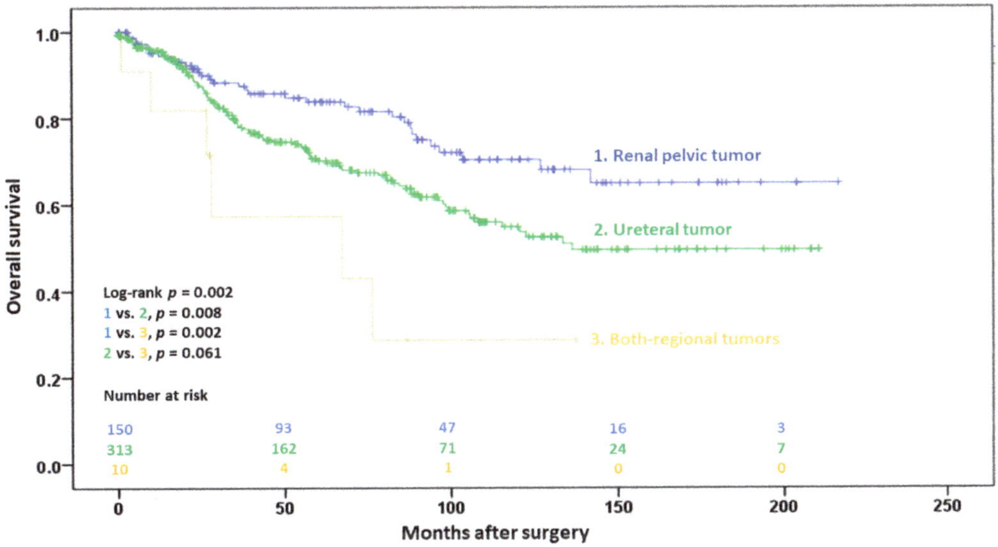

Figure 4. Kaplan–Meier estimates of overall survival in 476 patients following radical surgery for pT2 upper urinary tract urothelial carcinoma, with stratification by tumor location.

Table 4. Univariate and multivariate analysis predicting prognostic factors for overall survival in the patients with pT2 UTUC after radical surgery.

	Overall Survival			
	Univariate		Multivariate	
	HR (95% CI)	*p* Value	HR (95% CI)	*p* Value
Male gender (referent: female)	1.27 (0.91–1.76)	0.162		
Age (referent: <60 years)		<0.001		<0.001
60–70 years	2.38 (1.35–4.21)	0.003	2.63 (1.48–4.68)	0.001
70–80 years	2.88 (1.68–4.94)	<0.001	3.0 (1.72–5.23)	<0.001
>80	4.32 (2.29–8.16)	<0.001	4.04 (2.10–7.80)	<0.001
Contralateral UTUC (referent: absent)		0.860		
Previous	1.23 (0.60–2.52)	0.567		
Synchronous	1.47 (0.47–4.64)	0.507		
Metachronous	1.06 (0.60–1.89)	0.839		
Bladder cancer (referent: absent)				
Previous	2.24 (1.46–3.41)	<0.001	2.18 (1.40–3.40)	0.001
Synchronous	1.58 (1.08–2.31)	0.017	1.22 (0.81–1.83)	0.338
Metachronous	1.00 (0.71–1.41)	0.981		
Hydronephrosis grade (referent: grade 0)		0.280		
1	0.60 (0.27–1.33)	0.210		
2	1.02 (0.53–1.98)	0.954		
3	1.21 (0.64–2.30)	0.563		
4	1.17 (0.61–2.21)	0.640		
ASA score $\geq$ 3 (referent: ASA $\leq$ 2)	1.89 (1.33–2.70)	<0.001	1.40 (0.96–2.04)	0.084
Diagnostic ureteroscopy (referent: no)		0.301		
Ureteroscopic biopsy	1.16 (0.79–1.71)	0.447		
Ureteroscopy without biopsy	0.79 (0.51–1.23)	0.290		
Surgical approach (referent: open)		0.806		
Laparoscopic	0.91 (0.65–1.28)	0.596		
Robotic	1.17 (0.43–3.21)	0.757		
Ureterectomy procedure (referent: NU)	1.30 (0.72–2.35)	0.389		
Tumor location (referent: renal pelvis)		0.003		0.005
Ureter	1.69 (1.14–2.50)	0.009	1.62 (1.09–2.40)	0.018
Synchronous renal pelvis and ureter	3.67 (1.53–8.78)	0.003	3.84 (1.56–9.45)	0.003
Tumor grade (referent: low grade)	1.19 (0.52–2.69)	0.682		
Multifocal disease (referent: absent)	1.29 (0.91–1.83)	0.151		
Carcinoma in situ (referent: absent)	1.21 (0.85–1.72)	0.298		
Lymphovascular invasion (referent: absent)	1.33 (0.81–2.18)	0.263		
Positive surgical margin (referent: absent)	3.13 (1.59–6.17)	0.001	2.59 (1.27–5.25)	0.009
Chronic kidney disease [a] (referent: absent)	1.15 (0.76–1.75)	0.504		

Hydronephrosis grading scale, including grade 0—no caliceal or pelvic dilation, grade 1—pelvic dilatation only, grade 2—mild caliceal dilatation, grade 3—severe caliceal dilatation, and grade 4—renal parenchymal atrophy. [a] Chronic kidney disease was defined as estimated glomerular filtration rate less than 60 mL/min/1.73 m^2. UTUC: upper urinary tract urothelial carcinoma; HR: hazard ratio; CI: confidence interval; ASA: American Society of Anesthesiologists; NU: nephroureterectomy.

3.3. Subset Analysis

After excluding both-region cases, ureter tumor remained an unfavorable prognostic factor in the multivariate analysis for RFS (hazard ratio [HR] 1.85, 95% confidence interval [CI] 1.16–2.94; $p = 0.010$), CSS (HR 1.79, 95% CI 1.04–3.08; $p = 0.035$), and OS (HR 1.69, 95% CI 1.14–2.50; $p = 0.009$).

4. Discussion

Although many possible risk factors associated with recurrence and survival have been proposed [4], prognostic factors for patients with pT2 UTUC after radical surgery remain unclear. This may be due to the rare incidence of the disease and highly heterogeneous population enrolled in previous studies. Therefore, we only included patients with pT2N0M0 UTUC in this series. Although there are no data on the efficacy of postoperative chemotherapy or radiotherapy in terms of recurrence and mortality in patients with pT2N0M0 UTUC after radical surgery, our findings confirm the prognostic significance of several variables associated with disease recurrence and survival. Subsequent adjuvant therapy regimens and close follow-up in patients with poor prognostic factors are warranted despite complete pathological removal of the disease.

Previous studies have reported controversial results regarding the impact of primary tumor location on the outcome of UTUC treatment. Some studies failed to identify a difference in cancer-specific mortality between renal pelvic and ureteral tumors [17,18]. On the contrary, a retrospective study from multiple institutions, similar to our findings, showed a worse CSS for ureteral and both-region tumors than for renal pelvic tumors, even when adjusted for stage [19]. There are several possible explanations for the conflicting results between the present and previously published studies. In an international collaborative study from 13 centers worldwide, Raman et al. enrolled 1249 patients with UTUC managed by radical nephroureterectomy and assigned them into renal pelvic and ureteral groups [17]. After adjustment for pathologic tumor classification, grade, and lymph node status, tumor location did not independently predict cancer-specific mortality. Potential bias in this study may lie in the fact that tumors involving both the renal pelvis and ureteral regions were classified based on the dominant tumor location (in accordance with stage or size) under either the renal pelvic or ureteral group. In cases where renal pelvic and ureteral tumors are of the same stage, the tumor size is used to identify the tumor location. We believe this methodology can result in misclassification and bias, especially in an international retrospective study. Although the both-region group contained only 11 cases in this study, we postulate that tumors involving both the renal pelvis and ureter should be analyzed as distinct entities to avoid misclassification. In further analysis, tumor location remained a significant prognostic factor for RFS, CSS, and OS after excluding the both-region group. We also reported several important patient-related factors (e.g., history of previous bladder cancer, history of previous UTUC, and ASA score) and tumor-related factors (e.g., hydronephrosis, multifocality, CIS, lymphovascular invasion, and surgical margins) that were not assessed by Raman et al. [17]. In a similar report using administrative data from nine registries of the SEER database, Isbarn et al. identified 2824 patients treated with nephroureterectomy for UTUC and divided them into dichotomies according to primary tumor location [18]. Although the main findings were not different in terms of oncologic outcomes between patients with renal pelvic and ureteral tumors, data were collected by medical files review at participating institutions, thus introducing discrepancies in the interpretation of study variables. Overcoming these limitations, the study variables in the present study were reviewed by two independent urologists (YCH and HLL). Furthermore, this study was not a multi-institutional collaborative study, and practice patterns, including patients' access to care, disease management, surgical techniques, and follow-up after surgery, were relatively uniform at our institute.

The poor prognosis of ureteral involvement can be explained in several ways. Compared to renal pelvic tumor with the natural barriers of renal parenchyma, perirenal fat, and Gerota's fascia, ureteral involvement has a thin wall containing an extensive plexus of blood and lymphatic vessels, enabling easier invasion and spread of tumor cells [20]. Higher prevalence of hydronephrosis in ureteral involvement is also associated with more pronounced eGFR deterioration after radical nephroureterectomy [21], thereby restricting the use of postoperative cisplatin-based chemotherapy. Interestingly, a previous history of bladder cancer increased the risk of cancer-specific death by a 2.54-fold factor relative to no previous history of bladder cancer. Indeed, the proportion of multifocality and CIS was significantly higher in the group with a history of previous bladder cancer, which is a well-known predictor of poor outcomes after UTUC, than in the group with no previous history of bladder cancer, and this result is consistent with previous findings [22,23].

However, the effect of sex on the prognosis of UTUC after radical surgery remains unclear. Sikic et al. reported a 2.92-fold higher risk of cancer-specific death in female patients aged 59 years and older than in male patients [24]. Milojevic et al. found no significant difference in the CSS between female and male patients treated with radical nephroureterectomy [25]. In contrast, Wu et al. showed that male patients with UTUC were associated with more metachronous bladder cancer and higher cancer-specific mortality compared to female patients with UTUC [26]. Our observations that male patients with UTUC have worse cancer-specific mortality compared to female patients based on multivariate analysis are consistent with the previous findings. Multiple factors, including genetic background, environmental exposure, tumor biology, hormonal variation, and anatomical factors, may play a role in the reported sex differences. However, this finding is not in line with recently published data [27], and further epidemiologic and molecular research is required to address the impact of sex on the incidence, progression, and metastasis of patients with UTUC.

Unlike surgical margins, the effects of age on clinical outcomes in patients with UTUC have rarely been discussed. A large population-based study using the SEER database showed that older age is directly associated with a decrease in CSS after adjustment for stage, grade, and treatment type [28]. Reasons for this may be include changes in the biological potential of tumor cells, decreased host immunity with advancing age, or even different choices of treatment in elderly patients compared with younger patients [29]. In the current study, 3.2% of patients treated with segmental ureterectomy were aged < 60 years, and 13.0% were aged > 80 years, given the higher risk of residual disease [30]. Furthermore, elderly patients are less likely to undergo salvage chemotherapy for disease relapse [31], which has been shown to be associated with improved survival. These results indicate that treatment choice, at least in part, may account for the worse outcomes in older patients.

The current study had several limitations. First, due to the retrospective design of this study, biases are inevitable, as segmental ureteral resection in patients with distal ureteral tumors, with a serious renal insufficiency, or having a solitary kidney was chosen depending on patient preference after discussion with the treating urologist. Second, a centralized pathological review is lacking. The specimens being evaluated by various genitourinary pathologists over a long period could have led to discrepancies in the interpretation of the pathologic specimens. Third, the number of patients was too small to draw definite conclusions, particularly in the both-region group. Fourth, this study lacked data on adjuvant treatment. We could not confirm the effect of perioperative chemotherapy, immunotherapy, or radiotherapy on survival outcomes. Despite these limitations, our study was a relatively large cohort study focusing on the outcomes of pT2 UTUC after radical surgery. Our results indicate that patients with tumors located in the ureter or renal pelvis plus synchronous ureter could be candidates for additional treatment and closer follow-up after radical surgery. Prospective assessments to obtain a definitive role of adjuvant therapy in patients with pT2 UTUC are warranted.

5. Conclusions

Patients with pT2 UTUC and presence of ureteral involvement (ureteral and both-regional groups) had more frequent disease relapse and worse long-term oncological outcomes than other patients. Male sex, older age, history of previous bladder cancer, and positive surgical margins remain important unfavorable prognostic factors for recurrence and survival. Our findings support the need for more stringent follow-up strategies and subsequent adjuvant treatment in patients with those poor prognostic factors despite complete pathological removal of the disease. Prospectively large-scale studies investigating the role of tumor location in patients with pT2 UTUC are needed to obtain a definitive statement regarding this matter.

Author Contributions: Conceptualization, Y.-C.H., H.-J.W. and H.-L.L.; methodology, Y.-C.H. and H.-L.L.; software, H.-Y.L. and Y.-L.C.; validation, J.-M.L., C.-S.C., D.-R.H., C.-T.W. and M.-F.C.; formal analysis, Y.-C.H. and H.-L.L.; investigation, Y.-C.H.; resources, Y.-C.H., C.-S.C., C.-T.W., M.-F.C. and H.-J.W.; data curation, Y.-C.H. and H.-L.L.; writing—original draft preparation, Y.-C.H.; writing—review and editing, H.-L.L.; supervision, H.-J.W. and H.-L.L.; project administration, Y.-C.H. and H.-L.L.; funding acquisition, Y.-C.H. and H.-L.L. All authors have read and agreed to the published version of the manuscript.

Funding: The APC was funded by Chang Gung Medical Foundation, Taiwan (BMRPB51).

Institutional Review Board Statement: The study was conducted according to the guidelines of the Declaration of Helsinki and approved by the Institutional Review Board of Chang Gung Memorial Hospital on 28 May 2021 (IRB No. 202100779B0).

Informed Consent Statement: Patient consent was waived due to the retrospective nature of this study.

Data Availability Statement: The datasets generated during and/or analyzed during the current study are available from the corresponding author on reasonable request.

Acknowledgments: All individuals included in the section have consented to the acknowledgement. We would like to thank the Center for Shockwave Medicine and Tissue Engineering, Kaohsiung Chang Gung Memorial Hospital and Chang Gung University College of Medicine, Kaohsiung, Taiwan; Health Information and Epidemiology Laboratory, Chang Gung Memorial Hospital, Chiayi, Taiwan; and Chang Gung Medical Foundation for technical support and the Chin Pei Medical Foundation for partial funding support.

Conflicts of Interest: The authors declare no conflict of interest.

References

1. Siegel, R.L.; Miller, K.D.; Fuchs, H.E.; Jemal, A. Cancer statistics, 2022. *CA Cancer J. Clin.* **2022**, *72*, 7–33. [CrossRef]
2. Soria, F.; Shariat, S.F.; Lerner, S.P.; Fritsche, H.M.; Rink, M.; Kassouf, W.; Spiess, P.E.; Lotan, Y.; Ye, D.; Fernandez, M.I.; et al. Epidemiology, diagnosis, preoperative evaluation and prognostic assessment of upper-tract urothelial carcinoma (UTUC). *World J. Urol.* **2017**, *35*, 379–387. [CrossRef]
3. Catto, J.W.; Yates, D.R.; Rehman, I.; Azzouzi, A.R.; Patterson, J.; Sibony, M.; Cussenot, O.; Hamdy, F.C. Behavior of urothelial carcinoma with respect to anatomical location. *J. Urol.* **2007**, *177*, 1715–1720. [CrossRef]
4. Roupret, M.; Babjuk, M.; Burger, M.; Capoun, O.; Cohen, D.; Comperat, E.M.; Cowan, N.C.; Dominguez-Escrig, J.L.; Gontero, P.; Hugh Mostafid, A.; et al. European Association of Urology Guidelines on Upper Urinary Tract Urothelial Carcinoma: 2020 Update. *Eur. Urol.* **2021**, *79*, 62–79. [CrossRef]
5. Margulis, V.; Shariat, S.F.; Matin, S.F.; Kamat, A.M.; Zigeuner, R.; Kikuchi, E.; Lotan, Y.; Weizer, A.; Raman, J.D.; Wood, C.G.; et al. Outcomes of radical nephroureterectomy: A series from the Upper Tract Urothelial Carcinoma Collaboration. *Cancer* **2009**, *115*, 1224–1233. [CrossRef] [PubMed]
6. Flaig, T.W.; Spiess, P.E.; Agarwal, N.; Bangs, R.; Boorjian, S.A.; Buyyounouski, M.K.; Chang, S.; Downs, T.M.; Efstathiou, J.A.; Friedlander, T.; et al. Bladder Cancer, Version 3.2020, NCCN Clinical Practice Guidelines in Oncology. *J. Natl. Compr. Cancer Netw.* **2020**, *18*, 329–354. [CrossRef] [PubMed]
7. Birtle, A.; Johnson, M.; Chester, J.; Jones, R.; Dolling, D.; Bryan, R.T.; Harris, C.; Winterbottom, A.; Blacker, A.; Catto, J.W.F.; et al. Adjuvant chemotherapy in upper tract urothelial carcinoma (the POUT trial): A phase 3, open-label, randomised controlled trial. *Lancet* **2020**, *395*, 1268–1277. [CrossRef] [PubMed]
8. Leow, J.J.; Chong, Y.L.; Chang, S.L.; Valderrama, B.P.; Powles, T.; Bellmunt, J. Neoadjuvant and Adjuvant Chemotherapy for Upper Tract Urothelial Carcinoma: A 2020 Systematic Review and Meta-analysis, and Future Perspectives on Systemic Therapy. *Eur. Urol.* **2021**, *79*, 635–654. [CrossRef] [PubMed]
9. Tsai, M.S.; Lin, M.H.; Lee, C.P.; Yang, Y.H.; Chen, W.C.; Chang, G.H.; Tsai, Y.T.; Chen, P.C.; Tsai, Y.H. Chang Gung Research Database: A multi-institutional database consisting of original medical records. *Biomed. J.* **2017**, *40*, 263–269. [CrossRef]
10. Ito, Y.; Kikuchi, E.; Tanaka, N.; Miyajima, A.; Mikami, S.; Jinzaki, M.; Oya, M. Preoperative hydronephrosis grade independently predicts worse pathological outcomes in patients undergoing nephroureterectomy for upper tract urothelial carcinoma. *J. Urol.* **2011**, *185*, 1621–1626. [CrossRef]
11. Inker, L.A.; Eneanya, N.D.; Coresh, J.; Tighiouart, H.; Wang, D.; Sang, Y.; Crews, D.C.; Doria, A.; Estrella, M.M.; Froissart, M.; et al. New Creatinine- and Cystatin C-Based Equations to Estimate GFR without Race. *N. Engl. J. Med.* **2021**, *385*, 1737–1749. [CrossRef] [PubMed]

12. Delgado, C.; Baweja, M.; Crews, D.C.; Eneanya, N.D.; Gadegbeku, C.A.; Inker, L.A.; Mendu, M.L.; Miller, W.G.; Moxey-Mims, M.M.; Roberts, G.V.; et al. A Unifying Approach for GFR Estimation: Recommendations of the NKF-ASN Task Force on Reassessing the Inclusion of Race in Diagnosing Kidney Disease. *Am. J. Kidney Dis.* **2022**, *79*, 268–288.e1. [CrossRef] [PubMed]
13. Huang, Y.C.; Liu, Y.L.; Chen, M.F.; Chen, C.S.; Wu, C.T. Treatment Strategy for Dialysis Patient with Urothelial Carcinoma. *Diagnostics* **2021**, *11*, 1966. [CrossRef] [PubMed]
14. Liu, Y.L.; Wu, C.T.; Hsu, Y.C.; Chen, M.F.; Chen, C.S.; Shi, C.S.; Huang, Y.C. Perioperative Complications and Oncologic Outcomes after Radical Cystectomy in End-Stage Renal Disease Patients with Bladder Cancer Obtained Using a Standardized Reporting System. *Cancers* **2022**, *14*, 3512. [CrossRef] [PubMed]
15. Rink, M.; Ehdaie, B.; Cha, E.K.; Green, D.A.; Karakiewicz, P.I.; Babjuk, M.; Margulis, V.; Raman, J.D.; Svatek, R.S.; Fajkovic, H.; et al. Stage-specific impact of tumor location on oncologic outcomes in patients with upper and lower tract urothelial carcinoma following radical surgery. *Eur. Urol.* **2012**, *62*, 677–684. [CrossRef]
16. Hakimi, K.; Carbonara, U.; Djaladat, H.; Mehrazin, R.; Eun, D.; Reese, A.; Gonzalgo, M.L.; Margulis, V.; Uzzo, R.G.; Porter, J.; et al. Outcomes of Lymph Node Dissection in Nephroureterectomy in the Treatment of Upper Tract Urothelial Carcinoma: Analysis of the ROBUUST Registry. *J. Urol.* **2022**, *208*, 268–276. [CrossRef] [PubMed]
17. Raman, J.D.; Ng, C.K.; Scherr, D.S.; Margulis, V.; Lotan, Y.; Bensalah, K.; Patard, J.J.; Kikuchi, E.; Montorsi, F.; Zigeuner, R.; et al. Impact of tumor location on prognosis for patients with upper tract urothelial carcinoma managed by radical nephroureterectomy. *Eur. Urol.* **2010**, *57*, 1072–1079. [CrossRef]
18. Isbarn, H.; Jeldres, C.; Shariat, S.F.; Liberman, D.; Sun, M.; Lughezzani, G.; Widmer, H.; Arjane, P.; Pharand, D.; Fisch, M.; et al. Location of the primary tumor is not an independent predictor of cancer specific mortality in patients with upper urinary tract urothelial carcinoma. *J. Urol.* **2009**, *182*, 2177–2181. [CrossRef]
19. Ouzzane, A.; Colin, P.; Xylinas, E.; Pignot, G.; Ariane, M.M.; Saint, F.; Hoarau, N.; Adam, E.; Azemar, M.D.; Bensadoun, H.; et al. Ureteral and multifocal tumours have worse prognosis than renal pelvic tumours in urothelial carcinoma of the upper urinary tract treated by nephroureterectomy. *Eur. Urol.* **2011**, *60*, 1258–1265. [CrossRef]
20. Waseda, Y.; Saito, K.; Ishioka, J.; Matsuoka, Y.; Numao, N.; Fujii, Y.; Sakai, Y.; Koga, F.; Okuno, T.; Arisawa, C.; et al. Ureteral Involvement Is Associated with Poor Prognosis in Upper Urinary Tract Urothelial Carcinoma Patients Treated by Nephroureterectomy: A Multicenter Database Study. *Eur. Urol. Focus.* **2016**, *2*, 296–302. [CrossRef]
21. Hashimoto, T.; Ohno, Y.; Nakashima, J.; Gondo, T.; Nakagami, Y.; Namiki, K.; Horiguchi, Y.; Yoshioka, K.; Ohori, M.; Tachibana, M. Prediction of renal function after nephroureterectomy in patients with upper tract urothelial carcinoma. *Jpn. J. Clin. Oncol.* **2015**, *45*, 1064–1068. [CrossRef] [PubMed]
22. Youssef, R.F.; Shariat, S.F.; Lotan, Y.; Wood, C.G.; Sagalowsky, A.I.; Zigeuner, R.; Langner, C.; Montorsi, F.; Bolenz, C.; Margulis, V. Prognostic effect of urinary bladder carcinoma in situ on clinical outcome of subsequent upper tract urothelial carcinoma. *Urology* **2011**, *77*, 861–866. [CrossRef] [PubMed]
23. Nuhn, P.; Novara, G.; Seitz, C.; Gupta, A.; Matsumoto, K.; Kassouf, W.; Walton, T.J.; Fritsche, H.M.; Tritschler, S.; Martinez-Salamanca, J.I.; et al. Prognostic value of prior history of urothelial carcinoma of the bladder in patients with upper urinary tract urothelial carcinoma: Results from a retrospective multicenter study. *World J. Urol.* **2015**, *33*, 1005–1013. [CrossRef]
24. Sikic, D.; Wach, S.; Taubert, H.; Richterstetter, M.; Kunath, F.; Goebell, P.J.; Schick, S.; Olbert, P.; Huber, J.; Wullich, B.; et al. Female Gender Is an Age-dependent Negative Prognostic Factor for Patients with Upper Tract Urothelial Carcinoma. *Anticancer. Res.* **2015**, *35*, 4277–4281. [PubMed]
25. Milojevic, B.; Dzamic, Z.; Grozdic Milojevic, I.; Bumbasirevic, U.; Santric, V.; Kajmakovic, B.; Janicic, A.; Durutovic, O.; Dragicevic, D.; Bojanic, N.; et al. Prognostic value of Balkan endemic nephropathy and gender on upper tract urothelial carcinoma outcomes after radical nephroureterectomy: A cohort study. *Urol. Oncol.* **2021**, *39*, 786.e9–786.e16. [CrossRef]
26. Wu, Y.T.; Luo, H.L.; Wang, H.J.; Chen, Y.T.; Cheng, Y.T.; Chiang, P.H. Gender effect on the oncologic outcomes of upper urinary tract urothelial carcinoma in Taiwan. *Int. Urol. Nephrol.* **2020**, *52*, 1043–1048. [CrossRef]
27. Mori, K.; Mostafaei, H.; Enikeev, D.V.; Lysenko, I.; Quhal, F.; Kimura, S.; Karakiewicz, P.I.; Egawa, S.; Shariat, S.F. Differential Effect of Sex on Outcomes after Radical Surgery for Upper Tract and Bladder Urothelial Carcinoma: A Systematic Review and Meta-Analysis. *J. Urol.* **2020**, *204*, 58–62. [CrossRef] [PubMed]
28. Yap, S.A.; Schupp, C.W.; Chamie, K.; Evans, C.P.; Koppie, T.M. Effect of age on transitional cell carcinoma of the upper urinary tract: Presentation, treatment, and outcomes. *Urology* **2011**, *78*, 87–92. [CrossRef]
29. Shariat, S.F.; Godoy, G.; Lotan, Y.; Droller, M.; Karakiewicz, P.I.; Raman, J.D.; Isbarn, H.; Weizer, A.; Remzi, M.; Roscigno, M.; et al. Advanced patient age is associated with inferior cancer-specific survival after radical nephroureterectomy. *BJU Int.* **2010**, *105*, 1672–1677. [CrossRef] [PubMed]

30. Luo, H.L.; Chen, Y.T.; Cheng, Y.T.; Chiang, P.H. Re: Thomas Seisen, Benoit Peyronnet, Jose Luis Dominguez-Escrig; et al. Oncologic Outcomes of Kidney-sparing Surgery Versus Radical Nephroureterectomy for Upper Tract Urothelial Carcinoma: A Systematic Review by the EAU Non-muscle Invasive Bladder Cancer Guidelines Panel. Eur Urol 2016;70:1052-68: Preoperative Bladder Cancer History and Chronic Kidney Disease Are Associated with Occult Renal Pelvis Cancer in Preoperative Solitary Ureteral Cancer. *Eur. Urol.* **2017**, *71*, e109–e110. [CrossRef] [PubMed]
31. Ikeda, M.; Matsumoto, K.; Hirayama, T.; Koguchi, D.; Murakami, Y.; Matsuda, D.; Okuno, N.; Utsunomiya, T.; Taoka, Y.; Irie, A.; et al. Oncologic Outcomes of Salvage Chemotherapy in Patients with Recurrent or Metastatic Lesions after Radical Nephroureterectomy: A Multi-Institutional Retrospective Study. *Chemotherapy* **2020**, *65*, 134–140. [CrossRef] [PubMed]

cancers

MDPI

Review

Clinical and Biological Differences between Upper Tract Carcinoma and Bladder Urothelial Cancer, Including Implications for Clinical Practice

Félix Lefort [1,*], Yasmine Rhanine [1], Mathieu Larroquette [1,2], Charlotte Domblides [1,2], Luc Heraudet [1], Baptiste Sionneau [1], Simon Lambert [1], Matthieu Lasserre [1], Grégoire Robert [2,3], Alain Ravaud [1,2] and Marine Gross-Goupil [1]

1 Department of Medical Oncology, University Hospital of Bordeaux, 33000 Bordeaux, France; yasmine.rhanine@outlook.fr (Y.R.)
2 Faculty of Medicine, University of Bordeaux, 33000 Bordeaux, France; gregoire.robert@chu-bordeaux.fr
3 Department of Urology, University Hospital of Bordeaux, 33000 Bordeaux, France
* Correspondence: felix.lefort@chu-bordeaux.fr; Tel.: +33-(0)-556795808

Simple Summary: This review examines differences and similarities between upper tract urothelial carcinoma (UTUC) and bladder urothelial carcinoma (BUC) with respect to their epidemiological, clinical, pathological, and biological features and discusses the resulting therapeutic consequences. Systemic treatments for invasive and metastatic diseases are considered, and an overview of the expected developments in this field is provided.

Abstract: Upper tract urothelial carcinoma (UTUC) is a rare disease included, along with the much more frequent urothelial bladder cancer (BUC), in the family of urothelial carcinomas (UCs). However, while UTUCs and BUCs share several features, their epidemiological, clinical, pathological, and biological differences must be considered to establish an optimal therapeutic strategy. This review examines the clinical differences between UTUC and BUC, as well as the main results obtained by molecular screening of the two diseases. The findings of clinical trials, performed in peri-operative and metastatic settings and assessing systemic treatments in UC, are summarised. A comparison of the data obtained for UTUC and BUC suggests improved therapeutic approaches, both in regards to routine practice and future drug development.

Keywords: upper tract urothelial carcinoma (UTUC); invasive; metastatic; bladder carcinoma; systemic treatments

1. Introduction

Upper tract urothelial carcinoma (UTUC) is a rare cancer which is part of a much more frequent group of tumours known as urothelial carcinomas (UCs). Among the latter, bladder urothelial carcinoma (BUC) accounts for 90–95% of the cases [1]. While this grouping is based on the shared features of UTUC and BUC, the epidemiological, clinical, pathological, and biological differences between UTUC and BUC account for their description as "disparate twins" [2], impacting therapeutic strategies. Since the overwhelming majority of UCs are BUCs, studies leading to approved treatments for UTUC included very few UTUC patients. Thus, approval was granted by analogy with the guidelines proposed for BUC. Over the past few years, new molecules have been developed that have improved the prognosis of patients with BUC, but the data from the respective clinical trials should be more closely examined regarding the efficacy of these drugs for UTUC [3,4]. We begin this review with a comparison of the main characteristics of UTUC vs. BUC. We then analyse the data on recently approved molecules or emerging therapeutic targets in order to draw conclusions relevant to clinical practice and future research.

2. Epidemiology

The incidence of UTUC is approximately 2 per every 100,000 inhabitants/year [5], and that of BUC is about 18 per every 100,000 inhabitants/year [6]. The average age of UTUC and BUC patients at diagnosis is similar, around 73 years [7,8], but the male/female ratio differs: 2:1 for UTUC and 4:1 for BUC [7,9]. UTUC is more often diagnosed at an invasive stage than is BUC, with 56% and 25% of cases, respectively [7,10], a difference occurring due to the thinness of the ureteral wall, but also resulting from the more aggressive biology of UTUC. At the time of the initial diagnosis, the incidence of metastatic UTUC is only 12–16% [11], but ~30% of patients with localised UTUC will eventually develop metastases [10], a rate similar to that observed in BUC [12]. The risk of BUC recurrence is more frequent (22–47%) after UTUC [13,14] than is UTUC recurrence after BUC (2–6%) treatment [15]. This can be explained anatomically, as the ureteral meatus possesses an anti-reflux system that may prevent the dissemination of cancer cells from the bladder.

3. Risk Factors

Smoking is a major risk factor for UC. Studies of UTUC have estimated an increase in the relative risk from 2.5 to 7% [16–18], as also determined in BUC [19]. This risk varies according to smoking intensity and decreases after smoking cessation. Continued smoking after diagnosis is a poor prognostic factor [20]. Occupational exposure to aromatic amines, polycyclic aromatic hydrocarbons, and chlorinated solvents is also a risk factor for UTUC and BUC [21], as is chronic exposure to acrolein (an active metabolite of cyclophosphamide and ifosfamide) [22]. Chronic infections (bilharziasis) and inflammations are risk factors for both bladder and upper urinary tract cancers, but these lead, instead, to epidermoid carcinomas [21].) These common factors cause chronic aggression of the urothelium in both the upper urinary tract and the bladder, thus accounting for the development of cancer in both sites. However, other risks factors are specific for UTUC, providing evidence of its biological differences with BUC.

Aristolochic acid (AA) is the active element of the Aristolochiaceae family of herbaceous plants. Its accidental ingestion and its use in traditional pharmacopoeia are associated with the higher incidence of UTUC in the Balkans and on the Asian continent (Balkan endemic nephropathy, and Chinese herb nephropathy) [23]. Despite their better outcomes, patients with AA-associated UTUC are at higher risk of contralateral disease and BUC and thus, should be monitored closely [24]. A high incidence of UTUC (20–26.6% of all UCs) is also found on the southwest coast of Taiwan [25], where it is associated with peripheral vasculitis ("black foot disease"), related to the high concentration of arsenic in the water supplies [26].

Lynch syndrome, resulting from a constitutional mutation in one of the genes of the DNA mismatch repair system (*MLH1*, *MSH2*, *MSH6*, *PMS2*), predisposes patients to several cancers transmitted by autosomal dominant inheritance. In terms of its localisation, UTUC is the third most common (~5%) tumour on the spectrum of Lynch syndrome tumours, after colorectal and endometrial localisations [27]. A study of 115 UTUC patients screened for Lynch syndrome found a positivity rate of 5.2% [28]. The relative risk of developing a UTUC against in case of Lynch syndrome ranges from 14 to 22% vs. from 2.2 to 4.2% in the case of BUC [29]. The *MSH2* mutation is more commonly associated with the risk of UTUC [30].

4. Diagnosis

The diagnostic of UTUC, when not incidental, is mainly established because of haematuria (70–80% of the cases) [31]. Flank pain and systemic symptoms (deterioration of the general health status, fever) are frequently observed before UTUC diagnosis [32]. Ultrasonography is often performed as a descrambling examination to explore haematuria or flank pain. It allows for the detection of renal ureteral or bladder masses, as well as the measurement of hydronephrosis, but it shows a mild sensitivity and specificity; thus, it cannot replace computed tomography urography (CTU). In patients with metastatic disease, the diagnosis of BUC or UTUC relies on a biopsy taken at the most convenient site (primary tumour or metastasis site). In the early stages of the disease, however, the diagnosis of UTUC can be difficult due to its anatomic location, which will likely impact the therapeutic strategy.

For tumours discovered in the renal pelvis, UTUC must be distinguished from renal cell carcinomas. CTU is the reference imaging modality for the diagnostic workup of UTUC in patients with a creatinine clearance >30 mL/min. The entire urinary system is imaged through several acquisitions, obtained before and after the injection of contrast medium; a study during the excretory phase of contrast medium elimination should be included as well. Magnetic resonance urography can depict the entire urinary system, thus providing an alternative to CTU, especially if the latter is contraindicated [33].

Following the establishment of a diagnosis of UTUC, muscle invasion must be correctly assessed. Flexible ureterorenoscopy allows for the exploration of the entire upper urinary tract, as well as for direct visualisation and biopsy of the lesion. The sensitivity of biopsy in the diagnosis of UC is 89–95% [34]. Its reliability in predicting the tumour stage is low, with a high rate of underestimation (45% of Ta lesions are actually infiltrating tumours) [34]. Also, there is a rising concern that ureterorenoscopy increases the risk of intravesical recurrence [35], and a risk-stratified approach has been proposed to avoid this in high-risk cases [36]. Urinary cytology, based on cells obtained from the natural desquamation of the urothelial lining of the urinary tract, can be performed. Cytology is recommended in the diagnosis of UTUC, although it is less sensitive and less specific than when used in BUC. It should ideally be performed in situ (selective, during an endoscopic examination), before the injection of contrast medium. Cystoscopy is also recommended as part of the routine evaluation of UTUC because of the risk of synchronous and metachronous BUC, as described above.

5. Pathology

The WHO's histological classification and tumour grading system for bladder and upper urinary tract cancers are identical to those for bladder cancer. Urothelial carcinoma is the most common form of the disease, representing 90–95% of upper urinary tract cancers, whereas squamous cell carcinoma is rare (5–7%), and adenocarcinoma is even rarer (~1% of UTUCs). A variant histology (micropapillary, squamous, sarcomatoid) is found in ~25% of UTUCs [37] and BUCs [38], and is a poor prognostic factor in both.

6. Molecular Biology

A genomics comparison of UTUC and BUC provides the most striking example of the "disparate twins" concept [39]. Sfakianos et al. used next-generation sequencing to compare the genomics of patients with localised high-grade UTUC ($n = 83$) and BUC ($n = 102$) [40]. While many common genes were altered in BUC and UTUC, the respective prevalence differed, with a higher rate of alterations in UTUC than in BUC for *FGFR3* (35.6% vs. 21.6%, $p = 0.065$), *HRAS* (13.6% vs. 1.0%, $p = 0.001$), and *CDKN2B* (15.3% vs. 3.9%, $p = 0.016$) and higher rates in BUC than in UTUC for *TP53* and *ARID1A*. The authors also identified a trend of differences between UTUC and BUC in terms of potential therapeutic targets such as *TSC1* (11.9% vs. 3.9%, $p = 0.100$) and *PIK3CA* (10.2%vs. 21.6%, $p = 0.084$). Necchi et al. obtained similar results in a cohort of patients with advanced-stage UTUC ($n = 479$) and BUC ($n = 1984$) [41]. *FGFR3* mutations were more frequent in UTUC than in BUC (21% vs. 14%, $p = 0.002$), but the rates of amplifications (0.4% vs. 0.5%), rearrangements (3.3% vs. 3.9%), and multiple *FGFR3* alterations (1.3% vs. 1.0%) were similar. Interestingly, *FGFR3*-altered tumours showed concomitant *PI3KCA/RAS* alterations in 26.2% of UTUC patients and 26.5% of BUC patients. An increase in *HRAS* mutations was also reported (6.9% for UTUC; 2.8%, for BUC), with most of the *HRAS*-altered tumours arising from UTUC of the renal pelvis rather than from other anatomic sites. Among other targetable alterations, *ERBB2* (*HER2*) amplification was less frequent in UTUC (2.7%) than in BUC (7.9%). The homologous recombination repair pathway was frequently altered in both

UTUC (17%) and BUC (20%, $p = 0.2$), but the main actionable genes, such as *BRCA* 1 and 2, were altered in only 4.9% of BUC patients and 4.6% of UTUC patients.

As noted above, Lynch syndrome and micro-satellite instability (MSI)-high tumours are more likely to be found in patients with UTUC than in those with BUC. In the study of Necchi et al., patients with UTUC exhibited more frequent MSI-high tumours (3.4%) than did patients with BUC (0.8%; $p < 0.001$) [41]. Donahue et al. showed that Lynch-syndrome-associated UTUCs have a significantly higher tumour mutational burden (TMB) than do sporadic UTUCs, but the frequency of *FGFR* alterations is the same [42]. Interestingly, *FGFR3* alterations for Lynch-syndrome-associated UTUCs are mainly *R248C* mutations, suggesting the use of the latter as a biomarker for this population.

AA-associated UTUCs are linked with a higher TMB, including more frequent mutations in *TP53*, *NRAS*, and *HRAS* [24], whereas *FGFR* 3 mutations are rare, even in the early stages of the disease. The specific mutational signatures found in AA-associated UTUCs could help to identify individual exposure to this carcinogen [43].

Muscle-invasive BUCs have been classified according to their molecular subtype [44]. The 2017 TCGA classification recognises five molecular subtypes: luminal-papillary, luminal-infiltrated, luminal, basal/squamous, and neuronal [45]. Since the classification was developed without the inclusion of any patients with UTUC, Robinson et al. applied it to a cohort of 37 UTUC patients and found that most of the tumours were of the luminal-papillary type (62.5% vs. 27.3% for BUC in the TCGA study) [46].

Nectin-4 belongs to a family of cellular adhesion molecules and is found to be overexpressed in various tumours and is associated with cancer progression and poor prognosis [47]. Nectin-4 is the target protein for drugs such as the antibody-drug conjugate (ADC) enfortumab vedotin, and it is expressed in the majority of BUCs. In an immunohistochemical analysis, 83% of the biopsies from 524 BUC patients stained positive for Nectin-4 [48], whereas its expression rate in UTUC is probably lower. In a study of 99 patients with UTUC, Nectin-4 positivity was detected in 66% of the tumours examined by immunohistochemistry (IHC) [49].

The target protein for the ADC sacituzumab govitecan is Trop-2, a cell surface glycoprotein that acts as a transmembrane transducer of intracellular (IC) calcium signals [50]. TROP2 stimulates proliferation and cellular growth in human cervical and bladder cancer cells and was shown by IHC to be expressed at high rates in UTUC (94/99 patients) [51]. A study in which various cancers were immunostained for Trop-2 reported moderate to strong Trop-2 expression in 88.3% of UTUCs ($n = 62$) and 92% of high-grade invasive BUCs ($n = 735$) [52].

7. Treatment

The standard of surgical treatment for muscle-invasive, high-risk or recurrent low-risk, localised UTUC is radical nephroureterectomy (RNU) [33]. The choice of surgical technique (open, laparoscopy, robot) does not seem to affect efficacy outcomes [53]. RNU is often accompanied by lymphadenectomy, although the lymphatic drainage areas of the upper urinary tract are not clearly defined. Lymphadenectomy in combination with RNU enables better staging, guides therapeutic management (adjuvant chemotherapy), and may improve survival by reducing the risk of recurrence for tumours $\geq$ pT2 [54]. Conservative, kidney-preserving treatment can be considered for patients with low-risk lesions, defined as unifocal tumours, tumours with potential complete resection, low-grade tumours, and the absence of infiltration on imaging examinations [55]. This option must be followed by close endoscopic surveillance (flexible ureteroscopy).

7.1. Systemic Treatment in the Peri-Operative Setting

The standard of care for the peri-operative treatment of BUC is cisplatin-based neoadjuvant chemotherapy [56]. The same chemotherapy regimen is adopted for UTUC because of the risk of renal impairment after radical surgery. The benefit of neoadjuvant chemotherapy is well-established in BUC, with improvements in disease-free survival (DFS) and overall survival (OS), as well as an absolute improvement of ~8% in 5-year survival [57]. However, the three randomised clinical trials investigating this therapeutic strategy [58–60] excluded patients with UTUC; therefore, no conclusions for these patients can be drawn. Neoadjuvant chemotherapy for UTUC has been assessed only in retrospective comparative or single-arm prospective studies. In 2020, a meta-analysis collected 848 patients, 349 of whom had been treated with a neoadjuvant regimen (mainly cisplatin) and 449 who had been treated with surgery alone. The results showed a relative 56% OS benefit for the neoadjuvant chemotherapy group compared with the surgery alone group [hazard ratio (HR) = 0.44; 95% confidence interval (CI); 0.32–0.59, $p < 0.001$] [61]. Among the patients treated with neoadjuvant chemotherapy, a complete or partial (<ypT2N0M0) pathological response was determined in 11% and 42%, respectively. These relatively low rates raise concerns about potential progression during neoadjuvant treatment. For BUC, in the VESPER trial, 28% and 41% of patients treated with dd-MVAC exhibited a complete or partial (<ypT2N0M0) pathological response, respectively [62]. The benefit of neoadjuvant chemotherapy in UTUC thus remains inconclusive and must be investigated on a case-by-case basis. It is also important to note that the VESPER trial, which demonstrated the superiority of the dd-MVAC regimen over the GEMCIS regimen, included only patients with primary tumours of the bladder.

Beyond the question of benefit, a majority of UTUC patients are not eligible for neoadjuvant chemotherapy because of the unreliability of preoperative staging and histopathology, as well as the difficulty in proving the invasive nature of the tumour based on the biopsy. For BUC, conclusive evidence for the benefits of adjuvant chemotherapy is lacking, since all of the relevant trials showed significant methodological bias [63]. For UTUC, the phase III trial POUT randomised, after radical surgery, patients with localised pT2-T4 or pTany N+ UTUC [64], with 261 participants allocated to either the surveillance arm or the adjuvant chemotherapy arm. Chemotherapy was administered during the 90 days following radical surgery and consisted of four 21-day cycles of cisplatin (70 mg/m^2) and gemcitabine (GC) (1000 mg/m^2 on days 1 and 8 of each cycle) or carboplatin (AUC 4.5 or AUC5) and gemcitabine (GP). The results showed an improved DFS (HR = 0.45, 95% CI 0.30–0.68; $p = 0.0001$). At 3 years, 71% (95% CI: 61–78) and 46% (95% CI: 36–56) of patients receiving chemotherapy and surveillance, respectively, were event-free. This benefit was consistent across the subgroups, even for the 28% of patients who received GP [65]. This finding is critical for clinical practice, since cisplatin eligibility drops from 49% to 19% in UTUC after radical treatment [66]. An update of OS data (secondary endpoint) in 2021 showed that 67% of patients in the surveillance group were alive after 3 years versus 79% in the chemotherapy group, but reduction in the relative risk of death did not reach statistical significance (HR = 0.72; 95% CI: 0.47–1.08; $p = 0.11$).

Given the anti-tumour activity of immune checkpoint inhibitors (ICIs) in metastatic BUC, their efficacy has been assessed in the adjuvant setting. The phase 3 Checkmate 274 trial randomised patients with muscle-invasive UC who had undergone radical surgery to receive nivolumab or placebo every 2 weeks for one year [67]. The primary endpoint was DFS, among the intent-to-treat population, and expression by ≥1% of tumour cells, among patients with programmed death ligand 1 (PD-L1). The results showed a benefit of DFS for both groups. Nivolumab was approved by the European Medicines Agency (EMA) for patients with muscle-invasive UC with tumour cell PD-L1 expression ≥1% who are at high risk of recurrence after undergoing radical resection. This trial included a significant proportion (21%) of patients with UTUC, thus exceeding the usual ratio of 5%. Upon subgroup analysis, UTUC patients did not seem to benefit from adjuvant nivolumab, even after extended follow-up, as reported at the ASCO GU 2023 Symposium [68].

7.2. Future Perspectives

The question of peri-operative treatment for UTUC is being addressed in several ongoing clinical trials. As discussed above, the main issue regarding neoadjuvant regimens in UTUC is the need for biopsy-based proof of muscle invasion. Since most high-grade UTUCs at biopsy are found to show muscle invasion, the issue of whether tumour grade, when used as a criterion for neoadjuvant treatment, could lead to survival improvements remains to be determined. The phase II NAUTICAL trial (number of clinical trial (NCT) 04574960) randomises patients with high-grade UTUC to neoadjuvant or adjuvant chemotherapy. Another phase II/III trial (NCT04628767) also uses the criterion of high tumour grade to evaluate neoadjuvant chemotherapy, with or without durvalumab, in patients with localised UTUC. The ABACUS-2 phase 2 trial will assess the effect of neoadjuvant atezolizumab for patients with rare histological subtypes of bladder cancer or with UTUC who are at high risk of relapse (NCT04624399) [69].

The abovementioned anti-Nectin-4 antibody-drug conjugate enfortumab vedotin, shown to be effective in metastatic BUC [4], is currently being tested in the peri-operative setting. A specific phase II trial for UTUC (NCT05775471) will enrol patients at high risk of recurrence to receive neoadjuvant pembrolizumab and enfortumab vedotin and adjuvant pembrolizumab.

As also noted above, *FGFR* alterations are a more frequent feature of UTUC, especially in the early stages of the disease, and constitute a therapeutic target. The phase III PROOF 302 trial (NCT04197986) [70] includes patients with BUC and UTUC with *FGFR3* alterations and a high risk of recurrence who received neoadjuvant cisplatin or who are cisplatin-ineligible. Patients have been randomised to the placebo group or to receive anti FGFR infigratinib for up to one year in the adjuvant setting.

Since *HER2* overexpression is frequently found in UTUC (36% of score 2 or 3+ on the HercepTest) [71], a phase II trial (NCT05917158) is currently assessing the efficacy and safety of a recombinant humanised anti-HER2 antibody-drug conjugate and a PD-1 monoclonal antibody for the adjuvant treatment of HER2-positive UTUCs after RNU.

The main trials are summarised in Table 1.

Table 1. The main phase 3 trials for perioperative UTUC currently enrolling or for which results are pending.

Study Name and/or Number	Phase	Population	Experimental Arm	Comparator Arm	Primary Endpoint	Current Status
URANUS NCT02969083	Phase 2 Randomised Neoadjuvant Adjuvant	- cT2-pT4 cN0-N1 M0 - Randomisation between ARM A and B for eligible patients - RNU for ineligible patients	ARM A: RNU ARM B: neoadjuvant chemotherapy ARM C: adjuvant chemotherapy	NA	% of patients randomised	Recruiting
PROOF 302 NCT04197986 [70]	Phase 3 Randomised Adjuvant	- Invasive localised UTUC with FGFR3 alteration - If neoadjuvant chemotherapy, Stage ≥ ypT2 and/or yN+	Infigratinib	Placebo	DFS	Not recruiting
NCT05917158	Phase 2 Adjuvant	- pT2-pT4 pN0-3 M0 or pTany N1-3 M0 - Tissue immunohistochemistry HER2 2~3+	RC48-ADC (Anti Her2 ADC) + JS001 (anti-PD1)	NA	DFS	Recruiting
NAUTICAL NCT04574960	Phase 3 Randomised Neoadjuvant	- cT1-4 N0 M0 and high grade	Neoadjuvant chemotherapy	Adjuvant chemotherapy	DFS	Recruiting
NCT05775471	Phase 2 Neoadjuvant Adjuvant	- High-risk localised UTUC	Pembrolizumab + enfortumab Vedotin (néoadjuvant) followed by pembrolizumab (adjuvant)	NA	ORR	Not yet recruiting

ADC: antibody-drug conjugate; DFS: disease free survival; NA: not applicable; ORR: overall response rate; PD1: programmed cell death protein 1; RNU: radical nephroureterctomy; UC: urothelial carcinoma.

8. Systemic Treatment in the Metastatic Setting

8.1. Chemotherapy

For patients with advanced/metastatic disease, the standard method of care for those with BUC is a platinum-containing regimen, with a slight benefit for cisplatin over carboplatin. As the initial trials testing platinum did not include UTUC patients [72,73], platin regimens were applied in UTUC patients by complying with the BUC guidelines. Later, a retrospective analysis examined the impact of tumour location on survival outcomes in three RCTs that included UTUC patients: EORTC 30924 (M-VAC vs. high-dose M-VAC), EORTC 30986 (GC/carboplatin and methotrexate/carboplatin/vinblastine), and 30987 (GC-paclitaxel vs. GC, in patients fit for cisplatin). Among the 1039 patients, 161 (14.7%) suffered from UTUC. No difference in progression-free survival (PFS) or OS was observed [74], thus establishing the efficacy of the platinum regimen in UTUC.

In the second-line setting, mono-chemotherapy with taxanes was historically proposed for BUC patients, albeit based on retrospective studies, with few patients and deceptive results. In 2009, Bellmunt et al. published a phase III randomised trial comparing vinflunine (a vinca alkaloid) with best supportive care in the second line setting for 370 BUC patients. While the study did not find an OS benefit in the intent-to-treat population, a statistically significant benefit was identified when the 13 patients exhibiting significant protocol deviations were excluded. In that case, the median OS was 6.9 vs. 4.3 months (HR = 0.77; 95% CI 0.61–0.98) and the overall response rate (ORR) was 8.6%. Whether the study included patients with UTUC is unclear, as no data for this population are available.

In 2015, a prospective, observational study investigated the safety and efficacy of vinflunine in patients pre-treated with platinum-based chemotherapy [75]. Vinflunine was administered in the second line setting to 51 (66%) of the 77 patients. The median ORR was 23.4%, and the OS was 7.7 months. A 2017 subgroup analysis of the data from this study showed similar results for patients with UTUC (n = 18) and BUC (n = 59), with a median OS of 5.0 and 8.2 months and an ORR of 22.2% and 23.7%, respectively [76]. These results suggest the efficacy of vinflunine in UTUC, a treatment currently recommended in the second line setting, if immunotherapy is not feasible, or as a third- or subsequent-line treatment. A remaining question concerns the activity of vinflunine after immunotherapy, since it may potentiate the effect of subsequent chemotherapy [77]. A retrospective study of 105 patients who received vinflunine before (n = 44) or after (n = 61) immunotherapy showed an improved clinical benefit (51% and 25%, respectively, p = 0.020) and a trend toward OS improvement. This study included 23 (22%) patients with UTUC, but no conclusion could be drawn from this subgroup analyses.

8.2. Immunotherapy

In 2017, the KEYNOTE-045 study showed that, compared to mono chemotherapy, pembrolizumab significantly improved OS for BUC patients with disease progression after platinum-based chemotherapy (without avelumab maintenance) [78]. This trial included 75 (14%) UTUC patients. In the subgroup analyses, pembrolizumab was associated with a benefit over that of chemotherapy which appeared larger for UTUC (HR = 0.53; 95% CI: 0.28–1.01) than for BUC patients (HR = 0.77; 95% CI: 0.60–0.97). No data for the Lynch-syndrome status in UTUC patients were available to refine these results.

In 2020, the Javelin-100 trial randomised 700 patients without disease progression after first-line chemotherapy (4–6 cycles of GC or GP) to receive either maintenance avelumab or surveillance [79]. The study showed an OS benefit for avelumab maintenance (HR = 0.56; 95% CI: 0.40–0.79), which has since become the standard of care for BUC patients. In this trial, patients with UTUC were over-represented with 187 patients (27%), allowing for a comprehensive subgroup analysis [80], which showed a persistent trend (although less important) for OS benefit for the UTUC subgroup (HR = 0.63, 95% CI: 0.48–0.81, for patients with lower urinary tract tumours; HR = 0.90; 95% CI: 0.59–1.39, for patients with UTUC).

In the first-line setting, 374 cisplatin ineligible patients received pembrolizumab within the KEYNOTE-052 phase 2 trial. The ORR was 24% for the overall population, of which

19% of patients suffered from UTUC. The ORRs for UTUC and BUC were similar, at 22% and 28%, respectively. Based on these results and those from the KEYNOTE-361 trial, the US Food and Drug Administration (FDA), but not the EMA, approved pembrolizumab for patients with metastatic urothelial carcinoma (BUC or UTUC) who are not eligible for platinum-containing regimens.

The phase 2 IMvigor210 trial enrolled 119 patients with advanced UC who were ineligible for cisplatin to receive atezolizumab as a first-line therapy. The results led to FDA, but not EMA, approval of this regimen for cisplatin-ineligible patients with PD-L1-expressing UC or any patients who are platin-ineligible in the first-line setting, regardless of the tumour's anatomic site. While the study included à significant proportion of UTUC patients (28%), no subgroup analyses were published.

8.3. Targeted Therapies

In case of progression after chemotherapy and immunotherapy (maintenance or second-line), the anti-Nectin-4 ADC enfortumab vedotin is the standard of care for BUC patients. The phase 3 EV-301 trial randomised 608 patients with locally advanced or metastatic UC who had previously received platinum-containing chemotherapy, but who had experienced disease progression during or following PD-1/L1 inhibitor treatment to receive enfortumab vedotin or chemotherapy [4]. A significant improvement in OS was determined for the enfortumab vedotin group (HR = 0.70; 95% CI: 0.56–0.89) [4]. This study included 205 (34%) patients with UTUC, among whom enfortumab vedotin was associated with a benefit over chemotherapy, as determined in subgroup analyses. Recently, results of the EV 302 trial were presented at the 2023 ESMO Symposium [81]. In this trial, 886 patients with previously untreated metastatic BUC or UTUC were included. They were randomized to receive either enfortumab vedotin plus pembrolizumab or standard chemotherapy. The results showed a benefit in PFS (HR = 0.45; 95% CI: 0.38–0.45) and OS (HR = 0.47; 95% CI: 0.38–0.58) for the enfortumab vedotin plus pembrolizumab combination. This trial included a significant number of patients with UTUC (234 patients 27%). Subgroup analyses showed PFS and OS benefits for both BUC and UTUC, and indicated that pembrolizumab plus enfortumab vedotin should become the new standard in this setting.

Patients with metastatic UC harbouring an *FGFR2* or *FGFR3* alteration were shown to benefit from treatment with a pan-FGFR tyrosine kinase inhibitor. In a phase 2 study, 99 patients with UC (23 with UTUC) pretreated with chemotherapy received 8 mg of erdafitinib daily [82]. The study showed an ORR (primary endpoint) of 40% (39% for UTUC and 48% for BUC), with a median PFS of 5.5 months (95% CI: 4.2–6.0) in the overall population; no other data are available for the UTUC subgroup. The THOR phase III trial assessed erdafitinib vs. docetaxel or vinflunine in patients with advanced or metastatic UC. Patients must have shown progression after one or two prior treatments, including therapies with an anti-PD-(L)1 agent, and tumours must had pre-specified *FGFR* alterations [83]. Erdafitinib significantly increased the median OS compared with that of docetaxel or vinflunine (12.1 months vs. 7.8 months; HR = 0.64; 95% CI: 0.47–0.88). The study population included a high proportion of UTUC patients, as 89 out of 266 (33%) patients possessed a primary tumour in the upper urinary tract. An OS benefit achieved with erdafitinib was consistently observed across the subgroups, with a greater benefit in UTUC (HR = 0.34; 95% CI: 0.18–0.64) than in BUC (HR = 0.82; 95% CI: 0.56–1.18). Erdafitinib is currently approved by the EMA for patients with advanced or metastatic UC, characterised by *FGFR* alterations, that has progressed despite chemotherapy and immunotherapy, regardless of the primary site. Given the higher incidence of *FGFR* alterations in UTUC and the clinical activity observed in this population, erdafitinib can be considered as the treatment of choice for UTUC.

8.4. Future Perspectives

Clinical trials dedicated to metastatic UTUC are very rare, but several molecules are currently being studied in trials that include both BUC and UTUC patients. These trials are summarised in Tables 2 and 3.

8.4.1. Trop-2

In the phase 2 mono-arm TROPHY-U-01, 113 patients with metastatic UC and disease progression after prior platinum-based and anti PD(L)-1 therapies were allocated to receive sacituzumab govitecan, an anti-Trop2 antibody conjugated to SN-38 (an active metabolite of irinotecan) [84]. While the inclusion criteria allowed for the admission of patients with UTUC, no data for this population have been published. The phase 3 TROPiCS-04 is currently assessing the efficacy and safety of sacituzumab-govitecan in patients with metastatic UC and disease progression after prior platinum-based and anti PD(L)-1 therapies (NCT04527991) [85]. The study allowed for the admission of patients with UTUC and should provide results for this subgroup.

8.4.2. Immunotherapy

The results of the development of immunotherapy for UTUC and BC are currently indissociable, as there is no specific trial for UTUC. Ongoing trials with immunotherapy are evaluating several combinations of ICIs, or ICIs with other molecules, in the first-line setting as maintenance, or in the late stages of the disease (Table 2). The molecular differences between BUC and UTUC may one day allow for predictions of the ICI response and the development of biomarker-based clinical trials.

8.4.3. MSI-High Tumours

Contrary to the subgroup analyses of the neoadjuvant trial Checkmate 274, the outcomes were better for UTUC than for BUC in the KEYNOTE-045 trial. These differences reflected the presence among the UTUC population of patients with MSI-high tumours, known to be very good responders to ICIs [86]. To date, there is no large dataset for ICI efficacy in patients with MSI-high metastatic UTUC, but a report on a population of ten such patients treated with ICIs showed an impressive ORR of 90%, with 100% of the patients presenting without disease progression at 15 months [87]. In the future, such patients should be screened in a clinical trial to more fully understand the subgroup outcomes.

Some trials for UC in general are also of specific interest for UTUC because of its unique biology, as noted in previous sections. This issue is further examined below.

8.4.4. FGFR

The promising clinical activity of erdafitinib in UCs with *FGFR* alterations is particularly interesting for patients with UTUC, as *FGFR* alterations are more frequent in these tumours. New anti FGFR inhibitors, such as ICP-192 (gunagratinib) or TYRA-300, are currently being evaluated for UC in phase 2 trials (NCT04492293 and NCT05544552). Other anti-FGFR agents, such as AZD4547 in combination with tislelizumab (anti PD-1) and futibatinib in combination with pembrolizumab, are being tested in association with ICIs to enhance the anti-tumour effect in UC. Both are currently being evaluated in phase 2 trials (NCT05775874 and NCT04601857).

8.4.5. HER2

If HER2 amplifications are of low frequency in UC and even lower in UTUC, then the development of new antibody-drug conjugates targeting low-HER2 tumours may offer new treatment opportunities for UC. A recent study reported that 64% of 130 UTUC tumours analysed by IHC were at least HER2 1+ [88]. MRG002 (trastuzumab-vedotin) an antibody-drug conjugate targeting HER2 is being tested in the second- or third-line setting in a randomised phase 3 trial (NCT05754853) for patients with metastatic UC with HER2 positivity (IHC 3+ or IHC 2+).

8.4.6. The Homologous Recombination Repair (HRR) Pathway

The HRR pathway is frequently altered in both BUC and UTUC, suggesting the efficacy of poly(ADP-ribose) polymerase (PARP) inhibitors in these patients. In the mono-arm phase II TALASUR trial (NCT04678362), talazoparib was added to avelumab (regardless of HRR mutations) as a maintenance treatment in patients with metastatic UC without disease progression after chemotherapy consisting of a first-line platinum-regimen [89]. To improve patient selection, another mono-arm phase 2 trial selected patients with UC harbouring DNA damage response gene alterations and with disease progression, despite at least one prior line of treatment (NCT03448718). The results of these trials are likely to be very interesting for patients with AA-associated UTUC, which is often associated with HRR deficiency [90].

8.4.7. HRAS

HRAS mutations, although rare, are twice as frequent in UTUC than in BUC. Tipifarnib is a quinolinone that inhibits the enzyme farnesyl protein transferase and prevents the activation of *Ras* oncogenes. A phase 2 mono-arm trial is currently assessing tipifarnib in UCs harbouring *HRAS* or *STK11* mutations for patients pre-treated with platinum-based chemotherapy (NCT02535650). In preliminary results from 21 patients, the ORR was 24%, but there was no response for patients with tumours harbouring STK11 mutations [91].

8.4.8. TSC1

TSC1 mutations are three times more frequent in UTUC than in BC. Sapanisertib is a dual mTORC1/2 inhibitor that was tested in a phase 2 mono-arm trial (NCT03047213) in patients with metastatic UC. However, due to the absence of an objective response and poor tolerance of the drug, the trial was suspended [92].

Table 2. The main phase 2 trials for metastatic UTUC currently enrolling or for which results are pending.

Study Name and/or Number	Population	Experimental Arm	Comparator Arm	Primary Endpoint	Current Status
NCT05219435	- Stable after 4–6 cycles of first-line platinum based therapy	Nivolumab + ipilimumab	NA	PFS	Recruiting
NCT04678362 [89]	- Stable after 4–6 cycles of first-line platinum based therapy	Talazoparib + avelumab	NA	PFS	Recruiting
NCT03448718	- Progression despite one prior line of treatment for metastatic UC - Somatic alteration considered pathogenic/likely pathogenic in a predetermined list of DDR genes	Olaparib	NA	ORR	Active; not recruiting
NCT05775874	- Unresectable locally advanced or metastatic UC - *FGFR2/3* alterations	AZD4547 (Anti FGFR) + tislelizumab (Anti PD1)	NA	Safety index/ORR	Recruiting
NCT04601857 [93]	- First-line setting - Unfit for standard platinum-based chemotherapy. - Cohort A: *FGFR3* mutation or *FGFR1-4* fusion/rearrangement - Cohort B: all other patients with UC	Futibatinib (anti FGFR) + pembrolizumab	NA	ORR	Recruiting
BAYOU NCT03459846	- First-line setting - Ineligible for platinum-based chemotherapy - Known tumour HRR mutation	Arm 1: durval-umab/placebo Arm 2: durval-umab/olaparib	NA	PFS	Active; not recruiting
NCT02122172	- Prior platinum-based chemotherapy regimen - Second-line setting - Regardless of EGFR or HER2 expression	Afatinib	NA	PFS	Recruiting

Table 2. *Cont.*

Study Name and/or Number	Population	Experimental Arm	Comparator Arm	Primary Endpoint	Current Status
NCT03047213 [92]	- Prior platinum-based chemotherapy regimen or cisplatin unfit - Tumours harbouring a *TSC1* or *TSC2* mutation	Sapanisertib	NA	ORR (tsc1 patients)	Active; not recruiting
PRESERVE3 NCT04887831	- First line setting	Trilaciclib + gemcitabine + cisplatin or carboplatin followed by trilaciclib i avelumab maintenance	Gemcitabine + cisplatin or carboplatin followed by avelumab maintenance	PFS	Active; not recruiting

DDR: DNA damage response and repair; HRR: homologous recombination repair; NA: not applicable; ORR: overall response rate; PFS: progression-free survival; UC: urothelial carcinoma.

Table 3. The main phase 3 trials for metastatic UTUC currently enrolling or for which results are pending.

Study Name and/or Number	Population	Experimental Arm	Comparator Arm	Primary Endpoint	Current Status
NCT05911295	- Unresectable locally advanced or metastatic UC - First line setting - Patients platin-eligible - HER2 expression $\geq$ 1+ by immunohistochemistry	Disitamab vedotin + pembrolizumab	Gemcitabine + cisplatin or carboplatin	PFS	Recruiting
NCT05754853	- Progression following a platinum-containing regimen and (PD-1/PD-L1) therapy - HER2-positive (IHC 3+ or IHC 2+)	MRG002 (trastuzumab vedotin)	Physician's choice of treatment (docetaxel/paclitaxel/gemcitabine hydrochloride/pemetrexed disodium)		Recruiting
EV302 NCT04223856	- First-line setting	Arm A: enfortumab vedotin + pembrolizumab Arm C: enfortumab vedotin + pembrolizumab + cisplatin or carboplatin	Gemcitabine + cisplatin or carboplatin	PFS	Active; not recruiting
TROPICS-04 NCT04527991	- Progression following a platinum-containing regimen and (PD-1/PD-L1) therapy	Sacituzumab govitecan	Physician's choice of treatment (taxol/taxotere/vinflunin)	OS	Active; not recruiting
THOR trial NCT03390504	Cohort 1: - Prior treatment with anti-PD-(L)1 - No more than two prior lines of systemic treatment Cohort 2: - No prior treatment with an anti-PD-(L)1 agent - Only one line of prior systemic treatment	Erdafitinib	Vinflunine or docetaxel	OS	Active; not recruiting
NCT03898180	- Cisplatin-ineligible with a PD-L1-CPS $\geq$ 10 - Ineligible for any platinum-containing chemotherapy, regardless of CPS - First-line setting	Arm A: pembrolizumab + lenvatinib Arm B: pembrolizumab monotherapy	Pembrolizumab + placebo	PFS	Active; not recruiting

NA: not applicable; OS: overall survival; ORR: overall response rate; PFS: progression-free survival; PD(L)1: programmed cell death protein 1 (ligand); UC: urothelial carcinoma.

9. Discussion

While the common features of BUC and UTUC suggest shared therapeutic targets, the differences between these tumours should be taken into account in clinical practice and in trial design.

In the neoadjuvant setting, it is tempting to extrapolate the benefit of a neo adjuvant cisplatin-based regimen demonstrated in BUC to UTUC, especially because many patients will become cisplatin ineligible after nephroureterectomy. However, several issues specific to UTUC merit consideration. First, unlike BUC, there is no level 1 evidence for the benefit of neoadjuvant chemotherapy in UTUC. In 2022, a systematic review of 24 studies using neoadjuvant therapy in UTUC were analysed. Neoadjuvant treatment seemed to be associated with improved survival and better pathological response compared to the results for surgery alone. However, this result applied to retrospective or single arm trials, and there was no clear advantage when this method was compared to surgery followed by adjuvant treatment [94]. The lower ORR observed in UTUC when compared to those in BUC (determined in retrospective studies) raises concerns regarding the risk of tumour progression during neoadjuvant treatment and makes the side effects less acceptable. The use of biomarkers to predict the response to neoadjuvant treatment will improve patient selection. An analysis of the ORR for cisplatin-based chemotherapy, according to various molecular signatures (DNA repair genes, molecular subtypes, regulators of apoptosis, or genes involved in cellular efflux), failed to show that any were strong enough to be used in clinical practice [95]. The results of ongoing neoadjuvant trials should help to refine the indications for neoadjuvant therapy, especially for tumours harbouring targetable molecules.

The second main issue for neoadjuvant treatment in UTUC is the need to clearly identify muscle invasion, since the biopsies are much narrower and more difficult to perform than in BUC. A correlation with tumour grade was reported, as muscle invasive tumours at nephroureterectomy were found in 60% of patients with biopsies showing high-grade tumours [96]. Thus, several ongoing neoadjuvant trials proposed high-grade as an inclusion criterion. Nomograms using clinical biological and pathologic features, with an accuracy in predicting muscle invasive disease of ~80% [95,96], are available and could be useful tools for identifying candidates for clinical trials. Other predictive factors based on imaging and molecular biology studies mays also eventually help to predict muscle invasion more effectively.

In the adjuvant setting, the benefit of platin-based chemotherapy was well demonstrated in the POUT trial. The DFS benefit was significant for patients who received cisplatin or carboplatin, a crucial finding for clinical practice, since most patients exhibit renal impairment after nephroureterectomy. The Checkmate 274 trial showed that nivolumab improved DFS for the overall population in the adjuvant setting, but subgroup analyses showed no benefit for UTUC patients. Since most UTUCs are of the luminal-papillary molecular subtype, characterised by immune cell infiltration, they are probably less responsive to immunotherapy [45]. Further investigation is needed to determine the precise role of adjuvant immunotherapy for UTUC patients, especially because this indication competes with that used for adjuvant chemotherapy (as concluded in the POUT trial). A meta-analysis suggested a greater benefit of chemotherapy over immunotherapy in this setting [96]. Also, patients with UTUC associated with Lynch syndrome are more likely to benefit from immunotherapy, in which case, it may be more important to consider the MSI status than the primary site.

In the metastatic setting, the anatomic specificities of UTUC are a less informative determinant of the therapeutic strategy, and clinical trials have often mixed UTUC and BUC patients. However, the biological differences between the two entities, as discussed herein, can be useful in clinical practice. For instance, a higher proportion of UTUCs than BUCs are MSI-high tumours. The MSI-high status should then be assessed for UTUC, since it can predict immunotherapy efficacy, but also the screening of patients and their families for germline mutations should also be recommended. While several targetable gene alterations are over-represented in UTUC compared to BUC, they are nonetheless generally present in both diseases. Thus, the rarity of dedicated trials for metastatic UTUC is not an issue, if these patients can be included in trials gathering all UCs. Nevertheless, since the UTUC population is likely to exhibit distinct responses in clinical trials, the respective subgroup data and analyses should be systematically presented.

10. Conclusions

Although the similarities between UTUC and BUC have allowed for the rapid development and use of effective therapies in this rare group of diseases, the more recent understanding of the nature of these "disparate twins" raises critical issues concerning UTUC treatment. The lack of substantial evidence for neoadjuvant chemotherapy in UTUC has to be taken into account in routine practice, and there is an unmet need for dedicated trials in this setting. Comprehensive data from UTUC subgroup patients in mixed clinical trials should also be systematically published. Therapeutic strategies using molecular targets specific to UTUC could also lead to more precise medicine and improved outcomes for these patients.

Author Contributions: Writing—original draft preparation, F.L. and Y.R.; writing—review and editing, F.L., Y.R., A.R., M.L. (Mathieu Larroquette), M.L. (Matthieu Lasserre), B.S., S.L., L.H., G.R., C.D. and M.G.-G.; supervision, M.G.-G. and A.R. All authors have read and agreed to the published version of the manuscript.

Funding: This work received no external funding.

Conflicts of Interest: The authors declare no conflict of interest.

References

1. Siegel, R.L.; Miller, K.D.; Fuchs, H.E.; Jemal, A. Cancer Statistics, 2021. *CA Cancer J. Clin.* **2021**, *71*, 7–33. [CrossRef] [PubMed]
2. Green, D.A.; Rink, M.; Xylinas, E.; Matin, S.F.; Stenzl, A.; Roupret, M.; Karakiewicz, P.I.; Scherr, D.S.; Shariat, S.F. Urothelial Carcinoma of the Bladder and the Upper Tract: Disparate Twins. *J. Urol.* **2013**, *189*, 1214–1221. [CrossRef]
3. Bellmunt, J.; de Wit, R.; Vaughn, D.J.; Fradet, Y.; Lee, J.-L.; Fong, L.; Vogelzang, N.J.; Climent, M.A.; Petrylak, D.P.; Choueiri T.K.; et al. Pembrolizumab as Second-Line Therapy for Advanced Urothelial Carcinoma. *N. Engl. J. Med.* **2017**, *376*, 1015–1026 [CrossRef] [PubMed]
4. Powles, T.; Rosenberg, J.E.; Sonpavde, G.P.; Loriot, Y.; Durán, I.; Lee, J.-L.; Matsubara, N.; Vulsteke, C.; Castellano, D.; Wu, C.; et al Enfortumab Vedotin in Previously Treated Advanced Urothelial Carcinoma. *N. Engl. J. Med.* **2021**, *384*, 1125–1135. [CrossRef] [PubMed]
5. Soria, F.; Shariat, S.F.; Lerner, S.P.; Fritsche, H.-M.; Rink, M.; Kassouf, W.; Spiess, P.E.; Lotan, Y.; Ye, D.; Fernández, M.I.; et al Epidemiology, Diagnosis, Preoperative Evaluation and Prognostic Assessment of Upper-Tract Urothelial Carcinoma (UTUC) *World J. Urol.* **2017**, *35*, 379–387. [CrossRef] [PubMed]
6. Cancer of the Urinary Bladder—Cancer Stat Facts. Available online: https://seer.cancer.gov/statfacts/html/urinb.html (accessed on 9 July 2023).
7. Saginala, K.; Barsouk, A.; Aluru, J.S.; Rawla, P.; Padala, S.A.; Barsouk, A. Epidemiology of Bladder Cancer. *Med. Sci.* **2020**, *8*, 15 [CrossRef] [PubMed]
8. Wu, J.; Chen, S.; Wu, X.; Mao, W.; Wang, Y.; Xu, B.; Zheng, D.; Chen, M. Trends of Incidence and Prognosis of Upper Tract Urothelial Carcinoma. *Bosn. J. Basic Med. Sci.* **2021**, *21*, 607–619. [CrossRef]
9. Shariat, S.F.; Favaretto, R.L.; Gupta, A.; Fritsche, H.-M.; Matsumoto, K.; Kassouf, W.; Walton, T.J.; Tritschler, S.; Baba, S.; Matsushita, K.; et al. Gender Differences in Radical Nephroureterectomy for Upper Tract Urothelial Carcinoma. *World J. Urol.* **2011**, *29*, 481–486. [CrossRef]
10. Margulis, V.; Shariat, S.F.; Matin, S.F.; Kamat, A.M.; Zigeuner, R.; Kikuchi, E.; Lotan, Y.; Weizer, A.; Raman, J.D.; Wood, C.G.; et al Outcomes of Radical Nephroureterectomy: A Series from the Upper Tract Urothelial Carcinoma Collaboration. *Cancer* **2009**, *115*, 1224–1233. [CrossRef]
11. Hu, X.; Miao, J.; Qian, L.; Zhang, D.; Wei, H. The Predictors and Surgical Outcomes of Different Distant Metastases Patterns in Upper Tract Urothelial Carcinoma: A SEER-Based Study. *Front. Surg.* **2022**, *9*, 1045831. [CrossRef]
12. Mason, J.; Hasnain, Z.; Miranda, G.; Gill, K.; Djaladat, H.; Desai, M.; Newton, P.K.; Gill, I.S.; Kuhn, P. Prediction of Metastatic Patterns in Bladder Cancer: Spatiotemporal Progression and Development of a Novel, Web-Based Platform for Clinical Utility. *Eur. Urol. Open Sci.* **2021**, *32*, 8–18. [CrossRef]

13. Novara, G.; De Marco, V.; Dalpiaz, O.; Gottardo, F.; Bouygues, V.; Galfano, A.; Martignoni, G.; Patard, J.J.; Artibani, W.; Ficarra, V. Independent Predictors of Metachronous Bladder Transitional Cell Carcinoma (TCC) after Nephroureterectomy for TCC of the Upper Urinary Tract. *BJU Int.* **2008**, *101*, 1368–1374. [CrossRef]
14. Xylinas, E.; Rink, M.; Margulis, V.; Karakiewicz, P.; Novara, G.; Shariat, S.F. Upper Tract Urothelial Carcinoma Collaboration (UTUCC) Multifocal Carcinoma in Situ of the Upper Tract Is Associated with High Risk of Bladder Cancer Recurrence. *Eur. Urol.* **2012**, *61*, 1069–1070. [CrossRef] [PubMed]
15. Sanderson, K.M.; Cai, J.; Miranda, G.; Skinner, D.G.; Stein, J.P. Upper Tract Urothelial Recurrence Following Radical Cystectomy for Transitional Cell Carcinoma of the Bladder: An Analysis of 1069 Patients with 10-Year Followup. *J. Urol.* **2007**, *177*, 2088–2094. [CrossRef] [PubMed]
16. Dickman, K.G.; Fritsche, H.-M.; Grollman, A.P.; Thalmann, G.N.; Catto, J. Epidemiology and Risk Factors for Upper Urinary Urothelial Cancers. In *Upper Tract Urothelial Carcinoma*; Shariat, S.F., Xylinas, E., Eds.; Springer: New York, NY, USA, 2015; pp. 1–30. ISBN 978-1-4939-1501-9.
17. McLaughlin, J.K.; Silverman, D.T.; Hsing, A.W.; Ross, R.K.; Schoenberg, J.B.; Yu, M.C.; Stemhagen, A.; Lynch, C.F.; Blot, W.J.; Fraumeni, J.F. Cigarette Smoking and Cancers of the Renal Pelvis and Ureter. *Cancer Res.* **1992**, *52*, 254–257. [PubMed]
18. Crivelli, J.J.; Xylinas, E.; Kluth, L.A.; Rieken, M.; Rink, M.; Shariat, S.F. Effect of Smoking on Outcomes of Urothelial Carcinoma: A Systematic Review of the Literature. *Eur. Urol.* **2014**, *65*, 742–754. [CrossRef] [PubMed]
19. van Osch, F.H.; Jochems, S.H.; van Schooten, F.-J.; Bryan, R.T.; Zeegers, M.P. Quantified Relations between Exposure to Tobacco Smoking and Bladder Cancer Risk: A Meta-Analysis of 89 Observational Studies. *Int. J. Epidemiol.* **2016**, *45*, 857–870. [CrossRef] [PubMed]
20. Rink, M.; Xylinas, E.; Margulis, V.; Cha, E.K.; Ehdaie, B.; Raman, J.D.; Chun, F.K.; Matsumoto, K.; Lotan, Y.; Furberg, H.; et al. Impact of Smoking on Oncologic Outcomes of Upper Tract Urothelial Carcinoma After Radical Nephroureterectomy. *Eur. Urol.* **2013**, *63*, 1082–1090. [CrossRef] [PubMed]
21. Jubber, I.; Ong, S.; Bukavina, L.; Black, P.C.; Compérat, E.; Kamat, A.M.; Kiemeney, L.; Lawrentschuk, N.; Lerner, S.P.; Meeks, J.J.; et al. Epidemiology of Bladder Cancer in 2023: A Systematic Review of Risk Factors. *Eur. Urol.* **2023**, *84*, 176–190. [CrossRef]
22. Ouzzane, A.; Rouprêt, M.; Leon, P.; Yates, D.R.; Colin, P. Épidémiologie et facteurs de risque des tumeurs de la voie excrétrice urinaire supérieure: Revue de la littérature pour le rapport annuel de l'Association française d'urologie. *Prog. En Urol.* **2014**, *24*, 966–976. [CrossRef]
23. Wu, F.; Wang, T. Risk Assessment of Upper Tract Urothelial Carcinoma Related to Aristolochic Acid. *Cancer Epidemiol. Biomark. Prev. Publ. Am. Assoc. Cancer Res. Cosponsored Am. Soc. Prev. Oncol.* **2013**, *22*, 812–820. [CrossRef]
24. Castells, X.; Karanović, S.; Ardin, M.; Tomić, K.; Xylinas, E.; Durand, G.; Villar, S.; Forey, N.; Le Calvez-Kelm, F.; Voegele, C.; et al. Low-Coverage Exome Sequencing Screen in Formalin-Fixed Paraffin-Embedded Tumors Reveals Evidence of Exposure to Carcinogenic Aristolochic Acid. *Cancer Epidemiol. Biomark. Prev. Publ. Am. Assoc. Cancer Res. Cosponsored Am. Soc. Prev. Oncol.* **2015**, *24*, 1873–1881. [CrossRef] [PubMed]
25. Clinical and Epidemiological Features of Patients with Genitourinary Tract Tumour in a Blackfoot Disease Endemic Area of Taiwan—Tan—2008—BJU International—Wiley Online Library. Available online: https://bjui-journals-onlinelibrary-wiley-com.proxy.insermbiblio.inist.fr/doi/10.1111/j.1464-410X.2008.07565.x (accessed on 30 March 2023).
26. Arsenic in Drinking Water and Renal Cancers in Rural Bangladesh | Occupational&Environmental Medicine. Available online: https://oem.bmj.com/content/70/11/768 (accessed on 30 March 2023).
27. Koornstra, J.J.; Mourits, M.J.; Sijmons, R.H.; Leliveld, A.M.; Hollema, H.; Kleibeuker, J.H. Management of Extracolonic Tumours in Patients with Lynch Syndrome. *Lancet Oncol.* **2009**, *10*, 400–408. [CrossRef] [PubMed]
28. Metcalfe, M.J.; Petros, F.G.; Rao, P.; Mork, M.E.; Xiao, L.; Broaddus, R.R.; Matin, S.F. Universal Point of Care Testing for Lynch Syndrome in Patients with Upper Tract Urothelial Carcinoma. *J. Urol.* **2018**, *199*, 60–65. [CrossRef] [PubMed]
29. van der Post, R.S.; Kiemeney, L.A.; Ligtenberg, M.J.L.; Witjes, J.A.; Hulsbergen-van de Kaa, C.A.; Bodmer, D.; Schaap, L.; Kets, C.M.; van Krieken, J.H.J.M.; Hoogerbrugge, N. Risk of Urothelial Bladder Cancer in Lynch Syndrome Is Increased, in Particular among MSH2 Mutation Carriers. *J. Med. Genet.* **2010**, *47*, 464–470. [CrossRef] [PubMed]
30. Dominguez-Valentin, M.; Sampson, J.R.; Seppälä, T.T.; Ten Broeke, S.W.; Plazzer, J.-P.; Nakken, S.; Engel, C.; Aretz, S.; Jenkins, M.A.; Sunde, L.; et al. Cancer Risks by Gene, Age, and Gender in 6350 Carriers of Pathogenic Mismatch Repair Variants: Findings from the Prospective Lynch Syndrome Database. *Genet. Med.* **2020**, *22*, 15–25. [CrossRef]
31. Cowan, N.C. CT Urography for Hematuria. *Nat. Rev. Urol.* **2012**, *9*, 218–226. [CrossRef] [PubMed]
32. Baard, J.; Cormio, L.; Cavadas, V.; Alcaraz, A.; Shariat, S.F.; de la Rosette, J.; Laguna, M.P. Contemporary Patterns of Presentation, Diagnostics and Management of Upper Tract Urothelial Cancer in 101 Centres: The Clinical Research Office of the Endourological Society Global Upper Tract Urothelial Carcinoma Registry. *Curr. Opin. Urol.* **2021**, *31*, 354–362. [CrossRef]
33. Rouprêt, M.; Seisen, T.; Birtle, A.J.; Capoun, O.; Compérat, E.M.; Dominguez-Escrig, J.L.; Gürses Andersson, I.; Liedberg, F.; Mariappan, P.; Hugh Mostafid, A.; et al. European Association of Urology Guidelines on Upper Urinary Tract Urothelial Carcinoma: 2023 Update. *Eur. Urol.* **2023**, *84*, 49–64. [CrossRef]
34. Nison, L.; Bozzini, G.; Rouprêt, M.; Traxer, O.; Colin, P. Diagnostics clinique, urétéroscopique et photodynamique des tumeurs de la voie excrétrice urinaire supérieures: État-de-l'art pour le rapport scientifique annuel de l'Association française d'urologie. *Prog. En Urol.* **2014**, *24*, 977–986. [CrossRef]

35. Veeratterapillay, R.; Geraghty, R.; Pandian, R.; Roy, C.; Stenhouse, G.; Bird, C.; Soomro, N.; Paez, E.; Rogers, A.; Johnson, M.; et al. Ten-Year Survival Outcomes after Radical Nephroureterectomy with a Risk-Stratified Approach Using Prior Diagnostic Ureteroscopy: A Single-Institution Observational Retrospective Cohort Study. *BJU Int.* **2022**, *129*, 744–751. [CrossRef]
36. Loizzo, D.; Pandolfo, S.D.; Del Giudice, F.; Cerrato, C.; Chung, B.I.; Wu, Z.; Imbimbo, C.; Ditonno, P.; Derweesh, I.; Autorino, R. Ureteroscopy and Tailored Treatment of Upper Tract Urothelial Cancer: Recent Advances and Unmet Needs. *BJU Int.* **2022**, *130*, 35–37. [CrossRef]
37. Zamboni, S.; Foerster, B.; Abufaraj, M.; Seisen, T.; Roupret, M.; Colin, P.; De la Taille, A.; Di Bona, C.; Peyronnet, B.; Bensalah, K.; et al. Incidence and Survival Outcomes in Patients with Upper Urinary Tract Urothelial Carcinoma Diagnosed with Variant Histology and Treated with Nephroureterectomy. *BJU Int.* **2019**, *124*, 738–745. [CrossRef] [PubMed]
38. Chalasani, V.; Chin, J.L.; Izawa, J.I. Histologic Variants of Urothelial Bladder Cancer and Nonurothelial Histology in Bladder Cancer. *Can. Urol. Assoc. J.* **2009**, *3*, S193–S198. [CrossRef]
39. De Lorenzis, E.; Albo, G.; Longo, F.; Bebi, C.; Boeri, L.; Montanari, E. Current Knowledge on Genomic Profiling of Upper Tract Urothelial Carcinoma. *Genes* **2021**, *12*, 333. [CrossRef] [PubMed]
40. Sfakianos, J.P.; Cha, E.K.; Iyer, G.; Scott, S.N.; Zabor, E.C.; Shah, R.H.; Ren, Q.; Bagrodia, A.; Kim, P.H.; Hakimi, A.A.; et al. Genomic Characterization of Upper Tract Urothelial Carcinoma. *Eur. Urol.* **2015**, *68*, 970–977. [CrossRef] [PubMed]
41. Necchi, A.; Madison, R.; Pal, S.K.; Ross, J.S.; Agarwal, N.; Sonpavde, G.; Joshi, M.; Yin, M.; Miller, V.A.; Grivas, P.; et al. Comprehensive Genomic Profiling of Upper-Tract and Bladder Urothelial Carcinoma. *Eur. Urol. Focus* **2021**, *7*, 1339–1346. [CrossRef] [PubMed]
42. Donahue, T.F.; Bagrodia, A.; Audenet, F.; Donoghue, M.T.A.; Cha, E.K.; Sfakianos, J.P.; Sperling, D.; Al-Ahmadie, H.; Clendenning, M.; Rosty, C.; et al. Genomic Characterization of Upper-Tract Urothelial Carcinoma in Patients With Lynch Syndrome. *JCO Precis. Oncol.* **2018**, *2*, 1–13. [CrossRef]
43. Hoang, M.L.; Chen, C.-H.; Sidorenko, V.S.; He, J.; Dickman, K.G.; Yun, B.H.; Moriya, M.; Niknafs, N.; Douville, C.; Karchin, R.; et al. Mutational Signature of Aristolochic Acid Exposure as Revealed by Whole-Exome Sequencing. *Sci. Transl. Med.* **2013**, *5*, 197ra102. [CrossRef]
44. Lopez-Beltran, A.; Blanca, A.; Cimadamore, A.; Gogna, R.; Montironi, R.; Cheng, L. Molecular Classification of Bladder Urothelial Carcinoma Using NanoString-Based Gene Expression Analysis. *Cancers* **2021**, *13*, 5500. [CrossRef]
45. Robertson, A.G.; Kim, J.; Al-Ahmadie, H.; Bellmunt, J.; Guo, G.; Cherniack, A.D.; Hinoue, T.; Laird, P.W.; Hoadley, K.A.; Akbani, R.; et al. Comprehensive Molecular Characterization of Muscle-Invasive Bladder Cancer. *Cell* **2017**, *171*, 540–556.e25. [CrossRef] [PubMed]
46. Robinson, B.D.; Vlachostergios, P.J.; Bhinder, B.; Liu, W.; Li, K.; Moss, T.J.; Bareja, R.; Park, K.; Tavassoli, P.; Cyrta, J.; et al. Upper Tract Urothelial Carcinoma Has a Luminal-Papillary T-Cell Depleted Contexture and Activated FGFR3 Signaling. *Nat. Commun.* **2019**, *10*, 2977. [CrossRef] [PubMed]
47. Bouleftour, W.; Guillot, A.; Magne, N. The Anti-Nectin 4: A Promising Tumor Cells Target. A Systematic Review. *Mol. Cancer Ther.* **2022**, *21*, 493–501. [CrossRef] [PubMed]
48. Challita-Eid, P.M.; Satpayev, D.; Yang, P.; An, Z.; Morrison, K.; Shostak, Y.; Raitano, A.; Nadell, R.; Liu, W.; Lortie, D.R.; et al. Enfortumab Vedotin Antibody–Drug Conjugate Targeting Nectin-4 Is a Highly Potent Therapeutic Agent in Multiple Preclinical Cancer Models. *Cancer Res.* **2016**, *76*, 3003–3013. [CrossRef] [PubMed]
49. Tomiyama, E.; Fujita, K.; Rodriguez Pena, M.D.C.; Taheri, D.; Banno, E.; Kato, T.; Hatano, K.; Kawashima, A.; Ujike, T.; Uemura, M.; et al. Expression of Nectin-4 and PD-L1 in Upper Tract Urothelial Carcinoma. *Int. J. Mol. Sci.* **2020**, *21*, 5390. [CrossRef] [PubMed]
50. Wen, Y.; Ouyang, D.; Zou, Q.; Chen, Q.; Luo, N.; He, H.; Anwar, M.; Yi, W. A Literature Review of the Promising Future of TROP2: A Potential Drug Therapy Target. *Ann. Transl. Med.* **2022**, *10*, 1403. [CrossRef]
51. Tomiyama, E.; Fujita, K.; Nakano, K.; Kuwahara, K.; Minami, T.; Kato, T.; Hatano, K.; Kawashima, A.; Uemura, M.; Takao, T.; et al. Trop-2 in Upper Tract Urothelial Carcinoma. *Curr. Oncol. Tor. Ont* **2022**, *29*, 3911–3921. [CrossRef]
52. Dum, D.; Taherpour, N.; Menz, A.; Höflmayer, D.; Völkel, C.; Hinsch, A.; Gorbokon, N.; Lennartz, M.; Hube-Magg, C.; Fraune, C.; et al. Trophoblast Cell Surface Antigen 2 Expression in Human Tumors: A Tissue Microarray Study on 18,563 Tumors. *Pathobiology* **2022**, *89*, 245–258. [CrossRef]
53. Grob, G.; Rogers, D.; Pandolfo, S.D.; Vourganti, S.; Buscarini, M.; Mehrazin, R.; Grob, B.M.; Mir, M.C.; Perdonà, S.; Derweesh, I.H.; et al. Oncologic Outcomes Following Radical Nephroureterectomy for Upper Tract Urothelial Carcinoma: A Literature Review. *Transl. Androl. Urol.* **2023**, *12*, 1351–1362. [CrossRef]
54. Dominguez-Escrig, J.L.; Peyronnet, B.; Seisen, T.; Bruins, H.M.; Yuan, C.Y.; Babjuk, M.; Böhle, A.; Burger, M.; Compérat, E.M.; Gontero, P.; et al. Potential Benefit of Lymph Node Dissection During Radical Nephroureterectomy for Upper Tract Urothelial Carcinoma: A Systematic Review by the European Association of Urology Guidelines Panel on Non–Muscle-Invasive Bladder Cancer. *Eur. Urol. Focus* **2019**, *5*, 224–241. [CrossRef]
55. Babjuk, M.; Burger, M.; Capoun, O.; Cohen, D.; Compérat, E.M.; Dominguez Escrig, J.L.; Gontero, P.; Liedberg, F.; Masson-Lecomte, A.; Mostafid, A.H.; et al. European Association of Urology Guidelines on Non-Muscle-Invasive Bladder Cancer (Ta, T1, and Carcinoma in Situ). *Eur. Urol.* **2022**, *81*, 75–94. [CrossRef]

56. Powles, T.; Bellmunt, J.; Comperat, E.; Santis, M.D.; Huddart, R.; Loriot, Y.; Necchi, A.; Valderrama, B.P.; Ravaud, A.; Shariat, S.F.; et al. Bladder Cancer: ESMO Clinical Practice Guideline for Diagnosis, Treatment and Follow-Up☆. *Ann. Oncol.* **2022**, *33*, 244–258. [CrossRef]
57. Yin, M.; Joshi, M.; Meijer, R.P.; Glantz, M.; Holder, S.; Harvey, H.A.; Kaag, M.; Fransen van de Putte, E.E.; Horenblas, S.; Drabick, J.J. Neoadjuvant Chemotherapy for Muscle-Invasive Bladder Cancer: A Systematic Review and Two-Step Meta-Analysis. *Oncol.* **2016**, *21*, 708–715. [CrossRef] [PubMed]
58. Grossman, H.B.; Natale, R.B.; Tangen, C.M.; Speights, V.O.; Vogelzang, N.J.; Trump, D.L.; deVere White, R.W.; Sarosdy, M.F.; Wood, D.P.; Raghavan, D.; et al. Neoadjuvant Chemotherapy plus Cystectomy Compared with Cystectomy Alone for Locally Advanced Bladder Cancer. *N. Engl. J. Med.* **2003**, *349*, 859–866. [CrossRef] [PubMed]
59. International Collaboration of Trialists; Medical Research Council Advanced Bladder Cancer Working Party (now the National Cancer Research Institute Bladder Cancer Clinical Studies Group); European Organisation for Research and Treatment of Cancer Genito-Urinary Tract Cancer Group; Australian Bladder Cancer Study Group; National Cancer Institute of Canada Clinical Trials Group; Finnbladder; Norwegian Bladder Cancer Study Group; Club Urologico Espanol de Tratamiento Oncologico Group; Griffiths, G.; Hall, R.; et al. International Phase III Trial Assessing Neoadjuvant Cisplatin, Methotrexate, and Vinblastine Chemotherapy for Muscle-Invasive Bladder Cancer: Long-Term Results of the BA06 30894 Trial. *J. Clin. Oncol. Off. J. Am. Soc. Clin. Oncol.* **2011**, *29*, 2171–2177. [CrossRef]
60. Pfister, C.; Gravis, G.; Flechon, A.; Chevreau, C.; Mahammedi, H.; Laguerre, B.; Guillot, A.; Joly, F.; Allory, Y.; Harter, V.; et al. Multicenter Randomized Phase III Trial of Dose-Dense Methotrexate, Vinblastine, Doxorubicin, and Cisplatin (Dd-MVAC) or Gemcitabine and Cisplatin (GC) as Perioperative Chemotherapy for Muscle-Invasive Bladder Cancer (MIBC): Overall Survival (OS) Data at 5 Years in the GETUG/AFU V05 VESPER Trial. *J. Clin. Oncol.* **2023**, *41*, LBA4507. [CrossRef]
61. Leow, J.J.; Chong, Y.L.; Chang, S.L.; Valderrama, B.P.; Powles, T.; Bellmunt, J. Neoadjuvant and Adjuvant Chemotherapy for Upper Tract Urothelial Carcinoma: A 2020 Systematic Review and Meta-Analysis, and Future Perspectives on Systemic Therapy. *Eur. Urol.* **2021**, *79*, 635–654. [CrossRef] [PubMed]
62. Pfister, C.; Gravis, G.; Fléchon, A.; Soulié, M.; Guy, L.; Laguerre, B.; Mottet, N.; Joly, F.; Allory, Y.; Harter, V.; et al. Randomized Phase III Trial of Dose-Dense Methotrexate, Vinblastine, Doxorubicin, and Cisplatin, or Gemcitabine and Cisplatin as Perioperative Chemotherapy for Patients with Muscle-Invasive Bladder Cancer. Analysis of the GETUG/AFU V05 VESPER Trial Secondary Endpoints: Chemotherapy Toxicity and Pathological Responses. *Eur. Urol.* **2021**, *79*, 214–221. [CrossRef] [PubMed]
63. Burdett, S.; Fisher, D.J.; Vale, C.L.; Sternberg, C.N.; Clarke, N.W.; Parmar, M.K.B.; Bono, A.V.; Cognetti, F.; Collette, L.; Cote, R.J.; et al. Adjuvant Chemotherapy for Muscle-Invasive Bladder Cancer: A Systematic Review and Meta-Analysis of Individual Participant Data from Randomised Controlled Trials. *Eur. Urol.* **2022**, *81*, 50–61. [CrossRef]
64. Birtle, A.; Johnson, M.; Chester, J.; Jones, R.; Dolling, D.; Bryan, R.T.; Harris, C.; Winterbottom, A.; Blacker, A.; Catto, J.W.F.; et al. Adjuvant Chemotherapy in Upper Tract Urothelial Carcinoma (the POUT Trial): A Phase 3, Open-Label, Randomised Controlled Trial. *Lancet* **2020**, *395*, 1268–1277. [CrossRef] [PubMed]
65. Szarvas, T.; Módos, O.; Horváth, A.; Nyirády, P. Why Are Upper Tract Urothelial Carcinoma Two Different Diseases? *Transl. Androl. Urol.* **2016**, *5*, 63647. [CrossRef]
66. Bajorin, D.F.; Witjes, J.A.; Gschwend, J.E.; Schenker, M.; Valderrama, B.P.; Tomita, Y.; Bamias, A.; Lebret, T.; Shariat, S.F.; Park, S.H.; et al. Adjuvant Nivolumab versus Placebo in Muscle-Invasive Urothelial Carcinoma. *N. Engl. J. Med.* **2021**, *384*, 2102–2114. [CrossRef]
67. Extended Follow-Up Results from the CheckMate 274 Trial | Journal of Clinical Oncology. Available online: https://ascopubs.org/doi/abs/10.1200/JCO.2023.41.6_suppl.LBA443 (accessed on 12 July 2023).
68. Szabados, B.E.; Martinez, E.N.; Marquez, F.J.A.; Gauna, D.E.C.; Rodriguez-Vida, A.; de Espana, M.C.G.; Hussain, S.A.; Fernandez, C.A.; Linch, M.; Abella, T.B.; et al. 2363MO A Phase II Study Investigating the Safety and Efficacy of Neoadjuvant Atezolizumab in Non-Urothelial, Muscle Invasive Bladder Cancer (ABACUS-2). *Ann. Oncol.* **2023**, *34*, S1201–S1202. [CrossRef]
69. Pal, S.K.; Somford, D.M.; Grivas, P.; Sridhar, S.S.; Gupta, S.; Bellmunt, J.; Sonpavde, G.; Fleming, M.T.; Lerner, S.P.; Loriot, Y.; et al. Targeting FGFR3 Alterations with Adjuvant Infigratinib in Invasive Urothelial Carcinoma: The Phase III PROOF 302 Trial. *Future Oncol. Lond. Engl.* **2022**, *18*, 2599–2614. [CrossRef]
70. Soria, F.; Moschini, M.; Haitel, A.; Wirth, G.J.; Karam, J.A.; Wood, C.G.; Rouprêt, M.; Margulis, V.; Karakiewicz, P.I.; Briganti, A.; et al. HER2 Overexpression Is Associated with Worse Outcomes in Patients with Upper Tract Urothelial Carcinoma (UTUC). *World J. Urol.* **2017**, *35*, 251–259. [CrossRef] [PubMed]
71. Dogliotti, L.; Cartenì, G.; Siena, S.; Bertetto, O.; Martoni, A.; Bono, A.; Amadori, D.; Onat, H.; Marini, L. Gemcitabine plus Cisplatin versus Gemcitabine plus Carboplatin as First-Line Chemotherapy in Advanced Transitional Cell Carcinoma of the Urothelium: Results of a Randomized Phase 2 Trial. *Eur. Urol.* **2007**, *52*, 134–141. [CrossRef] [PubMed]
72. von der Maase, H.; Hansen, S.W.; Roberts, J.T.; Dogliotti, L.; Oliver, T.; Moore, M.J.; Bodrogi, I.; Albers, P.; Knuth, A.; Lippert, C.M.; et al. Gemcitabine and Cisplatin versus Methotrexate, Vinblastine, Doxorubicin, and Cisplatin in Advanced or Metastatic Bladder Cancer: Results of a Large, Randomized, Multinational, Multicenter, Phase III Study. *J. Clin. Oncol. Off. J. Am. Soc. Clin. Oncol.* **2000**, *18*, 3068–3077. [CrossRef] [PubMed]
73. Moschini, M.; Shariat, S.F.; Rouprêt, M.; De Santis, M.; Bellmunt, J.; Sternberg, C.N.; Tombal, B.; Collette, L. Impact of Primary Tumor Location on Survival from the European Organization for the Research and Treatment of Cancer Advanced Urothelial Cancer Studies. *J. Urol.* **2018**, *199*, 1149–1157. [CrossRef]

74. Retz, M.; de Geeter, P.; Goebell, P.J.; Matz, U.; de Schultz, W.; Hegele, A. Vinflunine in Routine Clinical Practice for the Treatment of Advanced or Metastatic Urothelial Cell Carcinoma—Data from a Prospective, Multicenter Experience. *BMC Cancer* **2015**, *15*, 455. [CrossRef] [PubMed]
75. Heers, H.; DE Geeter, P.; Goebell, P.J.; Matz, U.; DE Schultz, W.; Edlich, B.; Retz, M.; Hegele, A. Vinflunine in the Treatment of Upper Tract Urothelial Carcinoma—Subgroup Analysis of an Observational Study. *Anticancer Res.* **2017**, *37*, 6437–6442. [CrossRef]
76. Heraudet, L.; Delon, T.; Veillon, R.; Vergnenègre, C.; Lepetit, H.; Daste, A.; Ravaud, A.; Zysman, M.; Domblides, C. Effect of Prior Immunotherapy on the Efficacy of Chemotherapy in Advanced Non-Small Cell Lung Cancer: A Retrospective Study. *Thorac Cancer* **2022**, *13*, 1391–1400. [CrossRef]
77. Powles, T.; Park, S.H.; Voog, E.; Caserta, C.; Valderrama, B.P.; Gurney, H.; Kalofonos, H.; Radulović, S.; Demey, W.; Ullén, A. et al. Avelumab Maintenance Therapy for Advanced or Metastatic Urothelial Carcinoma. *N. Engl. J. Med.* **2020**, *383*, 1218–1230. [CrossRef]
78. Grivas, P.; Park, S.H.; Voog, E.; Caserta, C.; Gurney, H.; Bellmunt, J.; Kalofonos, H.; Ullén, A.; Loriot, Y.; Sridhar, S.S.; et al. Avelumab First-Line Maintenance Therapy for Advanced Urothelial Carcinoma: Comprehensive Clinical Subgroup Analyses from the JAVELIN Bladder 100 Phase 3 Trial. *Eur. Urol.* **2023**, *84*, 95–108. [CrossRef]
79. Powles, T.B.; Valderrama, B.P.; Gupta, S.; Bedke, J.; Kikuchi, E.; Hoffman-Censits, J.; Iyer, G.; Vulsteke, C.; Park, S.H.; Shin, S.J. et al. LBA6 EV-302/KEYNOTE-A39: Open-Label, Randomized Phase III Study of Enfortumab Vedotin in Combination with Pembrolizumab (EV + P) vs. Chemotherapy (Chemo) in Previously Untreated Locally Advanced Metastatic Urothelial Carcinoma (La/mUC). *Ann. Oncol.* **2023**, *34*, S1340. [CrossRef]
80. Loriot, Y.; Necchi, A.; Park, S.H.; Garcia-Donas, J.; Huddart, R.; Burgess, E.; Fleming, M.; Rezazadeh, A.; Mellado, B.; Varlamov, S. et al. Erdafitinib in Locally Advanced or Metastatic Urothelial Carcinoma. *N. Engl. J. Med.* **2019**, *381*, 338–348. [CrossRef]
81. Tagawa, S.T.; Balar, A.V.; Petrylak, D.P.; Kalebasty, A.R.; Loriot, Y.; Fléchon, A.; Jain, R.K.; Agarwal, N.; Bupathi, M.; Barthelemy P.; et al. TROPHY-U-01: A Phase II Open-Label Study of Sacituzumab Govitecan in Patients With Metastatic Urothelial Carcinoma Progressing After Platinum-Based Chemotherapy and Checkpoint Inhibitors. *J. Clin. Oncol. Off. J. Am. Soc. Clin. Oncol.* **2021**, *39* 2474–2485. [CrossRef]
82. Grivas, P.; Tagawa, S.T.; Bellmunt, J.; De Santis, M.; Duran, I.; Goebell, P.-J.; Necchi, A.; Sridhar, S.S.; Sternberg, C.N.; Aziz, M.U.; et al. TROPiCS-04: Study of Sacituzumab Govitecan in Metastatic or Locally Advanced Unresectable Urothelial Cancer That Has Progressed after Platinum and Checkpoint Inhibitor Therapy. *J. Clin. Oncol.* **2021**, *39*, TPS498. [CrossRef]
83. Le, D.T.; Uram, J.N.; Wang, H.; Bartlett, B.R.; Kemberling, H.; Eyring, A.D.; Skora, A.D.; Luber, B.S.; Azad, N.S.; Laheru, D.; et al. PD-1 Blockade in Tumors with Mismatch-Repair Deficiency. *N. Engl. J. Med.* **2015**, *372*, 2509–2520. [CrossRef] [PubMed]
84. Andreev-Drakhlin, A.; Shah, A.Y.; Adriazola, A.C.; Shaw, L.; Lopez, L.; James, M.; Matin, S.F.; Alhalabi, O.; Gao, J.; Siefker-Radtke, A.O.; et al. Efficacy of Immune Checkpoint Blockade in Patients with Advanced Upper Tract Urothelial Cancer and Mismatch Repair Deficiency or Microsatellite Instability (MSI). *J. Clin. Oncol.* **2021**, *39*, 487. [CrossRef]
85. Li, S.; Wu, X.; Yan, X.; Zhou, L.; Xu, H.; Li, J.; Liu, Y.; Tang, B.; Chi, Z.; Si, L.; et al. Prognostic Value of HER2 Expression Levels for Upper Tract Urothelial Carcinoma. *J. Clin. Oncol.* **2022**, *40*, 557. [CrossRef]
86. Coquan, E.; Clarisse, B.; Lequesne, J.; Brachet, P.-E.; Nevière, Z.; Meriaux, E.; Bonnet, I.; Castera, M.; Goardon, N.; Boutrois, J. et al. TALASUR Trial: A Single Arm Phase II Trial Assessing Efficacy and Safety of TALazoparib and Avelumab as Maintenance Therapy in Platinum-Sensitive Metastatic or Locally Advanced URothelial Carcinoma. *BMC Cancer* **2022**, *22*, 1213. [CrossRef]
87. Yang, K.; Yu, W.; Liu, H.; Lou, F.; Cao, S.; Wang, H.; He, Z. Mutational Pattern off Homologous Recombination Repair (HRR)-Related Genes in Upper Tract Urothelial Carcinoma. *Cancer Med.* **2023**, *12*, 15304–15316. [CrossRef] [PubMed]
88. Lee, J.; Kim, H.; Gualberto, A.; Scholz, C.R.; Park, S.H. Tipifarnib, a Farnesyltransferase Inhibitor, for Metastatic Urothelial Carcinoma Harboring HRAS Mutations. *J. Clin. Oncol.* **2020**, *38*, 5086. [CrossRef]
89. Kim, J.W.; Milowsky, M.I.; Hahn, N.M.; Kwiatkowski, D.J.; Morgans, A.K.; Davis, N.B.; Appleman, L.J.; Gupta, S.; Lara, P.; Lucky, N.; et al. Sapanisertib, a Dual mTORC1/2 Inhibitor, for TSC1- or TSC2-Mutated Metastatic Urothelial Carcinoma (mUC). *J. Clin. Oncol.* **2021**, *39*, 431. [CrossRef]
90. Koshkin, V.S.; Sonpavde, G.P.; Hwang, C.; Mellado, B.; Tomlinson, G.; Shimura, M.; Chisamore, M.J.; Gil, M.; Loriot, Y. Futibatinib plus Pembrolizumab in Patients (Pts) with Advanced or Metastatic Urothelial Carcinoma (mUC): Preliminary Safety Results from a Phase 2 Study. *J. Clin. Oncol.* **2022**, *40*, 501. [CrossRef]
91. Wu, Z.; Li, M.; Wang, L.; Paul, A.; Raman, J.D.; Necchi, A.; Psutka, S.P.; Buonerba, C.; Zargar, H.; Black, P.C.; et al. Neoadjuvant Systemic Therapy in Patients Undergoing Nephroureterectomy for Urothelial Cancer: A Multidisciplinary Systematic Review and Critical Analysis. *Minerva Urol. Nephrol.* **2022**, *74*, 518–527. [CrossRef]
92. Tse, J.; Ghandour, R.; Singla, N.; Lotan, Y. Molecular Predictors of Complete Response Following Neoadjuvant Chemotherapy in Urothelial Carcinoma of the Bladder and Upper Tracts. *Int. J. Mol. Sci.* **2019**, *20*, 793. [CrossRef] [PubMed]
93. Subiela, J.D.; Territo, A.; Mercadé, A.; Balañà, J.; Aumatell, J.; Calderon, J.; Gallioli, A.; González-Padilla, D.A.; Gaya, J.M.; Palou, J.; et al. Diagnostic Accuracy of Ureteroscopic Biopsy in Predicting Stage and Grade at Final Pathology in Upper Tract Urothelial Carcinoma: Systematic Review and Meta-Analysis. *Eur. J. Surg. Oncol. J. Eur. Soc. Surg. Oncol. Br. Assoc. Surg. Oncol.* **2020**, *46*, 1989–1997. [CrossRef]
94. Venkat, S.; Khan, A.I.; Lewicki, P.J.; Borregales, L.; Scherr, D.S. Novel Nomograms to Predict Muscle Invasion and Lymph Node Metastasis in Upper Tract Urothelial Carcinoma. *Urol. Oncol. Semin. Orig. Investig.* **2022**, *40*, 108.e11–108.e17. [CrossRef]

95. Petros, F.G.; Qiao, W.; Singla, N.; Clinton, T.N.; Robyak, H.; Raman, J.D.; Margulis, V.; Matin, S.F. Preoperative Multiplex Nomogram for Prediction of High-Risk Nonorgan-Confined Upper-Tract Urothelial Carcinoma. *Urol. Oncol.* **2019**, *37*, 292.e1–292.e9. [CrossRef]
96. Laukhtina, E.; Sari Motlagh, R.; Mori, K.; Katayama, S.; Rajwa, P.; Yanagisawa, T.; Quhal, F.; Mostafaei, H.; Grossmann, N.C.; König, F.; et al. Chemotherapy Is Superior to Checkpoint Inhibitors after Radical Surgery for Urothelial Carcinoma: A Systematic Review and Network Meta-Analysis of Oncologic and Toxicity Outcomes. *Crit. Rev. Oncol. Hematol.* **2022**, *169*, 103570. [CrossRef] [PubMed]

cancers

MDPI

Article

Prognostic Impact of Adjuvant Immunotherapy in Patients with High-Risk Upper Tract Urothelial Cancer: Results from the ROBUUST 2.0 Collaborative Group

Maxwell Otiato [1], Farshad Sheybaee Moghaddam [1], Alireza Ghoreifi [1], Riccardo Autorino [2], Gabriele Bignante [2], Chandru Sundaram [3], Daniel Sidhom [3], Ithaar H. Derweesh [4], Dhruv Puri [4], Vitaly Margulis [5], Benjamin Popokh [5], Firas Abdollah [6], Alex Stephens [6], Matteo Ferro [7], Giuseppe Simone [8], Gabriele Tuderti [8], Reza Mehrazin [9], Ahmed Eraky [9], Mark Gonzalgo [10], Omar Falik Nativ [10], Zhenjie Wu [11], Francesco Porpiglia [12], Enrico N. Checcucci [12], Andres Correa [13], Randall Lee [13], Alessandro Antonelli [14], Alessandro Veccia [14], Soroush Rais-Bahrami [15], Alireza Dehghanmanshadi [15], Nirmish Singla [16], Stephan Brönimann [16], Sisto Perdonà [17], Roberto Contieri [17], Takashi Yoshida [18], James Porter [19], Saum Ghodoussipour [20], Luca Lambertini [21], Andrea Minervini [21] and Hooman Djaladat [1,*]

1 Institute of Urology, University of Southern California, 1441 Eastlake Ave, Suite 7416, Los Angeles, CA 90089, USA; otiato@usc.edu (M.O.); farshad.sheybaeemoghaddam@med.usc.edu (F.S.M.); alireza.ghoreifi@med.usc.edu (A.G.)

2 Department of Urology, Rush University, Chicago, IL 60612, USA; riccardo_autorino@rush.edu (R.A.); gabriele.bignante@unito.it (G.B.)

3 Department of Urology, Indiana University, Indianapolis, IN 47405, USA; sundaram@iupui.edu (C.S.); sidhom@iupui.edu (D.S.)

4 Department of Urology, UC San Diego School of Medicine, La Jolla, CA 92093, USA; iderweesh@ucsd.edu (I.H.D.); dhruvpuri1997@gmail.com (D.P.)

5 Department of Urology, University of Texas Southwestern Medical Center, Dallas, TX 75390, USA; vitaly.margulis@utsouthwestern.edu (V.M.); benjamin.popokh@utsouthwestern.edu (B.P.)

6 Vattikuti Urology Institute, Henry Ford Hospital, Detroit, MI 48202, USA; firas.abdollah@gmail.com (F.A.); alexstephens@hfhs.org (A.S.)

7 Unit of Urology, Department of Health Science, University of Milan, ASST Santi Paolo e Carlo, 20172 Milan, Italy; drmatteoferro@gmail.com

8 Department of Urology, IRCCS "Regina Elena" National Cancer Institute, 00144 Rome, Italy; puldet@gmail.com (G.S.); gabriele.tuderti@gmail.com (G.T.)

9 Department of Urology, Icahn School of Medicine at Mount Sinai Hospital, New York, NY 10029, USA; reza.mehrazin@gmail.com (R.M.); ahmed.eraky@mountsinai.org (A.E.)

10 Desai Sethi Urology Institute, University of Miami Miller School of Medicine, Miami, FL 33136, USA; m.gonzalgo@med.miami.edu (M.G.); nativ@miami.edu (O.F.N.)

11 Department of Urology, Changhai Hospital, Naval Medical University, Shanghai 200433, China; wuzhenjie17@163.com

12 Department of Surgery, Candiolo Cancer Institute, FPO-IRCCS, 10060 Candiolo, Italy; porpiglia@libero.it (F.P.); checcu.e@hotmail.it (E.N.C.)

13 Fox Chase Cancer Center, Philadelphia, PA 19111, USA; andres.correa@fccc.edu (A.C.); randall.lee@fccc.edu (R.L.)

14 Department of Urology, University of Verona, 37129 Verona, Italy; alessandro_antonelli@me.com (A.A.); a.veccia88@gmail.com (A.V.)

15 Department of Urology, University of Alabama at Birmingham Heersink School of Medicine, Birmingham, AL 35294, USA; soroush@uab.edu (S.R.-B.); adehghanmanshadi@uabmc.edu (A.D.)

16 The James Buchanan Brady Urological Institute at John Hopkins, Baltimore, MD 21205, USA; nsingla2@jhmi.edu (N.S.); sbroniml@jh.edu (S.B.)

17 Department of Urology, Istituto Nazionale Tumori "Fondazione Pascale", 80131 Naples, Italy; s.perdona@istitutotumori.na.it (S.P.); contieri.ro@gmail.com (R.C.)

18 Department of Urology and Andrology, Kansai Medical University, Osaka 5708507, Japan; palmfiz2009@gmail.com

19 Swedish Medical Center, Seattle, WA 98122, USA; porter@swedishurology.com

20 Section of Urologic Oncology, Rutgers Cancer Institute, Rutgers Robert Wood Johnson Medical School, New Brunswick, NJ 08901, USA; sg1621@cinj.rutgers.edu

21 Oncologic Minimally Invasive Urology and Andrology Unit, Careggi Hospital, University of Florence, 50134 Florence, Italy; luca.lambertini@unifi.it (L.L.); andrea.minervini@unifi.it (A.M.)

* Correspondence: djaladat@med.usc.edu

Simple Summary: This study investigated the effect of immunotherapy on outcomes in patients with high-risk upper tract urothelial carcinoma (UTUC) following surgery. Using a large multi-institutional database, outcomes were compared between patients treated with immunotherapy and a matched group who received no additional therapy. Matching was based on tumor category, lymph node involvement, and prior chemotherapy. Results showed no significant improvement in recurrence-free or overall survival with immunotherapy. However, the presence of cancer in lymph nodes remained a strong predictor of poor survival. These findings suggest that immunotherapy may not provide added benefit in the current setting and highlight the need for better risk-based treatment strategies in high-risk UTUC.

Abstract: Background/Objective: The impact of adjuvant immunotherapy (IO) on the prognosis of patients with upper tract urothelial carcinoma (UTUC) remains unclear. This study examines the association of adjuvant IO with oncologic outcomes in patients with high-risk UTUC. **Methods**: This retrospective study reviewed patients with high-risk UTUC treated with adjuvant IO using the ROBotic surgery for Upper tract Urothelial cancer STudy (ROBUUST) database. Propensity-score-matched analysis (nearest-neighbor algorithm, caliper 0.1) was conducted to compare patients receiving adjuvant IO versus those who did not, with matching based on pathologic T and N category and receipt of neoadjuvant chemotherapy. Associations between adjuvant IO and urothelial recurrence-free survival (URFS), non-urothelial recurrence-free survival (NRFS), and overall survival (OS) were estimated using a Cox proportional hazards model. **Results**: Seventy-five patients received adjuvant IO following nephroureterectomy (median four cycles, including eleven (14.7%) nivolumab, thirty-one (41.3%) pembrolizumab, four (5.3%) atezolizumab, and twenty-nine (38.6%) other agents. These patients were matched to 68 patients without adjuvant therapy. Median follow-up times were 17 (IQR, 10–29) months and 20 (9–44) months for IO and no adjuvant therapy, respectively. Multivariable analysis revealed that adjuvant IO was not associated with URFS, NRFS, or OS. Pathologic nodal involvement (HR 7.52, $p < 0.001$) was the only independent predictor of worse OS. **Conclusions**: In this real-world retrospective data set, adjuvant IO does not have an impact on oncologic outcomes of UTUC patients following extirpative surgery.

Keywords: upper tract urothelial carcinoma; immunotherapy; outcomes; nephroureterectomy

1. Introduction

Upper tract urothelial carcinoma (UTUC) accounts for 5–10% of all urothelial tumors [1,2]. While radical nephroureterectomy (RNU) remains the standard curative treatment for localized and high-risk UTUC, surgical resection overall remains the only curative option for localized UTUC [3]. Adjuvant systemic therapy is currently recommended for high-stage UTUC patients following surgery [4,5]. Recent trials investigating adjuvant systemic chemotherapy in high-risk UTUC have continued to demonstrate improved outcomes [6].

A breakthrough in the discovery and adoption of immunotherapy (IO), targeted agents, and antibody–drug conjugates (ADCs) has transformed the systemic treatments of urothelial cancers across the disease continuum, including non-muscle-invasive bladder cancer (NMIBC) and muscle-invasive bladder cancer (MIBC). For NMIBC, intravesical Bacillus Calmette–Guérin (BCG) remains the gold standard for patients with high-risk disease. In cases unresponsive to BCG, pembrolizumab has been approved and has demonstrated efficacy, as highlighted in the KEYNOTE-057 trial. Additionally, emerging approaches, including novel intravesical gene therapies and combination intravesical chemotherapies, have shown promising early results [7–9]. For MIBC, neoadjuvant cisplatin-based chemotherapy followed by radical cystectomy remains standard, with immune checkpoint inhibitors now being incorporated into perioperative treatment settings. For metastatic disease, platinum-based chemotherapy continues to serve as the first-line treatment; however, the combination of enfortumab vedotin and pembrolizumab has brought forth unprecedented survival benefits, offering great promise to a new standard of care. ADCs such as enfortumab vedotin and sacituzumab govitecan, along with FGFR inhibitors like erdafitinib for tumors with FGFR2/3 alterations, are now established as later lines of therapy [9–15].

For UTUC, the role of immunotherapy is still emerging. Currently, adjuvant nivolumab therapy is an option for patients with UTUC who have undergone neoadjuvant platinum-based chemotherapy or for those who are ineligible or refuse perioperative cisplatin [7,16]. The results of the CheckMate 274 trial showed adjuvant nivolumab significantly improves disease-free survival (DFS) compared to placebo in patients with locally advanced urothelial carcinoma after cystectomy or nephroureterectomy [17,18]. Similarly, the AMBASSADOR trial demonstrated that adjuvant pembrolizumab significantly improves DFS in patients with high-risk muscle-invasive urothelial carcinoma (MIUC), including those with UTUC, after radical surgery [19]. In contrast, the IMvigor 010 study found that adjuvant atezolizumab did not significantly enhance DFS compared to observation in patients with high-risk MIUC, also including those with UTUC [13]. While current literature provides evidence for MIUC, powered evidence specifically evaluating the role of adjuvant IO therapies in UTUC remains limited. Real-world data may offer valuable insights into the effectiveness and safety of adjuvant IO in UTUC, especially given the rarity of the disease and the limited availability of randomized trials. The impact of other adjuvant IOs on prognosis and survival in UTUC patients remains understudied.

This study aims to examine the association between adjuvant IO and oncological outcomes in patients with high-risk UTUC, evaluate clinical and pathological factors and treatment patterns as predictors of response to adjuvant IO, and offer perspectives into the role of adjuvant IO and its integration into existing management protocols for high-risk UTUC.

2. Materials and Methods

This retrospective cohort study utilized data from the ROBotic surgery for Upper Tract Urothelial cancer STudy (ROBUUST) database, a multi-institutional registry of patients undergoing surgery for UTUC across 17 centers worldwide. Data-sharing agreements were established with each center and Institutional Review Board (IRB) approval was obtained at all participating centers (IRB No. 161197). The inclusion criteria were patients with high-risk UTUC, according to European Association of Urology guidelines, who underwent curative robotic nephroureterectomy or segmental ureterectomy and were treated with adjuvant IO between January 2015 and December 2022 [20]. Patients with unknown pathologic stage, unknown receipt of adjuvant IO, and missing survival data were excluded. Four groups were identified based on adjuvant therapy use: IO, chemotherapy, a combination of IO and chemotherapy, and no adjuvant therapy. Of note, patients received adjuvant systemic therapy according to each center's multidisciplinary decision.

The study collected data on demographic, clinicopathological, pathological, and survival variables. Demographic and baseline characteristics included age, gender, body mass index (BMI), American Society of Anesthesiologists (ASA) score, Eastern Cooperative Oncology Group (ECOG) status, history of type 2 diabetes mellitus, history of bladder cancer, tumor size, tumor location, and type of surgery. Pathological variables consisted of pathological TNM staging, grade, tumor necrosis, lymphovascular invasion, tumor multifocality, and margin status.

The primary outcome, urothelial recurrence-free survival (URFS), was calculated from the date of surgery to the date of first documented clinical recurrent disease in the bladder, contralateral ureter, or contralateral renal pelvis, as diagnosed by biopsy. If the patient did not have recurrence documented, the outcome was calculated as the date of last follow-up or death, indicating the patient was considered recurrence-free up until that time. Secondary outcomes included non-urothelial recurrence-free survival (NRFS) and overall survival (OS). NRFS was defined as survival without recurrent disease identified by clinical or paraclinical investigations including imaging outside the bladder or the contralateral upper tract.

Data analysis was conducted using IBM SPSS v25 (IBM Corp, Armonk, NY, USA), with statistical significance defined as $p < 0.05$. Baseline characteristics of treatment groups were compared using χ^2 tests for categorical variables and ANOVA for continuous variables. Categorical variables were reported as frequencies and percentages, while continuous variables were presented as medians with interquartile ranges (IQRs).

Propensity scores were estimated using logistic regression models that included pathological T and N category and the receipt of neoadjuvant chemotherapy. The IO group was matched to the no adjuvant therapy group using a 1:1 nearest-neighbor algorithm without replacement (caliper width = 0.1 SD).

URFS, NRFS, and OS were compared between the IO group and the no adjuvant therapy group using an adjusted Kaplan–Meier method. A multivariable Cox proportional hazards regression model was performed to assess baseline and pathological variables as independent factors associated with survival outcomes.

3. Results

Among the 1911 patients initially included in the ROBUUST registry, 219 (11%) patients received adjuvant chemotherapy, 27 (1.4%) patients received a combination of chemotherapy and IO, and 1590 (83%) patients were not treated with any systemic therapy. A total of 75 (3.9%) patients received IO alone (mean (IQR) age, 73 (67–79) years; 65% male). Pembrolizumab was the most common type of adjuvant IO (31 patients (41.3%)), followed by nivolumab (13 patients (17.3%)), atezolizumab and avelumab (2 patients (2.67%) each), and durvalumab (1 patient (1.3%)). The remaining 25 patients (33.3%) received an unspecified immunotherapy.

Baseline and clinical features (before and after propensity score matching (PSM)) for the treatment groups are shown in Table 1. Based on PSM including pathological T and N category and the receipt of neoadjuvant chemotherapy, there were 75 patients who received adjuvant IO and 68 patients who did not receive adjuvant therapy. The median time to follow-up was 17 (IQR, 10–29) months and 20 (9–44) months for the IO and no adjuvant therapy groups, respectively. There were no significant differences in demographic characteristics or pathologic features between the two groups. In the IO cohort, 51 patients (69.9%) had pathologic T category greater than T2, 45 patients (61.6%) had multifocal tumors, and 37 patients (50.7%) had received prior neoadjuvant therapy. Regarding nodal status, 26 patients (36.6%) were classified as pN0, while 19 patients (26.8%) and 26 patients (36.6%) were classified as pN+ and pNx, respectively (Table 1).

Table 1. Demographic and Clinical Characteristics of UTUC Patients Among Treatment Groups.

	Before PSM			After PSM		
	Immunotherapy	**No Adjuvant Therapy**	***p*-Value**	**Immunotherapy**	**No Adjuvant Therapy**	***p*-Value**
N	75	1590	N/A	75	68	N/A
Age, median, (IQR), y	73 (67–79)	72 (65–79)	<0.001	73 (67–79)	73 (67.25–80)	0.686
Tumor Size, median, (IQR), cm	3.4 (2–4.6)	3 (2–5)	0.671	3.4 (2–4.62)	3.7 (2.15–6)	0.254
Sex, n (%)						
Male	49 (65.3)	932 (58.6)	0.227	49 (65.3)	40 (58.8)	0.423
Female	26 (34.7)	658 (41.4)		26 (34.7)	28 (41.2)	
N/A	0 (0)	0 (0)				
Histology, n (%)						
Urothelial	66 (97)	1465 (93)	0.26	66 (97)	63 (93)	0.47
Variant	2 (3)	69 (5)		2 (3)	4 (6)	
N/A	7 (0)	56 (0)		7 (0)	0 (0)	
Grade, n (%)						
Low	2 (2.7)	331 (22.3)	<0.001	2 (2.7)	3 (4.5)	0.547
High	73 (97.3)	1155 (77.7)		73 (97.3)	63 (95.5)	
N/A	0 (0)	104 (0)		0 (0)	0 (0)	
Pathologic T Stage (pT), n (%)						
$p \leq$ T2	22 (30.1)	992 (66.4)	<0.001	22 (30.1)	20 (29.4)	0.925
$p >$ T2	51 (69.9)	501 (72.3)		51 (69.9)	48 (70.6)	
N/A	73 (0)	97 (0)		2 (0)	0 (0)	
Pathologic N Stage (pN), n (%)						
N0	26 (36.6)	472 (32)	<0.001	26 (36.6)	27 (39.7)	0.921
N+	19 (26.8)	123 (8.4)		19 (26.8)	18 (26.5)	
Nx	26 (36.6)	878 (59.6)		26 (36.6)	23 (33.8)	
N/A	4 (0)	117 (0)		4 (0)	0 (0)	
Neoadjuvant Therapy, n (%)						
Yes	37 (50.7)	161 (10.2)	<0.001	37 (50.7)	35 (51.5)	0.926
No	36 (49.3)	1423 (89.8)		36 (49.3)	33 (48.5)	
N/A	2 (0)	6 (0)		2 (0)	0 (0)	
Recurrence, n (%)						
Yes	34 (45.3)	463 (30.7)	<0.001	41 (54.7)	41 (63.1)	0.314
No	41 (54.7)	1045 (69.3)		34 (45.3)	24 (36.9)	
N/A	0 (0)	82 (0)		0 (0)	3 (0)	
Metastasis, n (%)						
Yes	41 (54.7)	1190 (86.1)	<0.001	41 (54.7)	20 (31.3)	0.006
No	34 (45.3)	192 (13.9)		34 (45.3)	44 (68.8)	
N/A	0 (0)	208 (0)		0 (0)	4 (0)	
Death, n (%)						
Yes	23 (30.7)	221 (14.7)	<0.001	23 (30.7)	13 (36.1)	0.136
No	52 (69.3)	1280 (85.3)		52 (69.3)	53 (80.3)	
N/A	0 (0)	89 (0)		0 (0)	2 (0)	

The OS rate at 1 year for the adjuvant IO vs. non-IO groups was 83% vs. 84% ($p = 0.06$), indicating no significant difference. Similarly, the URFS rate at 1 year for the adjuvant IO vs. non-IO groups was 24% vs. 29% ($p = 0.52$), showing no significant difference. Compared with the cohort with no adjuvant therapy, the cohort with IO had a higher proportion of non-urothelial recurrences observed within 9 months after PSM (IO, 41 (54.7%); no adjuvant therapy, 20 (31.3%); $p = 0.006$). However, when time-to-event was accounted for using Kaplan–Meier analysis, the 1-year survival probability was 18% vs. 30% for the adjuvant IO and non-IO groups ($p = 0.14$), with no detected differences (Figure 1).

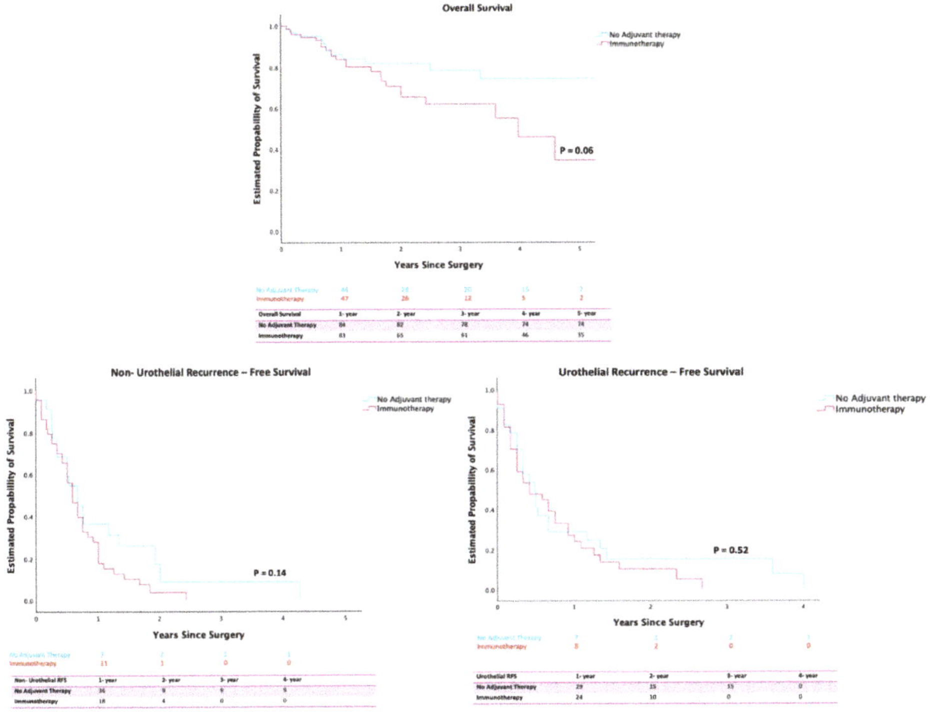

Figure 1. Kaplan–Meier Analysis of Estimated Probability for Oncologic Outcomes.

The presence of pathologic nodal disease (pN+) was associated with significantly worse OS (HR, 7.52; 95% CI, 2.67–21.2) following multivariable Cox regression analysis. No other pathological factors were found to be independent predictors of URFS, NRFS, and OS (Figure 2).

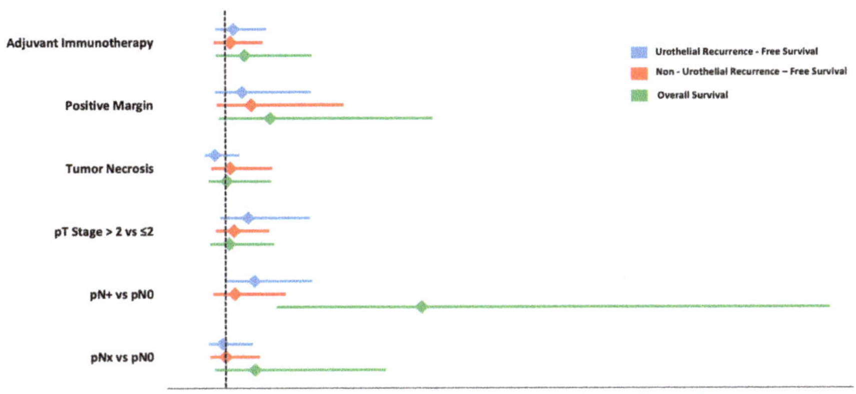

Figure 2. Multivariable Cox Regression Forest Plot of Variables Associated with Oncologic Outcomes.

4. Discussion

This retrospective study evaluated the association between IO and survival outcomes among patients with UTUC following surgery with curative intent from centers worldwide. The diverse cohort study of data found no evidence of a survival or oncologic benefit from adjuvant IO in this patient population.

While the adjuvant IO group demonstrated a higher proportion of non-urothelial recurrence within the study period, Kaplan–Meier analysis did not detect a statistically significant difference in NRFS between groups at 1 year. The greater number of recurrences in the IO group (54.7% vs. 31.3%) may reflect clustering of early events in our cohort. However, survival analysis revealed that overall recurrence risk over time was not significantly different. Our results suggest that, while IO-treated patients may experience earlier non-urothelial recurrence, their risk of long-term recurrence is not statistically different from those who received no adjuvant therapy.

In recent years, indications for adjuvant IO in patients with urothelial cancer have been evolving, driven by an increasing number of studies [21,22]. However, research dedicated to the investigation of this topic in UTUC remains limited, with most powered evidence derived from studies on locally advanced or metastatic urothelial carcinoma of the bladder. This may be due in part to the rarity of UTUC and the heterogeneity of the disease, making it difficult to conduct large-scale, UTUC-specific trials with adjuvant immunotherapies beyond nivolumab, pembrolizumab, and atezolizumab [23].

Current evidence from trials presents mixed findings regarding the evolving role of immunotherapy in UTUC [16]. The CheckMate 274 trial demonstrated a median DFS of 20.8 months with nivolumab, compared to 10.8 months with placebo (HR, 0.70; 98.22% CI, 0.55–0.90; $p < 0.001$), in patients with high-risk MUIC. The expanded analysis confirmed DFS benefits across various subgroups, including UTUC, and highlighted that adjuvant nivolumab significantly improves DFS, particularly among patients with higher PD-L1 expression [17,18].

Similarly, the AMBASSADOR trial, which compared adjuvant pembrolizumab to observation in patients with high-risk MUIC, reported a median DFS of 29.6 months with pembrolizumab compared to 14.2 months with observation (HR, 0.73; 95% CI, 0.59–0.90; $p = 0.003$), indicating adjuvant pembrolizumab significantly confers a DFS advantage for patients, including patients with UTUC [18]. However, a systematic review and meta-analysis by Sayyid et al. showed no observed DFS benefit in patients with UTUC when treated with pembrolizumab and other adjuvant immune checkpoint inhibitors (HR, 1.19; 95% CI, 0.86–1.64) [24]. The differences in disease-free survival outcomes between this trial and our study may be attributed to variations in patient selection, trial design, biomarker stratification, and duration of follow-up.

The IMvigor 010 trial, which randomized patients with postoperative MUIC to receive either adjuvant atezolizumab or observation, found no significant DFS improvement (19.4 vs. 16.6 months; HR, 0.89; 95% CI, 0.74–1.08; $p = 0.24$). The study also found adverse events were more frequent in the atezolizumab group, with serious adverse events occurring in 31% of patients compared to 18% in the observation group [25].

Additionally, a comprehensive meta-analysis by Laukhtina et al. reported that adjuvant chemotherapy is associated with a significantly lower likelihood of disease progression in UTUC than observation/placebo [26]. IOs, such as atezolizumab and nivolumab, did not demonstrate a similar benefit but had a comparable risk of adverse effects to that of the observation/placebo group. These findings support the use of adjuvant chemotherapy over IOs in the treatment of high-risk UTUC following extirpative surgery and align with results from the POUT trial, which showed DFS benefit with adjuvant platinum-based chemotherapy in high-risk UTUC patients [6,26]. However, current clinical guidelines

(AUA, EAU, NCCN) continue to recommend neoadjuvant chemotherapy based primarily on data from MIBC, highlighting the need for additional evidence and treatment options specifically tailored to the adjuvant setting in UTUC [16,18].

Consistent with these findings, our study found that different types of adjuvant IO did not improve nor compromise survival outcomes, even after adjusting for demographic and pathological factors. There still remains a lack of powered evidence regarding the specific role of adjuvant IO therapies in UTUC, compared to MIUC. The role of IOs in UTUC treatment remains uncertain, and adjuvant chemotherapy appears to provide a more consistent prognostic and survival benefit for high-risk UTUC patients following surgery [26]. However, further research is necessary to fully explore all other treatment agents and combinations.

A key strength of this study is the detailed and comprehensive characterization of both demographic and pathological variables, which adds a level of real-world granularity often missing in previous studies. Our analysis includes a broad range of clinically relevant variables such as age, gender, BMI, ASA score, ECOG status, and comorbidities like type 2 diabetes mellitus and history of bladder cancer. Tumor-specific factors—including tumor size, location, multifocality, and margin status—alongside robust pathological variables such as TNM staging, grade, necrosis, and lymphovascular invasion, provide a multidimensional view of patient and disease profiles. This data allows for a more nuanced interpretation of outcomes and enhances the clinical relevance of our findings, distinguishing our work from prior literature that often relies on less detailed, registry-level inputs.

Multivariate Cox regression analysis identified pathologic nodal disease as the sole independent factor negatively impacting overall survival. This finding suggests that patients with nodal involvement (pN+) after nephroureterectomy are at a much higher risk of poor outcomes compared with those without nodal disease (pN0), highlighting the critical role that nodal status plays in predicting long-term survival. Hakimi et al. previously found that patients who underwent nephroureterectomy alone with positive lymph nodes had substantially worse 2-year OS and RFS compared to those with negative lymph nodes (42% vs. 86% for OS, 35% vs. 61% for RFS) [27]. Similarly, a study by Kagawa et al. also highlighted that patients with pN+ status had notably worse cancer-specific survival (CSS), RFS, and OS compared to those with pN0, even when receiving adjuvant IO [28]. Identifying pathologic nodal disease as an independent prognostic factor in our study further emphasizes the role of lymph node dissection in predicting outcomes for patients, while also highlighting the potential role of biomarkers—such as ctDNA—in identifying patients at highest risk for non-organ-confined disease [29,30]

While these findings may help inform treatment paradigms for UTUC, they are exploratory and should not define clinical practice standards. Further studies are warranted to validate the role of adjuvant IO in high-risk UTUC and ongoing trials may provide more definitive guidance.

These findings should be considered in the context of several limitations. The retrospective design excluded patients with unavailable survival status or unknown follow-up data, potentially introducing selection bias. Another limitation of the study is the relatively short median follow-up duration for the primary and secondary outcomes, 29 s. Given the natural progression of the disease, a longer follow-up period may provide a more accurate assessment of survival differences between groups. It is possible that, with extended follow-up, significant time-dependent differences in OS, URS, and NRFS may emerge. Future studies with longer observation periods may be worthwhile to better capture long-term survival trends and potential late recurrences. Additionally, the data may be prone to confounding effects, as not all variables may have been fully adjusted through PSM. The

ROBUUST database also does not capture or account for detailed information on specific IO regimens, including their duration and doses. Patients within the cohort may have received suboptimal IO treatments, which could have obscured the benefit of the therapy. Given there is an absence of powered prospective trials for UTUC, further investigation through a robust PSM-driven retrospective study or randomized control trial (RCT) should be considered to understand the role that different IO types and durations may play in survival following nephroureterectomy for UTUC.

5. Conclusions

Using a large multi-institutional database for patients who underwent RNU, these findings suggest that adjuvant IO is not associated with improved oncologic outcomes of UTUC patients following extirpative surgery. Further consideration should be given to conducting randomized controlled trials and investigating the role of adjuvant immunotherapy in this subset of patients.

Author Contributions: M.O.: Conceptualization, Methodology, Investigation, Data curation, Writing—original draft preparation, Validation, Writing—review and editing, Visualization, Supervision. F.S.M.: Methodology, Investigation, Formal analysis, Writing—original draft preparation, Validation, Writing—review and editing, Visualization, Supervision. A.G.: Conceptualization, Methodology, Investigation, Formal analysis, Validation, Writing—review and editing, Supervision. R.A.: Writing—review and editing, Validation, Investigation, Data curation. G.B.: Writing—review and editing, Validation, Investigation, Data curation. C.S.: Writing—review and editing, Validation, Investigation, Data curation. D.S.: Writing—review and editing, Validation, Investigation, Data curation. I.H.D.: Writing—review and editing, Validation, Investigation, Data curation. D.P.: Writing—review and editing, Validation, Investigation, Data curation. V.M.: Writing—review and editing, Validation, Investigation, Data curation. B.P.: Writing—review and editing, Validation, Investigation, Data curation. F.A.: Writing—review and editing, Validation, Investigation, Data curation. A.S.: Writing—review and editing, Validation, Investigation, Data curation. M.F.: Writing—review and editing, Validation, Investigation, Data curation. G.S.: Writing—review and editing, Validation, Investigation, Data curation. G.T.: Writing—review and editing, Validation, Investigation, Data curation. R.M.: Writing—review and editing, Validation, Investigation, Data curation. A.E.: Writing—review and editing, Validation, Investigation, Data curation. M.G.: Writing—review and editing, Validation, Investigation, Data curation. O.F.N.: Writing—review and editing, Validation, Investigation, Data curation. Z.W.: Writing—review and editing, Validation, Investigation, Data curation. F.P.: Writing—review and editing, Validation, Investigation, Data curation. E.N.C.: Writing—review and editing, Validation, Investigation, Data curation. A.C.: Writing—review and editing, Validation, Investigation, Data curation. R.L.: Writing—review and editing, Validation, Investigation, Data curation. A.A.: Writing—review and editing, Validation, Investigation, Data curation. A.V.: Writing—review and editing, Validation, Investigation, Data curation. S.R.-B.: Writing—review and editing, Validation, Investigation, Data curation. A.D.: Writing—review and editing, Validation, Investigation, Data curation. N.S.: Writing—review and editing, Validation, Investigation, Data curation. S.B.: Writing—review and editing, Validation, Investigation, Data curation. S.P.: Writing—review and editing, Validation, Investigation, Data curation. R.C.: Writing—review and editing, Validation, Investigation, Data curation. T.Y.: Writing—review and editing, Validation, Investigation, Data curation. J.P.: Writing—review and editing, Validation, Investigation, Data curation. S.G.: Writing—review and editing, Validation, Investigation, Data curation. L.L.: Writing—review and editing, Validation, Investigation, Data curation. A.M.: Writing—review and editing, Validation, Investigation, Data curation. H.D.: Conceptualization, Methodology, Investigation, Validation, Writing—Review and Editing. All authors have read and agreed to the published version of the manuscript.

Funding: This research received no external funding.

Institutional Review Board Statement: The study was conducted in accordance with the principles of the Declaration of Helsinki. Ethics Committee Name: Rush University Institutional Review Board. Approval Code: 22111001-IRB01-AM04. Date of Approval: 30 January 2023.

Informed Consent Statement: Informed consent was obtained from all subjects involved in the study.

Data Availability Statement: The original contributions presented in this study are included in the article. Further inquiries can be directed to the corresponding author.

Conflicts of Interest: The authors declare no conflicts of interest.

Abbreviations

The following abbreviations are used in this manuscript:

IO	immunotherapy
UTUC	upper tract urothelial carcinoma
ROBUUST	ROBotic surgery for Upper tract Urothelial cancer STudy
URFS	urothelial recurrence-free survival
NFRS	non-urothelial-free survival
OS	overall survival
MIUC	muscle-invasive urothelial carcinoma
CSS	cancer-specific survival
RNU	radical nephroureterectomy (RNU)
NMIBC	non-muscle-invasive bladder cancer
MIBC	muscle-invasive bladder cancer
ADC	antibody–drug conjugate
BCG	Bacillus Calmette–Guérin

References

1. Roberts, J.L.; Ghali, F.; Aganovic, L.; Bechis, S.; Healy, K.; Rivera-Sanfeliz, G.; Autorino, R.; Derweesh, I. Diagnosis, management, and follow-up of upper tract urothelial carcinoma: An interdisciplinary collaboration between urology and radiology. *Abdom. Radiol.* **2019**, *44*, 3893–3905. [CrossRef]
2. Rouprêt, M.; Seisen, T.; Birtle, A.J.; Capoun, O.; Compérat, E.M.; Dominguez-Escrig, J.L.; Gürses Andersson, I.; Liedberg, F.; Mariappan, P.; Hugh Mostafid, A.; et al. European Association of Urology Guidelines on Upper Urinary Tract Urothelial Carcinoma: 2023 Update. *Eur. Urol.* **2023**, *84*, 49–64. [CrossRef]
3. Lughezzani, G.; Sun, M.; Perrotte, P.; Shariat, S.F.; Jeldres, C.; Budaus, L.; Alasker, A.; Duclos, A.; Widmer, H.; Latour, M.; et al. Should bladder cuff excision remain the standard of care at nephroureterectomy in patients with urothelial carcinoma of the renal pelvis? A population-based study. *Eur. Urol.* **2010**, *57*, 956–962. [CrossRef] [PubMed]
4. Birtle, A.; Johnson, M.; Chester, J.; Jones, R.; Dolling, D.; Bryan, R.T.; Harris, C.; Winterbottom, A.; Blacker, A.; Catto, J.W.F.; et al. Adjuvant chemotherapy in upper tract urothelial carcinoma (the POUT trial): A phase 3, open-label, randomised controlled trial. *Lancet* **2020**, *395*, 1268–1277. [CrossRef] [PubMed]
5. Di Bello, F.; Jannello, L.M.I.; Siech, C.; de Angelis, M.; Rodriguez Peñaranda, N.; Tian, Z.; Goyal, J.A.; Ruvolo, C.C.; Califano, G.; Creta, M.; et al. Adjuvant Systemic Therapy Improved Survival After Radical Nephroureterectomy for Upper Tract Urothelial Carcinoma. *Ann. Surg. Oncol.* **2024**, *31*, 7229–7236. [CrossRef] [PubMed]
6. Birtle, A.J.; Jones, R.; Chester, J.; Lewis, R.; Biscombe, K.; Johnson, M.; Blacker, A.; Bryan, R.T.; Catto, J.W.F.; Choudhury, A.; et al. Improved Disease-Free Survival with Adjuvant Chemotherapy After Nephroureterectomy for Upper Tract Urothelial Cancer: Final Results of the POUT Trial. *J. Clin. Oncol.* **2024**, *42*, 1466–1471. [CrossRef]
7. Coleman, J.A.; Clark, P.E.; Bixler, B.R.; Buckley, D.I.; Chang, S.S.; Chou, R.; Hoffman-Censits, J.; Kulkarni, G.S.; Matin, S.F.; Pierorazio, P.M.; et al. Diagnosis and Management of Non-Metastatic Upper Tract Urothelial Carcinoma: AUA/SUO Guideline. *J. Urol.* **2023**, *209*, 1071–1081. [CrossRef]
8. Necchi, A.; Roumiguié, M.; Kamat, A.M.; Shore, N.D.; Boormans, J.L.; Esen, A.A.; Lebret, T.; Kandori, S.; Bajorin, D.F.; Krieger, L.E.M.; et al. Pembrolizumab monotherapy for high-risk non-muscle-invasive bladder cancer without carcinoma in situ and unresponsive to BCG (KEYNOTE-057): A single-arm, multicentre, phase 2 trial. *Lancet. Oncol.* **2024**, *25*, 720–730. [CrossRef]

9. López-Beltrán, A.; Cookson, M.S.; Guercio, B.J.; Cheng, L. Advances in diagnosis and treatment of bladder cancer. *BMJ Clin. Res. Ec* **2024**, *384*, e076743. [CrossRef]
10. Cigliola, A.; Beccia, V.; Anghelone, A.; Panebianco, M.; Ciccarese, C.; Iacovelli, R. 2023 ASCO Genitourinary Cancers Symposiur A focus on urothelial carcinoma. *Expert Rev. Anticancer. Ther.* **2023**, *23*, 1123–1126. [CrossRef]
11. Flaig, T.W.; Spiess, P.E.; Abern, M.; Agarwal, N.; Bangs, R.; Buyyounouski, M.K.; Chan, K.; Chang, S.S.; Chang, P Friedlander, T.; et al. NCCN Guidelines® Insights: Bladder cancer, version 3.2024. *J. Natl. Compr. Cancer Netw.* **2024**, *22* 216–225. [CrossRef]
12. Yajima, S.; Masuda, H. Immune checkpoint inhibitors and antibody-drug conjugates in urothelial carcinoma: Current landscap and future directions. *Cancers* **2025**, *17*, 1594. [CrossRef] [PubMed]
13. Piombino, C.; Tonni, E.; Oltrecolli, M.; Pirola, M.; Pipitone, S.; Baldessari, C.; Dominici, M.; Sabbatini, R.; Vitale, M.G. Immunother apy in urothelial cancer: Current status and future directions. *Expert Rev. Anticancer. Ther.* **2023**, *23*, 1141–1155. [CrossRef [PubMed]
14. Thomas, V.M.; Jo, Y.; Tripathi, N.; Roy, S.; Chigarira, B.; Narang, A.; Gebrael, G.; Chehade, C.H.; Sayegh, N.; Fortuna, G.G.; et a Treatment patterns and attrition with lines of therapy for advanced urothelial carcinoma in the US. *JAMA Netw. Open* **2024** *7*, e249417. [CrossRef]
15. Zhang, M.; Zuo, Y.; Chen, S.; Li, Y.; Xing, Y.; Yang, L.; Wang, H.; Guo, R. Antibody-drug conjugates in urothelial carcinoma Scientometric analysis and clinical trials analysis. *Front. Oncol.* **2024**, *14*, 1323366. [CrossRef] [PubMed]
16. Kolawa, A.; D'Souza, A.; Tulpule, V. Overview, Diagnosis, and Perioperative Systemic Therapy of Upper Tract Urothelia Carcinoma. *Cancers* **2023**, *15*, 4813. [CrossRef]
17. Galsky, M.D.; Bajorin, D.F.; Witjes, J.A.; Gschwend, J.E.; Tomita, Y.; Nasroulah, F.; Li, J.; Collette, S.; Valderrama, B.P. Grimm, M.O.; et al. Disease-free Survival Analysis for Patients with High-risk Muscle-invasive Urothelial Carcinoma fror the Randomized CheckMate 274 Trial by PD-L1 Combined Positive Score and Tumor Cell Score. *Eur. Urol.* **2023**, *83*, 432–44C [CrossRef]
18. Bajorin, D.F.; Witjes, J.A.; Gschwend, J.E.; Schenker, M.; Valderrama, B.P.; Tomita, Y.; Bamias, A.; Lebret, T.; Shariat, S.F. Park, S.H.; et al. Adjuvant Nivolumab versus Placebo in Muscle-Invasive Urothelial Carcinoma. *N. Engl. J. Med.* **2021**, *384* 2102–2114. [CrossRef]
19. Apolo, A.B.; Ballman, K.V.; Sonpavde, G.; Berg, S.; Kim, W.Y.; Parikh, R.; Teo, M.Y.; Sweis, R.F.; Geynisman, D.M. Grivas, P.; et al. Adjuvant Pembrolizumab versus Observation in Muscle-Invasive Urothelial Carcinoma. *N. Engl. J. Med* **2025**, *392*, 45–55. [CrossRef]
20. Bitaraf, M.; Ghafoori Yazdi, M.; Amini, E. Upper Tract Urothelial Carcinoma (UTUC) Diagnosis and Risk Stratification: A Comprehensive Review. *Cancers* **2023**, *15*, 4987. [CrossRef]
21. Powles, T.; Park, S.H.; Voog, E.; Caserta, C.; Valderrama, B.P.; Gurney, H.; Kalofonos, H.; Radulović, S.; Demey, W. Ullén, A.; et al. Avelumab Maintenance Therapy for Advanced or Metastatic Urothelial Carcinoma. *N. Engl. J. Med.* **2020**, *383* 1218–1230. [CrossRef] [PubMed]
22. Bellmunt, J.; de Wit, R.; Vaughn, D.J.; Fradet, Y.; Lee, J.L.; Fong, L.; Vogelzang, N.J.; Climent, M.A.; Petrylak, D.P. Choueiri, T.K.; et al. Pembrolizumab as Second-Line Therapy for Advanced Urothelial Carcinoma. *N. Engl. J. Med.* **2017** *376*, 1015–1026. [CrossRef]
23. Califano, G.; Ouzaid, I.; Verze, P.; Hermieu, J.F.; Mirone, V.; Xylinas, E. Immune checkpoint inhibition in upper tract urothelial carcinoma. *World J. Urol.* **2021**, *39*, 1357–1367. [CrossRef]
24. Sayyid, R.K.; Bernardino, R.; Chavarriaga, J.; Kumar, R.; Randhawa, H.; Wettstein, M.S.; Cockburn, J.G.; Klaassen, Z. Fleshner, N.E. Adjuvant immune checkpoint inhibitors for urothelial carcinoma: Systematic review and Meta-analysis *World J. Urol.* **2024**, *42*, 418. [CrossRef]
25. Bellmunt, J.; Hussain, M.; Gschwend, J.E.; Albers, P.; Oudard, S.; Castellano, D.; Daneshmand, S.; Nishiyama, H. Majchrowicz, M.; Degaonkar, V.; et al. Adjuvant atezolizumab versus observation in muscle-invasive urothelial carcinoma (IMvigor010): A multicentre, open-label, randomised, phase 3 trial. *Lancet Oncol.* **2021**, *22*, 525–537. [CrossRef] [PubMed]
26. Laukhtina, E.; Sari Motlagh, R.; Mori, K.; Katayama, S.; Rajwa, P.; Yanagisawa, T.; Quhal, F.; Mostafaei, H.; Grossmann, N.C. König, F.; et al. Chemotherapy is superior to checkpoint inhibitors after radical surgery for urothelial carcinoma: A systematic review and network meta-analysis of oncologic and toxicity outcomes. *Crit. Rev. Oncol./Hematol.* **2022**, *169*, 103570. [CrossRef]
27. Hakimi, K.; Carbonara, U.; Djaladat, H.; Mehrazin, R.; Eun, D.; Reese, A.; Gonzalgo, M.L.; Margulis, V.; Uzzo, R.G.; Porter, J.; et al Outcomes of Lymph Node Dissection in Nephroureterectomy in the Treatment of Upper Tract Urothelial Carcinoma: Analysis of the ROBUUST Registry. *J. Urol.* **2022**, *208*, 268–276. [CrossRef] [PubMed]
28. Kagawa, H.; Urabe, F.; Kiuchi, Y.; Katsumi, K.; Yamaguchi, R.; Suhara, Y.; Yoshihara, K.; Goto, Y.; Sadakane, I.; Yata, Y.; et al Real-world outcomes of adjuvant immunotherapy candidates with upper tract urothelial carcinoma: Results of a multicenter cohort study. *Int. J. Clin. Oncol.* **2024**, *29*, 55–63. [CrossRef]

29. Holzbeierlein, J.; Bixler, B.R.; Buckley, D.I.; Chang, S.S.; Holmes, R.S.; James, A.C.; Kirkby, E.; McKiernan, J.M.; Schuckman, A. Treatment of Non-Metastatic Muscle-Invasive Bladder Cancer: AUA/ASCO/SUO Guideline (2017; Amended 2020, 2024). *J. Urol.* **2024**, *212*, 3–10. [CrossRef]
30. Huelster, H.L.; Gould, B.; Schiftan, E.A.; Camperlengo, L.; Davaro, F.; Rose, K.M.; Soupir, A.C.; Jia, S.; Zheng, T.; Sexton, W.J.; et al. Novel Use of Circulating Tumor DNA to Identify Muscle-Invasive and Non-Organ-Confined Upper Tract Urothelial Carcinoma. *Eur. Urol.* **2024**, *85*, 283–292. [CrossRef]

MDPI AG
Grosspeteranlage 5
4052 Basel
Switzerland
Tel.: +41 61 683 77 34

Cancers Editorial Office
E-mail: cancers@mdpi.com
www.mdpi.com/journal/cancers

www.ingramcontent.com/pod-product-compliance
Lightning Source LLC
Chambersburg PA
CBHW062039220926
51850CB00010B/2604
* 9 7 8 3 7 2 5 8 4 7 2 7 3 *